To all nursing students,

Your commitment to becoming successful and your dedication to the profession of nursing will bring never-ending rewards!

SAUNDERS

STRATEGIES *for* TEST SUCCESS

Passing Nursing School
and the NCLEX® Examination

SAUNDERS

STRATEGIES *for* TEST SUCCESS

Passing Nursing School
and the NCLEX® Examination

LINDA ANNE SILVESTRI, MSN, RN, PhD(c)
Instructor of Nursing
Salve Regina University
Newport, Rhode Island

President
Nursing Reviews, Inc.
and
Professional Nursing Seminars, Inc.
Charlestown, Rhode Island

Instructor
NCLEX-RN® and NCLEX-PN® Review Courses

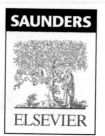

SAUNDERS

ELSEVIER

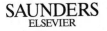

3251 Riverport Lane
St. Louis, Missouri 63043

SAUNDERS STRATEGIES FOR TEST SUCCESS: ISBN: 978-1-4160-6202-8
PASSING NURSING SCHOOL AND THE NCLEX® EXAMINATION

NOTICE

Knowledge and best practice in this field are constantly changing. As new research and experience broaden our knowledge, changes in practice, treatment, and drug therapy may become necessary or appropriate. Readers are advised to check the most current information provided (i) on procedures featured or (ii) by the manufacturer of each product to be administered to verify the recommended dose or formula, the method and duration of administration, and contraindications. It is the responsibility of the practitioner, relying on their own experience and knowledge of the patient, to make diagnoses, to determine dosages and the best treatment for each individual patient, and to take all appropriate safety precautions. To the fullest extent of the law, neither the Publisher nor the Author assumes any liability for any injury and/or damage to persons or property arising out of or related to any use of the material contained in this book.

Previous edition copyrighted 2005

NCLEX® is a registered trademark and service mark of the National Council of State Boards of Nursing, Inc.

Nursing diagnoses from **Nursing Diagnoses—Definitions and Classification 2009-2011** © 2009, 2007, 2005, 2003, 2001, 1998, 1996, 1994 NANDA International. **Used by arrangement with Wiley-Blackwell Publishing, a company of John Wiley & Sons, Inc.**

Library of Congress Cataloging-in-Publication Data

Silvestri, Linda Anne.
    Saunders strategies for test success : passing nursing school and the NCLEX examination / Linda Anne Silvestri.—2nd ed.
       p. ; cm.
    Includes bibliographical references and index.
    ISBN 978-1-4160-6202-8 (pbk. : alk. paper)
    1. Nursing—Examinations, questions, etc. I. Title. II. Title: Strategies for test success.
    [DNLM: 1. Nursing, Practical—Examination Questions. WY 18.2 S587st 2010]
    RT55.S4875 2010
    610.73076—dc22

                                                    2009028648

Director, Review and Testing: Loren S. Wilson
Senior Editor: Kristin Geen
Developmental Editor: Todd McKenzie
Publishing Services Manager: Anne Altepeter
Senior Project Manager: Doug Turner
Designer: Charlie Siebel

Printed in the United States of America

Last digit is the print number: 9 8 7 6 5 4 3 2 1

About the Author

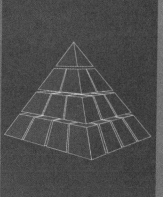

As a child, I always dreamed of becoming either a nurse or a teacher. Initially I chose to become a nurse because I really wanted to help others, especially those who were ill. Then I realized that both of my dreams could come true: I could be both a nurse and a teacher. So I pursued my dreams.

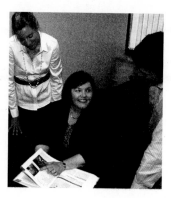

I received my diploma in nursing at Cooley Dickinson Hospital School of Nursing in Northampton, Massachusetts. Afterward, I worked at Baystate Medical Center in Springfield, Massachusetts. While there, I cared for clients in acute medical-surgical units, the intensive care unit, the emergency department, pediatric units, and other acute care units. Later I received an associate degree from Holyoke Community College in Holyoke, Massachusetts, my BSN from American International College in Springfield, Massachusetts, and my MSN from Anna Maria College in Paxton, Massachusetts, with a dual major in Nursing Management and Patient Education. Currently I am working on my PhD in Nursing at the University of Nevada, Las Vegas, and I am doing research related to success on the NCLEX examination. I am also a member of the Honor Society of Nursing, Sigma Theta Tau International, Phi Kappa Phi, the Western Institute of Nursing, the Eastern Nursing Research Society, and the Golden Key International Honour Society.

As a native of Springfield, Massachusetts, I began my teaching career as an instructor of medical-surgical nursing and leadership-management nursing at Baystate Medical Center School of Nursing in 1981. In 1989, I relocated to Rhode Island and began teaching medical-surgical nursing and psychiatric nursing to RN and LPN students at the Community College of Rhode Island. Later in 1994, I began teaching nursing at Salve Regina University in Newport, Rhode Island, and remain there as an adjunct faculty member.

My experiences as a student, nursing educator, and item writer for the NCLEX exams aided me as I developed a comprehensive review course to prepare nursing students and graduates for the NCLEX examination. In 1991, I established Professional Nursing Seminars, Inc., and in 2000, I started Nursing Reviews, Inc. Both companies are dedicated to conducting review courses for the NCLEX-RN and the NCLEX-PN examinations and assisting nursing graduates to achieve their goals of becoming Registered Nurses and/or Licensed Practical/Vocational Nurses.

Today, I conduct review courses for NCLEX examinations throughout New England and am the author of numerous successful review products. I am so pleased that you have decided to let me join you in your journey to success in testing for nursing examinations and for the NCLEX examination!

Reviewers

Jacqueline B. Arnett, RN, BSN, CPN

Staff Development Coordinator
Life Care Centers of America
Tucson, Arizona

Mary M. Fabick, MSN, MEd, RN, CEN

Associate Professor of Nursing
Milligan College
Milligan College, Tennessee

Donna Elise Wilsker, MSN, RN

Assistant Professor of Nursing
Lamar University
Beaumont, Texas

Student Reviewers

Sarah E. Hollenberg

University of Missouri—St. Louis
St. Louis, Missouri

Angela Silvestri

Salve Regina University
Newport, Rhode Island

Lindsay S. Walsh

Truman State University
Kirksville, Missouri

Preface

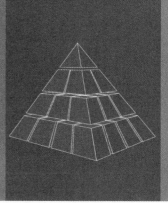

Welcome to *Saunders Pyramid to Success!*

Saunders Strategies for Test Success: Passing Nursing School and the NCLEX® Examination is one in a series of products designed to assist you in achieving your goal of passing your nursing courses and becoming a licensed nurse. This product provides you with test-taking strategies that will help you pass your nursing examinations and the NCLEX examination.

ORGANIZATION

Saunders Strategies for Test Success: Passing Nursing School and the NCLEX® Examination contains four parts spread out over 19 chapters and 7 appendices. The chapters that describe the test-taking strategies include several sample questions that illustrate how to use each test-taking strategy. The sample questions represent all types of question formats including multiple choice, fill-in-the-blank, multiple response, prioritizing (ordered response), and questions that contain a figure or illustration. In addition to the sample questions in the chapters, a total of 500 practice questions accompany this book. There are 200 practice questions in the book, and the software contains the 200 practice questions from the book along with an additional 300 practice questions. All of the practice questions reflect the framework and the content identified in the most current NCLEX test plans. The practice questions in this book relate to each Client Needs category and each Integrated Process of the NCLEX exam. The Client Needs categories include Safe and Effective Care Environment, Health Promotion and Maintenance, Psychosocial Integrity, and Physiological Integrity. The Integrated Processes include Caring, Communication and Documentation, Nursing Process, and Teaching and Learning.

PART I: Study and Test Preparation

Chapter 1: Preparing for Nursing Examinations

The information contained in this chapter focuses on the exams that you will take during your nursing program and provides you with information on how to prepare for these exams. Topics include the purpose of nursing exams, what you can expect on nursing exams, how nursing exams are different from other exams, and the types of questions on nursing exams. Additional topics include preparing for a nursing exam using your textbook, classroom notes, flash cards, study guides, and study groups.

Chapter 2: Developing Study Skills

This chapter discusses several topics related to study skills and study habits. It provides you with information on how to develop or refine study skills and how to develop good study habits so that you will be well prepared for your nursing exams. Included are the top 10 *Pyramid Points* and study habits. Also, study skills such as listening, note-taking, reading, remembering content, and critical thinking skills are discussed.

Chapter 3: Reducing Test Anxiety

This chapter focuses on the important points related to test anxiety. In this chapter you are provided with self-assessment points to determine if you experience test anxiety. Additionally, the causes of test anxiety, how to prevent test anxiety, and how to control test anxiety before an exam are discussed. Points about maintaining a positive attitude and what you can do when you experience test anxiety are presented in this chapter.

Chapter 4: NCLEX® Preparation

This chapter focuses on preparing for the NCLEX exam—the exam that you must take and pass after you graduate from nursing school in order to become a licensed nurse. This chapter emphasizes the important point that NCLEX preparation begins the moment that you enter your nursing program. Specific to the NCLEX, it provides you with the steps for preparing for the NCLEX, self-assessment points to determine your readiness, and a plan for preparation.

PART II: Strategies for Success

Chapter 5: How to Avoid "Reading Into the Question"

One of the pitfalls that can cause a problem when answering a question is "reading into the question." What "reading into the question" means is that you are considering issues beyond the information that is presented in the question. This chapter describes the strategies to use when answering a question to prevent this from happening and includes topics such as how to read a question, strategic words, the subject of the question, and how to use the process of elimination.

Chapter 6: Positive and Negative Event Queries

This chapter describes the differences between a positive and a negative event query in a question. Reading the question carefully and noting the type of query used is important to assist in answering a question correctly. This chapter also identifies the strategic words or phrases that indicate whether the question contains a positive or negative event query.

Chapter 7: Questions Requiring Prioritization

Some of the test questions on your nursing exams and on the NCLEX will require you to use the skill of prioritizing nursing actions. These types of questions can be difficult because when a question requires prioritization, all of the options may be correct and you will need to determine the correct order of action. This chapter describes the test-taking strategies that you can use to answer prioritizing questions correctly. Some of these strategies include the ABCs (airway, breathing, and circulation), Maslow's Hierarchy of Needs theory, and the steps of the nursing process. Also included in this chapter are the strategies for determining the need to contact the physician.

Chapter 8: Leading and Managing, Delegating, and Assignment-Making Questions

Some test questions that you will need to answer will relate to the nurse's responsibilities regarding delegating care and assignment making and the supervisory role of these responsibilities. This chapter reviews the guidelines and principles related to delegating and assignment making, two very important roles of the nurse as a leader and manager. It also provides you with information about the tasks and activities that can be delegated and assigned to a nursing assistant, licensed practical/vocational nurse, and registered nurse. Guidelines for time management are also reviewed, because managing time efficiently is a key factor for completing activities and tasks within a given time period.

Chapter 9: Communication Questions

Communication is a process through which information is exchanged, either verbally or nonverbally, between two or more individuals and is an extremely important role of the nurse. This chapter reviews the guidelines to follow when answering communication questions and identifies various cultural aspects to consider when communicating and caring for clients. Additionally, therapeutic and nontherapeutic communication techniques are presented.

Chapter 10: Pharmacology Questions

Pharmacology is one of the most difficult nursing content areas to master and feel comfortable with. One reason that it is so difficult is because of the enormous number of medications available. Another reason is that there is a vast amount of information to know about each medication. It is important for you to spend ample time studying and reviewing pharmacology in preparation for your nursing exams and for the NCLEX and to use this knowledge to answer pharmacology questions. However, you may be presented with pharmacology questions on your exams that present medications that you are unfamiliar with, in which case you will need to make an educated guess to answer the question. This chapter provides you with the strategies and general guidelines to use for making an educated guess to answer pharmacology questions correctly.

Chapter 11: Additional Pyramid Strategies

This chapter reviews additional helpful strategies that will assist in answering a test question correctly. Also included in this chapter are strategies that are useful for answering questions related to medication and intravenous calculations, laboratory values, client positioning, and therapeutic diets. Strategies that will be helpful when answering questions related to disasters are also presented in this chapter.

PART III: Practice Test

Part III comprises a 200-question test that provides you the opportunity to practice using various test-taking strategies when answering exam questions. The questions in this test are grouped together based on their content area so that you can easily locate practice test questions that relate to the content area that you are studying in nursing school. These content areas include fundamental skills, adult health, mental health, maternity, child health, pharmacology, delegating and prioritizing, and leadership and management. The correct answer, rationale for correct and incorrect options, a test-taking strategy, a tip for the beginning nursing student, question codes, and a reference text with a page number are provided for each question.

PART IV: Appendices

Part IV contains Appendices A through G.

SPECIAL FEATURES OF THE BOOK

Pyramid Points ⬥

Pyramid Points are the bullets that are placed at specific areas throughout the chapters. The *Pyramid Points* identify content that is important in preparation for the NCLEX examination.

Tip for the Beginning Nursing Student

A tip for the beginning nursing student can be located with each sample question located in the chapters in the book. Additionally, a tip for the beginning nursing student accompanies each question in the practice test located in Part III and on the accompanying software. This tip provides the beginning nursing student with a description of the content or disorder addressed in the question.

NCLEX® Tip ✓

NCLEX tips are located through the chapters in the book. These tips relate to NCLEX information and detail important points that are associated with the content addressed.

Practice Test Questions

The chapters in this book contain several practice questions that illustrate specific test-taking strategies. In addition to the practice questions integrated into the chapters, there is a 200-question practice test in the book. The software that accompanies the book contains a total of 500 questions

(200 questions from the practice test and 300 additional questions). The 200-question practice test in the book and all of the questions on the CD provide the correct answer, a rationale for correct and incorrect options, a test-taking strategy, a tip for the beginning nursing student, question codes, and a reference text with a page number.

Alternate Item Format Test Questions

In addition to multiple-choice questions, alternate item format test questions are included throughout the book, the practice test located in Part III, and on the accompanying software. The alternate item format questions include fill in the blank, multiple response, prioritizing (ordered response), and questions that contain a figure or illustration.

Answer Section for Practice-Test Questions

The answer sections for each practice-test question in Part III and on the accompanying software include the correct answer, rationale, tip for the beginning nursing student, test-taking strategy, question categories, and reference source. The structure for the answer section is unique and provides the following information:

The Rationale: The rationale provides you with the significant information regarding both correct and incorrect options.

Tip for the Beginning Nursing Student: A tip for the beginning nursing student accompanies each question in the practice test located in Part III and on the accompanying software. This tip provides the beginning nursing student with a description of the content or disorder addressed in the question.

Test-Taking Strategy: The test-taking strategy provides you with the logical path in selecting the correct option and assists you in selecting an answer to a question on which you must guess. This feature reinforces what you learned in the book about the use of test-taking strategies. Specific suggestions for review are identified in the test-taking strategy.

Question Categories: Each question is identified based on the categories used by the NCLEX test plan. Additional content categories are provided with each question to help you identify areas in need of review. The categories identified with each practice question include Level of Cognitive Ability, Client Needs, Integrated Process, and the specific nursing Content Area. All categories are identified by their full names so that you do not need to memorize codes or abbreviations.

Reference: A reference, including a page number, is provided so you can easily find the information that you need to review in your undergraduate nursing textbooks.

Software

Packaged in this book you will find a CD containing NCLEX review software. This software contains 500 practice questions in the multiple-choice format or in the alternate item format such as fill in the blank, multiple response, prioritizing (ordered response), and questions that contain a figure or illustration. This Windows- and Macintosh-compatible program offers three testing modes for review:

Study: All questions in a specific selected area. The answer, rationale, tip for the beginning nursing student, test-taking strategy, question categories, and reference source appear after answering each question.

Quiz: Ten questions in a specific selected area. The answer, rationale, tip for the beginning nursing student, test-taking strategy, question category, reference source, and results appear after you answer all 10 questions.

Examination: Seventy-five questions in a specific selected area. The answer, rationale, tip for the beginning nursing student, test-taking strategy, question categories, reference source, and results appear after you answer all 75 questions.

Content Areas on the Software

When you use the software, you will be able to select practice questions based on a Client Needs area or a content area. The Client Needs areas include Safe and Effective Care Environment, Health Promotion and Maintenance, Psychosocial Integrity, and Physiological Integrity. The content areas include the following:

CONTENT AREAS

Fundamental Skills
Maternity
Child Health
Mental Health
Delegating/Prioritizing
Leadership/Management
Pharmacology
Adult Health

HOW TO USE THIS BOOK

Saunders Strategies for Test Success: Passing Nursing School and the NCLEX® Examination is especially designed to help you with your successful journey to the peak of the *Saunders Pyramid to Success*, becoming a licensed nurse. This book focuses on test-taking strategies that will help you pass both the nursing examinations that you need to take in nursing school and the NCLEX examination. You should begin your process through the *Saunders Pyramid to Success* by reading all of the chapters in this book to learn the strategies that you can use to answer test questions. Be sure to read the NCLEX tips located throughout the chapters and the tip for the beginning nursing student located with each sample question. While in nursing school, answer the questions in the practice test located in Part III and on the accompanying software that relate to the content area you are studying.

When using the software, it is best to begin by selecting the Study Mode because you will receive immediate feedback regarding the answer, rationale, tip for the beginning nursing student, test-taking strategies, question codes, and reference source. Therefore, you will be provided with immediate information about your strengths and weaknesses. Once you have answered the practice-test question, read the rationale, tip for the beginning nursing student, and the test-taking strategy. The rationale provides you with the significant information regarding both the correct and incorrect options. The tip provides you with a description of the content or disorder addressed in the question. The test-taking strategy offers you the logical path to selecting the correct option. The strategy also identifies content area that you need to review if you had difficulty with the question. Use the reference source listed to easily find the information that you need to review.

It is very important to identify your strengths and weaknesses with regard to nursing content areas. Additionally, it is also important to strengthen any weak areas in order to be successful on your nursing exams and on the NCLEX examination. Several products in *Saunders Pyramid to Success* can be used to strengthen any weak areas. These additional products in *Saunders Pyramid to Success* can be obtained by calling 1-800-545-2522 or visiting www.elsevierhealth.com. These products are described next.

RN Products

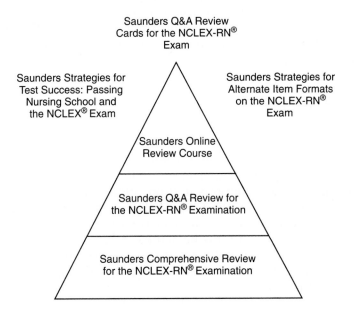

Saunders Comprehensive Review for the NCLEX-RN® Examination

This is an excellent resource to use both while you are in nursing school and in preparation for the NCLEX examination. This book contains 20 units and 76 chapters, and each chapter is designed to identify specific components of nursing content. The book and accompanying software contain more than 4200 practice questions and include alternate item format questions. The software also contains a 75-question assessment test that generates an individualized study calendar.

Saunders Q&A Review for the NCLEX-RN® Examination

This book and accompanying software provide you with more than 5200 practice questions based on the NCLEX-RN test plan. The chapters in this book are uniquely designed and are based on the NCLEX-RN examination test plan framework, including Client Needs and Integrated Processes.

Alternate item format questions are included. With practice questions focused on the Client Needs and the Integrated Processes, you can assess your level of competence.

Saunders Online Review Course for the NCLEX-RN® Examination

The online NCLEX-RN review course addresses all areas of the test plan identified by the National Council of State Boards of Nursing, Inc. The course gives you a systematic and individualized method for preparing to take the NCLEX examination. It contains a pretest that provides feedback regarding your strengths and weaknesses and generates an individualized study schedule in a calendar format. Content review with practice questions and case studies, figures and illustrations, a glossary, and animations and videos are included. A cumulative examination and a computerized adaptive exam (CAT) are also key components of the online review course. There are thousands of questions in this program, and the types of practice questions in this course include multiple choice, fill in the blank, multiple response, prioritizing (ordered response), and questions containing figures that may require you to use the computer mouse to answer.

Saunders Alternate Item Formats on the NCLEX-RN® Examination

The *Saunders Alternate Item Formats on the NCLEX-RN® Examination* focuses specifically on the alternate item format questions that will appear on your nursing examinations and on the NCLEX-RN examination. This resource is organized by the Client Needs component of the test plan, is accompanied by a CD, and includes more than 275 alternate item format questions, including fill-in-the-blank, multiple-response, prioritizing (ordered response), figure/illustration (hot spot), and chart/exhibit questions. A total of 15 audio (heart and lung sound) questions are also included on the CD.

Saunders Q&A Review Cards for the NCLEX-RN® Exam

The *Saunders Q&A Review Cards for the NCLEX-RN® Exam* provides you with 1000 NCLEX-RN review questions, including all types of alternate item format questions, in a convenient flashcard format. This is the perfect portable study resource that you can use anytime and anywhere. Review questions are on the front of each card and are organized by Client Needs, consistent with the current NCLEX-RN test plan. Answers are included on the back of the card, along with rationales, test-taking strategies, and Integrated Process categories.

PN Products

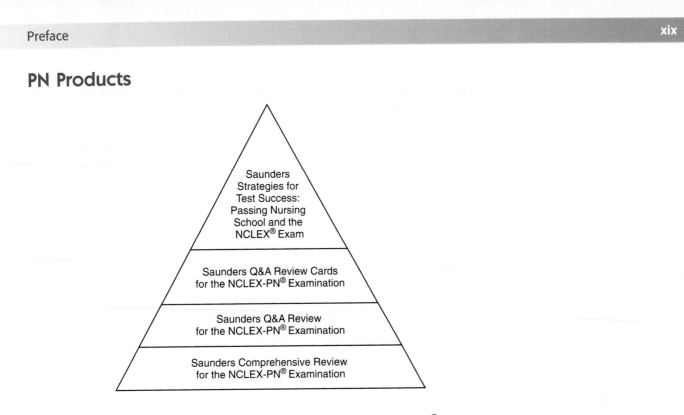

Saunders Comprehensive Review for the NCLEX-PN® Examination

This is an excellent resource to use both while you are in nursing school and in preparation for the NCLEX examination. This book contains 20 units and 66 chapters, and each chapter is designed to identify specific components of nursing content. The book and accompanying software contain 3700 practice questions and include alternate item format questions. The software also contains a 75-question assessment test that generates an individualized study calendar.

Saunders Q&A Review for the NCLEX-PN® Examination

This book and accompanying software provide you with more than 3200 practice questions based on the NCLEX-PN test plan. The chapters in this book are uniquely designed and are based on the NCLEX-PN examination test plan framework, including Client Needs and Integrated Processes. Alternate item format questions are included. With practice questions focused on the Client Needs and the Integrated Processes, you can assess your level of competence.

Saunders Review Cards for the NCLEX-PN® Examination

The *Saunders Review Cards for the NCLEX-PN® Examination* provides you with more than 900 practice test questions, including multiple-choice questions and alternate item format questions, such as fill-in-the-blank, multiple-response, prioritizing (ordered response), and image (hot spot) questions. The practice question is located on one side of the review card. The reverse side of the review card contains the correct answer, rationale, and question categories for the practice question on the front of the card.

Good luck with your journey through the *Saunders Pyramid to Success*. I wish you continued success throughout your nursing program and in your new career as a nurse!

Linda Anne Silvestri, MSN, RN, PhD(c)

Acknowledgments

Sincere appreciation and warmest thanks are extended to the many individuals who in their own way have contributed to the publication of this book.

First, I want to thank all of my nursing students at the Community College of Rhode Island in Warwick, who approached me in 1991 and persuaded me to assist them in preparing to take the NCLEX examination. Their enthusiasm and inspiration led to the commencement of my professional endeavors in conducting NCLEX review courses for nursing students. I also thank the numerous nursing students who have attended my review courses for their willingness to share their needs and ideas. Their input has certainly added a special uniqueness to this publication.

I wish to acknowledge all of the nursing faculty who have taught in my NCLEX review courses. Their commitment, dedication, and expertise have certainly assisted nursing students in achieving success with the NCLEX examination. Additionally, I want to acknowledge Laurent W. Valliere for his commitment and dedication in helping my nursing students prepare for the NCLEX exam from a nonacademic point of view.

I sincerely acknowledge and thank two very important individuals from Elsevier who are dedicated to my work in creating NCLEX products for nursing students. I thank Kristin Geen, senior editor, for her continuous assistance, enthusiasm, and support as I prepared this publication. And I thank Todd McKenzie, developmental editor, for his support and assistance, ideas for the product, maintaining organization for manuscript production, and for his patience with me as I completed this publication.

I also want to acknowledge all of the staff at Elsevier for their tremendous assistance throughout the preparation and production of this publication. A special thank you to all.

I thank Loren S. Wilson, vice president and publisher. I also thank all of the special people in the production department—Doug Turner, senior project manager; Anne Altepeter, production services manager; Dave Rushing, multimedia producer; and Charlie Seibel, designer, who all played such significant roles in finalizing this publication.

I want to acknowledge all of the staff in the marketing department, especially Bob Boehringher, executive marketing director; Susan Copeland, associate marketing manager; Dan Hughes, Evolve Reach marketing manager; and Kathy Mantz, executive marketing manager, for their support and creative ideas for this publication.

I sincerely want to thank Cindy Geiss and the artists at Graphic World in St. Louis, Missouri, for preparing the cartoons for this book and for their attention to detail and their assistance in the production of this book.

I would also like to acknowledge Patricia Mieg, former educational sales representative, who encouraged me to submit my ideas about the *Pyramid to Success* to the W.B. Saunders Company.

I want to acknowledge my parents, who opened my door of opportunity in education. I thank my mother, Frances Mary, for all of her love, support, and assistance as I continuously worked to achieve my professional goals. I thank my father, Arnold Lawrence, who always provided insightful words of encouragement. My memories of his love and support will always remain in my heart.

I also thank my sister, Dianne Elodia; my brother, Lawrence Peter; and my nieces and nephew, Gina Marie, Angela, and Nicholas; and my fiancé, Larry, all of whom were continuously supportive, giving, and helpful during my research and preparation of this publication. And, a special thank you to my niece Angela, who is a nursing student, for providing ideas for this publication.

I also need to thank Salve Regina University for the opportunity to educate nursing students in the baccalaureate nursing program and for its support during my research and writing of this publication. I would like to especially acknowledge my colleagues, Dr. Peggy Matteson, Dr. Ellen McCarty, Dr. JoAnn Mullaney, and Dr. Bethany Sykes for all of their support and encouragement.

I wish to acknowledge the Community College of Rhode Island, which provided me the opportunity to educate nursing students in the Associate Degree of Nursing Program, and a special thank you to Patricia Miller, MSN, RN, and Michelina McClellan, MS, RN, from Baystate Medical Center, School of Nursing, in Springfield, Massachusetts, who were my first mentors in nursing education.

Lastly, a very special thank you to all my nursing students, past, present and future. You light up my life! And, your curiosity, enthusiasm for learning, and desire to become successful are so inspiring.

Linda Anne Silvestri, MSN, RN, PhD(c)

Contents

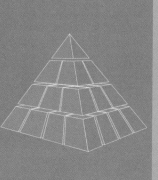

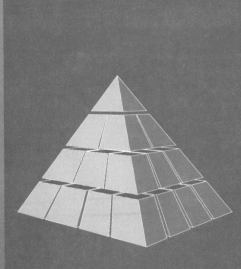

Part 1

Study and Test Preparation

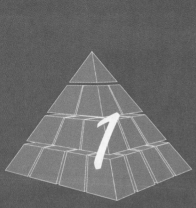

1 Chapter

Preparing for Nursing Examinations

WHEN AND WHY ARE NURSING EXAMS ADMINISTERED?

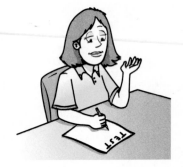

Nursing exams are administered at various points throughout each nursing course. Your nursing faculty administers these exams to you to test your knowledge of the content taught in a course and to test your ability to analyze and apply concepts learned to care for clients in various situations. The exams that you take in your nursing courses are also designed to prepare you for the NCLEX exam, the examination that you need to take and pass after you graduate in order to become a licensed nurse. Additional purposes for administering exams are listed in the box below.

PURPOSES FOR ADMINISTERING EXAMS

1. To test knowledge of the content taught in a course
2. To test the ability to analyze and apply concepts learned to care for clients in various situations
3. To ensure the development of a professional nurse who can safely and competently care for clients served in the profession
4. To ensure the development of a critical thinker who can make sound judgments and decisions based on evidence-based practice
5. To make certain that the student is a successful NCLEX exam candidate who will pass the NCLEX exam on his or her first sitting

---

THE BEGINNING NURSING STUDENT: WHAT SHOULD YOU THINK ABOUT?

What Is a Beginning Nursing Student?

If you have just completed your support courses (e.g., anatomy and physiology, microbiology, chemistry) and are entering your first nursing course, then you are a beginning nursing student. Your first nursing course is most likely titled "Fundamentals in Nursing" or something similar, and in this course you will learn all the safe and basic concepts necessary for caring for a client.

The NCLEX® Exam: Why Do You Need to Think About It Now?

You may think that the NCLEX exam is far off, and it is; however, it is critical that you think about it the moment you enter your first nursing class. You may ask, "Why is this important?" To be successful on the NCLEX exam, you need to become as familiar as possible with what it is all about as early as possible in the nursing program. You need to know that taking the NCLEX exam will be a reality once you graduate and that this exam must be passed in order to become a licensed nurse. Often students are concerned with the "here and now" of what they want to and need to accomplish and are not concerned about the future, the NCLEX exam. Students say, "I will worry about the NCLEX exam when the time comes." At this point, it is much too late. So think about this exam early; visit the National Council of State Boards of Nursing (NCSBN) Web site at www.ncsbn.org, and download the detailed test plan for the NCLEX exam. This test plan provides a wealth of information about the exam and lists the content areas that will be tested on it. Use these lists as your study guides for preparing for exams for each nursing course. Consider that, by doing this, you are not only preparing for your nursing exams but also preparing for the NCLEX exam at the same time. You will be ready when the NCLEX exam becomes a reality for you!

Planning: Why Is It So Important?

Much of your success in nursing school has to do with how you plan and organize your time. You will have a very busy schedule and will need to plan ahead to best prepare for your exams, clinical experiences, and other assignments that are due. Get an organizer with a calendar or another type of calendar that you feel will suit your needs, and use this as your planning guide for everything that you will need to do. Make notes about both your short-term goals and your long-term goals. For your short-term goals, note your classes and times, school meetings and appointments, study session times, assignment due dates, exam times, and any other obligations related to school. For your long-term goals, note what you plan to accomplish each year until your projected graduation date. Look at your calendar daily to meet any day-to-day obligations, and look ahead at your long-term goals to be sure that you are ready for graduation.

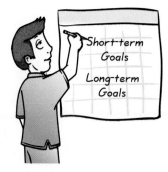

WHAT CAN YOU EXPECT ON NURSING EXAMS?

How Do Nursing Exams Differ From Other Exams?

When you enter your first nursing course, you need to remember that your exam experience in college up to this point has related to testing in support courses, such as anatomy and physiology, microbiology, and chemistry. In these courses, test questions on exams have been primarily at the cognitive level of knowledge or comprehension. These support courses have required not only a great deal of reading but also memorization in order to answer the exam questions correctly. So basically, your test-taking skills to this point may be quite good but are based on knowledge, some comprehension, and memorization.

Nursing exams differ greatly from the exams that you have been used to taking. Memorization will not get you through a nursing exam. There may be some memorization necessary in nursing, such as memorizing certain laboratory values or memorizing formulas for calculating a medication dosage or an intravenous fluid solution. However, the exam questions on a nursing exam will be at a higher cognitive level than that requiring memorization and will require that you analyze information in a test question or take the information in a test question and apply the information to a situation. You will not be able to rely only on recall skills to answer test questions on a nursing exam. Now you need to understand pathophysiology related to certain nursing content and disease processes and to analyze, apply, and use critical thinking skills to answer exam questions. Do not let that first nursing exam "blow you away" or "throw you for a loop," as some may say. Be ready for it, and you will do great and pass!

Beware of Nursing Exams!

What Types of Questions Can You Expect on Nursing Exams?

Nursing exams are administered to test your competency to care for clients safely and competently in the clinical setting. They are also administered to prepare you for the NCLEX exam. Most questions that you will encounter on nursing exams will be multiple choice in which there will be a question and four possible options. You are probably very familiar with these types of questions from your support courses, but again what you need to remember is that nursing exam questions will require that you think critically. There are other types of questions that may be included in nursing exams, known as alternate item formats, because these alternate types of questions are used in the NCLEX exam. These types include multiple response, fill-in-the-blank, prioritizing (ordered response), chart/exhibit, or a question that includes a picture or illustration. The total number of questions on an exam will vary depending on a variety of factors, such as instructor's preference, the amount of nursing content being tested, and the amount of time for testing. Your nursing instructor determines the number of questions that will be included in an exam.

✓ **NCLEX® Exam Tip**

On the NCLEX exam, most of the questions will be in the multiple-choice format. You will also have questions known as alternate item formats. These types of questions include multiple response, fill-in-the-blank, prioritizing (ordered response), chart/exhibit, or a question that includes a picture or illustration.

Are Test-Taking Strategies Important?

Test-taking strategies are important points that will help you to determine what the question is asking, how to select the correct answer, or how to narrow your choices when you must guess at an answer. Use of test-taking strategies is critical when taking a nursing exam, because in many of the exam questions, all options may be correct, but depending on the way the question is worded, you may need to prioritize to select the correct answer. In addition, many times you may be able to narrow your choices down to two options and then you may struggle with making a selection. In these situations the use of test-taking strategies is critical. Therefore it is important to become skillful in the use of test-taking strategies. Chapters 5 through 11 of this book provide specific test-taking strategies for answering nursing exam questions. In addition, Appendix A provides a guide to test-taking strategies for answering nursing exam questions.

YOUR COURSE SYLLABUS: WHY IS IT IMPORTANT?

Your course syllabus is your map of the course. It provides your course objectives, course and program policies and procedures, required readings and other activities, class schedule including your exam schedule, and other information related to the course. Your course objectives are the goals that you need to meet in order to pass the course, so be sure to read and understand them. In addition, your exam questions directly reflect your course objectives. Your required reading and other activities and your class and exam schedule are important to note, because you need to plan ahead and prepare ahead for these requirements. So be sure that you pay attention to what is stated in your course syllabus.

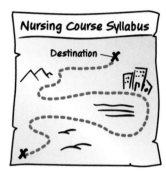

HOW CAN YOU BEST USE YOUR TEXTBOOK TO GET READY FOR A NURSING EXAM?
Required Reading

In a nursing program, you can expect that you will need to do a tremendous amount of reading. Your course syllabus will list the required reading, and it is important to do the reading before the scheduled class. For example, if a class is scheduled and the content listed is "Standard and Other Precautions," you need to read the associated reading assignment before class. Reading the material before class is vital for a number of reasons. First, faculty expects that you read the material before coming to class so that you will be prepared for the lecture. Next, reading before class provides you with the opportunity to identify areas that you do not understand and can ask about during class. So jot down questions that come to your mind as you are reading and bring this list of questions to class. Finally, many faculty will administer pop quizzes, which are unannounced quizzes administered at the beginning of class that include questions about the material that was to be read. So to be best prepared, read before class!

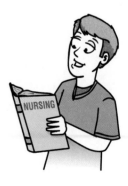

> Do not fall behind with your reading assignments!

It is important to keep current with your reading assignments, because if you fall behind it will be very difficult to catch up. During a reading session you may find that you are having difficulty focusing and concentrating. In other words you read a page of a textbook, get to the bottom of the page, and cannot even remember what you read. This happens to everyone because of not focusing. This is the time when you need to stop reading and take on another activity. Get up out of your chair, move around, and take some deep breaths. Taking a walk or some other form of exercise will help to clear your mind and get you back on track so that you can focus. You will learn what your individual concentration tolerance is and what activity helps to get you back on track and use this as a guide for planning your reading sessions. If you find that after 45 minutes your concentration level diminishes, then plan on breaks and a different activity every 45 minutes.

As you read your chapters, try to identify what you think will be asked on your nursing exam. Note the chapter headings and bolded vocabulary, and read the information in boxes, charts, and graphs located throughout the chapters in your textbook. In addition to highlighting key points, make margin notes for yourself for study.

Reading the Preface of the Textbook

Many times students skip the preface of the textbook, because they are anxious and excited to learn nursing information. It is understandable that you are excited to get going on learning all about nursing, but remember that you have an enormous amount of reading in your textbook and that you need to make the best use of your time to accomplish everything that you need to. The preface of your textbook is going to provide valuable information about how to best use the book. It will also provide information about the special student resources available to you for preparing for exams. You may find that a Web site is available that provides practice exam questions that correlate with each chapter in your textbook. Take advantage of this valuable resource to prepare yourself for your exams. Practice as many study questions as you can in preparation for the exam.

Practice Exam Questions

The questions on nursing exams are written in very identifiable and structured ways, which are outlined in later chapters of this book. Remember that "practice makes perfect!" So practice as many questions as you can in preparation for your exams. Simply knowing how the question will be structured and becoming familiar and comfortable with what you will encounter will assist you in passing an exam. Get your hands on as many study questions as possible, because this will help you to be successful not only on nursing examinations, but also on the NCLEX exam!

Many nursing textbooks provide practice exam questions at the end of a content chapter and provide a CD that contains practice exam questions, so be sure to look for these in your textbook and practice answering these questions. Next, be sure to check the preface in your textbook to locate the Web site for access to additional practice questions. Finally, use your NCLEX review book and review the content and practice questions that correlate with what you will be tested on. An additional key point to keep in mind is, after you answer practice questions, to be sure to read the accompanying rationale and test-taking strategy for each question to understand the content and the logical path for answering correctly.

Practice makes perfect!

Highlighting Key Points in the Chapter

As you read, highlight key points. Key points will include any information in the text that has to do with the nurse caring for the client. For example, key points would include signs and symptoms of a disorder and nursing interventions. Highlighting key points is extremely helpful when it is time to review before an exam. When reviewing for an exam you will be able to reread only what you have highlighted rather than the entire chapter. Highlighting is also helpful to identify points that may require clarification from your instructor.

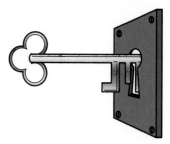

Flash Cards

Once you have highlighted key points, make some flash cards. Flash cards serve as a study guide, are portable and easy to carry in your backpack, and will help you with studying and reviewing for an exam. For example, you can list signs and symptoms of a disorder or various laboratory values on a flash card.

CLASSROOM NOTES: HOW CAN YOU BEST USE THEM?

How to Take Notes in Class

Taking good notes is an important part of preparing for an exam. How you take notes in college may differ greatly from how you took them in high school. For example, you may be accustomed to copying notes from a blackboard, because this was the way that notes were taken in high school. This will differ in college, and notes will not be written on a blackboard for you to copy. Now you need to make note of the significant points made by your instructor during lectures. Some instructors may provide various types of handouts or other materials to be used as guides during lectures; even so, these do not replace the need for you to take notes during a lecture. However, regardless of whether handout materials are provided, one important point to remember is that you will not be able to write down every word that the instructor says, so work at developing your own personal method of shorthand and abbreviations

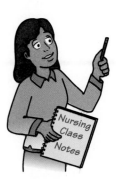

that you will understand. Reading your textbook assignments before class will be extremely helpful with the note-taking process, because you will be familiar with the significant points. During the lecture you can take notes on the significant points made by your instructor, and you will know what these points are if you read the assigned content before going to class.

Using Nursing Class Notes to Prepare for an Exam

After your lecture, read and organize your class notes. Combine your lecture notes with the reading notes that you made when you read your chapters. You will better understand the information if you merge the key points. You can make flash cards for any content area that seems difficult for you; for example, make a flash card that lists the steps in a procedure or the signs and symptoms of a disease. The worst thing that you can do is to put your class notes aside until it is time for an exam. You need to read your class notes on a daily basis so that you are learning and understanding as the course progresses. Plan a time to have your own mini–study sessions each day to read your notes. One week before the exam spend more time in your mini–study sessions so that you will be ready. You do not want to cram exam content into your head the night before an exam!

STUDY GUIDES

Two possible types of study guides may be available in nursing courses. The first is an ancillary book that accompanies your textbook. This study guide will correlate with the chapters of your textbook and provide all sorts of practice exercises and questions that will help you to reinforce content from the textbook. You may be assigned to complete these chapters in the study guide, and it is important that you do even if your course instructor does not monitor completion of them and even if you do not receive any credit for completing them. Completing the study guide will reinforce content from the textbook. In addition, often some questions and information in the study guide will be placed on your exams as test questions. So take the time to complete your study guides.

The second type of study guide that may be available is a study guide provided by your course instructor. This type of study guide is extremely helpful and lists content areas that you need to be sure that you understand. In nursing studies, you will receive a vast amount of information from classroom handouts, classroom notes, and the chapter(s) of your textbook. You need to understand all this information. It can be extremely overwhelming to weed through all the information and determine what is important. Therefore study guides can be extremely helpful to assist in preparing for an exam, because they provide you with a focus or direction of study. So be sure to review the points listed on the study guide. If your instructor listed a certain point in the study guide, then it must be important!

If your course instructor does not provide a study guide, then make your own. As you read the assigned chapters in your textbook, list the important points that you are highlighting. Also, as you review your class notes add the important points to your self-created study guide. These will be the points that your instructor emphasized or may have said in class, "Be sure that you remember this!"

▲ STUDY GROUPS

Study groups are very helpful for some students but not for all students, so you need to think about whether they will be helpful to you. The type of learner that you are will guide you in deciding whether a study group will work for you. You may be the type of learner who requires quiet and alone time to absorb the material, or you may be the type of learner who learns best by reviewing content aloud with others. One strategy that you may want to consider is to do your quiet and alone studying and once you feel that you have mastered the content then join a study group to reinforce information. Just be sure that you meet your needs, and do not be persuaded to join a study group if it will not work for you. Whether you study alone or with a group, try to anticipate what the instructor may ask on the exam. Also, it is helpful to create your own exam questions for review.

STANDARDIZED TESTING: WHY IS IT SO IMPORTANT?

You may be administered a standardized test at the end of each nursing course. This depends on the preference of your nursing program. These tests are administered primarily to assess your knowledge of the content that you learned in the nursing course. Another valuable purpose of a standardized test is that it provides a detailed report of your strengths and weaknesses and content areas that you need to improve on. These reports will help you to plan both short-term and long-term goals and provide you with valuable information for planning for the NCLEX exam. So take these standardized exams seriously and prepare for them, even if they carry no weight with regard to course grading. These are your personalized and individualized study guides for future nursing courses and the NCLEX exam. So get a three-ring binder, label it "My NCLEX Study Guide," and place all your detailed standardized reports in this binder. When it comes time to focus on future exams, primarily the NCLEX exam, you will have what you need to begin and direct your review and study.

REFERENCES

Silvestri, L. (2010). *Saunders comprehensive review for the NCLEX-PN® examination* (4th ed.). St. Louis: Saunders.

Silvestri, L. (2008). *Saunders comprehensive review for the NCLEX-RN® examination* (4th ed.). St. Louis: Saunders.

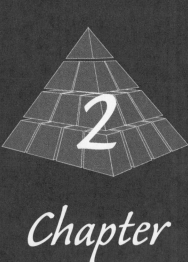

Developing Study Skills

Chapter 2

WHAT ARE GOOD STUDY SKILLS?

Good study skills mean that you have developed good study habits and adhered to a study schedule in which you have incorporated methods for learning and understanding nursing content. Good study habits develop by organizing your time and disciplining yourself to keep to your study schedule. It is important to remember that success comes from working hard, so do not just think about studying; instead, actually incorporate study into your daily school pattern.

Time management is an important factor in developing good study habits and skills. In the nursing program, you will be very busy with classes, laboratory sessions, and clinical experiences. You will need to complete a great deal of reading and assignments and take and pass exams. There are only 24 hours in a day, and you will have a limited number of hours in each day to spend on studying, so you need to use this time as effectively and as efficiently as possible. To help you get started, this chapter discusses some important points for developing these habits and skills. Chapter 1 gives additional study habits and skills as they relate specifically to nursing exams.

HOW DO YOU IDENTIFY AND PLAN YOUR STUDY TIMES?

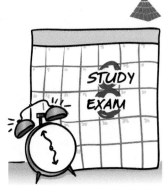

An important part of identifying time for study is using a calendar. The calendar can come in the form of an electronic calendar or the more traditional paper type of calendar. Whatever you prefer to use will work for you. Choose the type that best fits your needs, and let it be your academic life-guide.

At the beginning of each semester, enter your class schedule into your calendar. Once you receive your course syllabus for each course, read it carefully and pay close attention to due dates for assignments and exam dates. Enter these dates in the calendar. In addition, enter into your calendar any other important dates, such as extracurricular activities or other personal activities that you have scheduled. Carry your calendar with you when you go to class. The instructor may change an assignment due date or an exam date, so you want to be sure that you can immediately make that change in your calendar. Once all this information has been added to your calendar you can plan your study times.

Your calendar or academic life-guide is critical to your success in effectively managing your time and developing a study plan for the semester. Be sure to look at your calendar every day to plan for the following day. Look ahead to the next week, and note what is scheduled (e.g., an exam) or due to be handed in (e.g., an assignment). If you are diligent about entering your semester schedule and course requirements into your calendar and reviewing your calendar daily, you can easily manage your time in a busy semester.

WHAT STUDY HABITS DO YOU NEED TO DEVELOP?

A habit is a pattern of behavior that an individual establishes through repetition of the behavior. Habits can be good ones or bad ones, and you need to focus on developing good habits for studying. If you develop good habits and stick to them, you will be successful in the nursing program. There are many study habits that you can develop for yourself, and you may already have some study habits in place that you developed while in high school. If you do and they worked, then integrate these study habits into your college study plan. In addition, use the following top-10 pyramid points and study habits to help plan your study sessions.

Top-10 Pyramid Points and Study Habits

Pyramid point and study habit 1: Plan daily specific times for studying.

Look at your calendar to identify daily times that are free of any other commitments, such as class or clinical obligations, and make these your study times. Block these times off in your calendar as your study times. If you have breaks between classes, use them for study. For example, if you have a class from 8:00 AM to 10:00 AM and do not have another class until 1:00 PM, block out time between these classes as study time. Set regular study time sessions for each day because this will help to establish a routine that becomes part of your school life, and remember that it is acceptable to revise your study time sessions if necessary. In other words, if you find that a particular study time is not working, then select another time to take its place. During your study time be sure that your time is spent on something related to your nursing course work.

Pyramid point and study habit 2: Try not to do too much studying at one time.

It is better to plan more than one study time per day rather than to plan a lengthy block of study time. In other words, plan more than one study session daily. If you try to do too much studying at one time, you will easily tire and you will not be able to concentrate and retain the information. Your study time will be more effective if you space it over shorter periods of time.

Pyramid point and study habit 3: Set goals for your study time.

Think about what you want to accomplish during each study time. Set your goal in writing. This will help you to keep focused and concentrate on your task at hand. Then work at meeting your goal. If for whatever reason you are unable to meet your set study time goal, do not become discouraged. Just look at where you left off, revise your goals for your next study session, and keep moving forward on your plan!

Pyramid point and study habit 4: Avoid procrastination.

Stick to your study schedule, and start studying as you planned to do. It is very easy to get off track and procrastinate because "I just do not feel like studying" or "the content or assignment is difficult" or "I would rather be doing something else." If you procrastinate you will not meet your goals and will need to rush at a later time to complete your work. This places unnecessary stress on you and then you will end up having to cram, so start studying when you planned to do so. You will feel great after your study session knowing that you accomplished a goal.

Pyramid point and study habit 5: Study the most difficult material when you are most alert.

Some students do best with studying in the early-morning hours, some do better during the daytime hours, and some do best during the evening hours. You need to determine which time is best for you and when you are most rested and alert and have the most mental energy. Once you have determined this, use this time to work on your most difficult material. If you have the mental energy and stamina, this difficult task will be easier to grasp.

Pyramid point and study habit 6: Find a special study place that is free of external distractions.

Your special study area should be quiet and comfortable. It can be your dormitory room, a study lounge, the library, a special room at home, or any other quiet area that works for you. Do not plan to study in a crowded or noisy room, such as a student social lounge, cafeteria, or cafe. Find your special area of tranquility, and post a "do not disturb" sign. Be sure that your cell phone is off and that any other phone or the television is off or far enough away from you so that you will not be distracted.

Your study area should be adequate and roomy enough to support your necessary books, notes, and other essentials required to make the study session a success. The lighting in your special study area should be soft and provide the right amount of light to allow easy reading. Remember that temperature control is also critical to your comfort. If it is too hot, you may become sleepy. If it is too cold, you may begin to shiver and have difficulty concentrating. So find a room temperature that is comfortable for you. Remember that your special study area should be quiet and comfortable.

Pyramid point and study habit 7: Seek help when you do not understand the material.

If you are having difficulty understanding the material, seek help. Remember that in many cases "two heads are better than one." You can ask another student to help explain a difficult content area that you do not understand, and do not ever hesitate to ask your instructor to explain the information to you. During your study session, if you are "stuck" and are not able to understand the information using the resources that are immediately available to you, move on to the next topic. Do not waste your valuable study time. Make note of the information that you do not understand, and seek clarification later. Start the next topic to make the most of the study time you have planned.

Pyramid point and study habit 8: Plan study breaks.

Study breaks are important to keep your mind fresh and alert. All people differ in terms of the length of time that they can sit and study and maintain focus to concentrate. How will you know when you need a study break? If you are having difficulty focusing and are moving through content but are not grasping the material, then you need a study break. If you read a page of content but at the end of the page you do not remember what you read, then you need a study break. If you are experiencing "mind chatter" or are thinking about other things except the task that you are supposed to be focusing on, then you need a study break. If you are feeling sleepy or hungry, you need a study break.

Pyramid point and study habit 9: Eat a healthy diet, and exercise regularly.

Eating a healthy diet will build and maintain your energy level and your stamina to meet your set goals. Did you know that eating fatty types of foods will slow you down? Yes they will; so you need to avoid fatty foods. As you will learn in nursing school, nutrition is important for the functioning of every cell in your body. A nurse is also a teacher, and you will be teaching your clients about the importance of eating healthy. So practice what you will be preaching!

Breakfast is an extremely important meal because it starts your day with the fuel that you need to think and perform all the activities ahead of you; but be sure to eat a healthy breakfast. Stay away from bacon, sausage, and high-sugar syrups. Instead, for example, eat a bagel with some peanut butter or cereal, eat fruit, and drink some juice. Eat lighter meals and eat more frequently to keep your body fueled and energized. Include complex carbohydrates and protein in your diet for energy. In addition, carry snacks in your backpack for between meals or for your study breaks; but again be sure that these snacks are healthy ones. Also, be careful not to include too much caffeine in your daily diet. Caffeine will make you jittery and nervous and cause you to have difficulty focusing and concentrating. Remember that a motor vehicle needs gas or it will not run; so think about your body as the motor vehicle needing healthy food to move along and progress efficiently through the day!

Exercising regularly is another extremely important habit to develop. Exercise will enhance or maintain your *physical fitness* and strength and your overall *health.* Regular physical exercise also boosts the immune system, helps prevent disease, and improves your mental health. So get into the habit of exercising regularly. As with healthy eating, you will be teaching your clients about the importance of regular exercise. Again, practice what you will be preaching! What type of exercise should you do? That depends on what you like to do. It can be anything from walking or running to working out at a gym. Even simply getting into the habit of walking to class rather than driving to class will help. Exercise is also a great outlet when you take a study break; take a walk during your break. This will get your circulation flowing, and you will find that your mind will clear and you are able to focus and concentrate.

Pyramid point and study habit 10: Get an adequate amount of sleep every night.

Sleep is like food, air, or water. You need it to think and function adequately, and you need it to survive. Lack of an adequate amount of sleep will cause mental, emotional, and physical fatigue and irritability. Think about it—do you want to go into a classroom to take an exam feeling irritable or mentally, emotionally, or physically fatigued? Of course not, because then you are placing yourself at risk for failure. If you develop a schedule for studying and stick to it then you will not have to worry about being up all night preparing for an exam the next day. One of the worst things that you can do is to cram the night before an exam and stay up all night studying. If you do this it will be very difficult to focus and concentrate while taking the exam. If you have developed a structured study plan and stuck to it, the night before the exam will require simply a review of the content. So get into the habit of going to bed at night at a specific time that will provide you with an adequate amount (6 to 8 hours) of quality sleep.

Do you have difficulty falling asleep? If you do, this is probably because you are lying in bed thinking about all sorts of things, such as everything that you need to get done over the next day, the next week, and the remainder of the semester; or you may have other sorts of things on your mind. Whatever it may be that is keeping you awake needs to be eliminated from your mind. How do you do this? This may be a trial and error sort of task that will require implementing various measures or strategies to help you fall asleep until you find the one that will work for you. Remember that a measure that works for someone else may not work for you; but, if you determine what will work for you and get into the habit of implementing this measure repetitively, you will find that you will easily be able to fall asleep at night. Some measures to help you fall asleep are listed in the box below.

MEASURES TO PROMOTE SLEEP

Develop a time schedule for when you will go to bed at night.
Avoid taking naps during the day.
Avoid consuming caffeine-containing drinks and foods.
Eat healthy, and exercise regularly (avoid exercise within 3 or 4 hours of bedtime because activity increases metabolism and alertness for a few hours).
Avoid eating heavily close to bedtime.
Adjust the room temperature to meet your physical needs; a cool environment is best.
Keep the lights off in the room at bedtime.
Ensure a quiet environment; place a "sleeping" sign on your door, and use comfortable earplugs if necessary.
Turn your clock around or place it in a drawer so that you cannot see it.
Perform a relaxation technique, such as reading; slow, deep breathing; or meditating.
Use a natural sleep remedy, such as drinking a cup of warm milk or caffeine-free tea.

 NCLEX® Exam Tip

When you graduate from nursing school and are preparing to take the NCLEX exam, remember that you have been successful up to this point. Therefore the study habits and study skills that you used during your nursing education were effective. Use these same study habits and study skills to prepare for the NCLEX exam!

WHAT STUDY SKILLS ARE IMPORTANT?

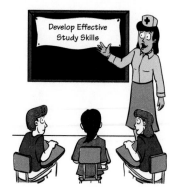

Effective study skills develop once you have your study schedule in place and begin to implement your plan of study. Effective study skills also develop from good study habits. You may already have effective study skills in place that you developed when you were in high school; if you do and these worked for you, then continue with these study skills during your nursing education. Remember that everyone is different and what may work for someone else may not work for you. So it is important to know what works for you! This chapter provides some of the many study skills that you can implement.

Good Listening Skills

It is vital to your success that you become a good listener. Listen, and get to know your instructor. Listen carefully for verbal indicators made by your instructor that will alert you to what is important to note. Some verbal indicators are statements that begin with the words: "Never forget ...," "Please understand ...," or "This is definitely on the NCLEX exam." Listen to the inflection of your instructor's voice, and if he or she suddenly accents some content area, take that note. If your instructor becomes more animated during part of the lecture, pay attention and take note of that content. Finally, whatever the instructor reviews in class is worth highlighting because it will likely be on the next exam as an exam question.

If you are going to succeed as a good listener you must get your mind prepared before arriving to class. You must leave the daydreaming and "mind chatter" at home and come to class ready to pay close attention to every word the instructor speaks. You may not always find the content being discussed interesting, but keep in mind that you will be tested on the material and it is your responsibility to listen and learn.

Always pay attention to what your instructor may write on the blackboard or provide in a handout. If the instructor takes the time to write or diagram something on the blackboard or in a handout, you can be fairly certain that this information will turn up on the exam as an exam question.

Effective Note Taking

You cannot go to class and take notes without pens, pencils, and a note pad in a binder. It does not matter whether you use pen or pencil; you decide which one works best for you. Make sure that the pen or pencil fits your hand comfortably and has a smooth writing tip. Also, remember that pencils contain lead that can break and pens can run out of ink, so pack more than one of each in your backpack. Your note pad should have index inserts to that you will be able to label sections as necessary, and the binder needs to be secure enough to hold the note pad and any handout material that the instructor distributes to the class.

Good note taking is a talent that requires practice and good listening skills. First, remember that you are taking notes, not writing a novel. You cannot write down every word that the instructor says. Develop a personal shorthand that will help you transcribe the important points of your instructor's lecture. For example, the instructor may say, "The signs and symptoms include nausea, vomiting, and diarrhea." Your shorthand note could read, "S&S = N/V/D." With practice you can develop an abbreviated note-taking style that will work successfully for you. Also, most students find that rewriting their notes after class is a good study habit, because it clarifies and reinforces what they have read and learned in class. You may find this strategy valuable to add to your study regimen. Some additional points related to effective note-taking are provided in Chapter 1.

Reading Skills

In nursing, reading involves active involvement with your textbook. Plan to do detailed reading in order to extract information accurately. In other words, do not scan or skim the content in the textbook chapter. In addition, always have a medical/nursing dictionary with you when you study; when you come across a word that you never heard of (e.g., edema, which means swelling), look it up and make note of it in your notebook as a new vocabulary word. Chapter 1 provides strategies to implement when you are reading your textbook. Some additional strategies include the following:

1. Read one section at a time under each major heading. Highlight the key points. Develop some questions that come to mind, and write these questions in your notebook. Find the answers to the questions, and if necessary plan to bring the question to class for further clarification.
2. After you finish reading some of the sections under major headings, look again at the questions that you developed and think about the answers. If you were not able to recall the answers, review these sections in the text again. Then continue reading the chapter.
3. After you have read the entire chapter, review all the highlighted key points and any notes that you made, and review the questions that you have developed to see if you can answer them. If not, then review these areas in the chapter again. It may also be helpful to make a flash card for any information that is difficult.

Remembering Content

Remembering what you have listened to in class and remembering what you read are essential for your success in passing exams, success in future nursing courses, and success on the NCLEX exam. If you are unable to remember what you learned, then you will be unable to apply the information in future nursing courses, in the clinical setting, or on the NCLEX exam. Some strategies for remembering content include rewriting class notes, reading your class notes every day, doing the required reading before coming to class, highlighting key points in your textbook as you read, completing study guides provided for you, and creating flash cards for the material that is difficult for you. Chapter 1 provides points related to these strategies.

An additional strategy that you can use to remember content is to develop an acronym, a mnemonic, or easily remembered letters, words, or phrases for difficult information. Many times your instructor will identify ways to remember difficult information, but you can develop these on your own or with your classmates. Three examples of these are listed in the box that follows.

EXAMPLES OF ACRONYMS/MNEMONICS FOR REMEMBERING DIFFICULT CONTENT

RN—When mixing regular and NPH insulin in the same syringe, draw up the *R*egular insulin first, followed by the *N*PH insulin. Remember the acronym *RN* when mixing both these types of insulin in the same syringe. *Tip for the beginning nursing student:* Insulin is a medication that is prescribed for some clients with diabetes mellitus. Many times it is necessary to administer both regular and NPH insulin, and these insulins need to be mixed in the same syringe. There is a procedure for mixing these insulins, and it is important to draw the regular insulin into the syringe first. You will learn about this procedure when you study medication administration. You will also learn about this procedure in your medical-surgical nursing course when you study endocrine disorders.

Decorticate posturing versus decerebrate posturing—In de*cort*icate posturing the upper extremities (arms, wrists, fingers) are flexed with adduction of the arms. In other words, the upper extremities are brought to the *core* of the body; whereas in decerebrate posturing, the upper extremities are stiffly extended and adducted with internal rotation and pronation of the palms. Therefore, when trying to distinguish the characteristics of each type of posturing, remember that in de*cort*icate, the upper extremities are brought to the *core* of the body. *Tip for the beginning nursing student:* Posturing is an abnormal position assumed by a client with a neurological disorder and indicates deterioration in the client's condition. You will learn about posturing in your medical-surgical nursing course when you study neurological disorders.

Monoamine oxidase inhibitors (MAOIs)—MAOIs are antidepressants and include the following medications:

Phenelzine sulfate (*N*ardil)

Tranylcypromine sulfate (*P*arnate)

Isocarboxazid (*M*arplan)

Remembering the acronym *NPM* as meaning *N*ot *P*leasant *M*edications will assist in remembering the medications that belong in the MAOI classification. *Tip for the beginning nursing student:* MAOIs are antidepressants that are used to treat depression. There are adverse effects associated with this classification of medications, and clients must follow specific dietary measures when taking these medications. Therefore it is important to know which medications are in the classification of MAOIs. You will learn about MAOIs in your pharmacology and your psychiatric/mental health—nursing courses.

Critical Thinking Skills

Critical thinking skills involve an intellectual process of actively analyzing information. It is essential that you develop good critical thinking skills, because you will be making very important decisions in the clinical setting when you care for clients. In the clinical setting, you will gather information and then will need to analyze and apply this information, make decisions, and evaluate the outcome.

Critical thinking skills take time to develop, but if you are mindful of the fact that you need to develop these skills then you can set some goals for yourself regarding becoming a critical thinker. So what can you do to develop critical thinking skills? One strategy that you can begin with is to consistently ask yourself questions as you read nursing content. Write these questions in your notebook, and then present them in class for discussion. This discussion will generate critical thinking among your classmates. Another strategy to develop critical thinking skills is to learn content from an analytical perspective. In other words, be creative. Look at a collection of information that you are learning, and instead of simply learning the facts, think about the information in an investigative manner. For example, if you are learning about standard precautions (a basic level of infection control that should be used in the care of all clients all of the time to reduce the risk of transmission of microorganisms), do not simply remember that handwashing must be done before and after contact with a client or that gloves are worn when coming in contact with blood or body fluid excretions and secretions. Think about this content critically, and question *why* these procedures need to be followed. Critical thinking takes more time and energy than simply learning facts and content, but it is an essential part of the learning process in nursing. So work at it, and make it a habit to think about things critically.

▲ WHEN SHOULD YOU START TO STUDY FOR AN EXAM?

Studying for an exam begins the moment your course begins and you start reading your textbooks, attend class, and take notes. Plan and schedule daily study sessions for yourself, and read your class notes taken up to that point, with a particular focus on your new notes, the notes taken that day. This is an important part of preparing for an exam so that you will not be faced with cramming the night before. Procrastinating and waiting until the last minute to prepare an exam are two of the worst things that you can do, because these place unnecessary pressure on you and set the stage for developing test anxiety. So start preparing right away. One week before a scheduled exam, increase the time that you spend in your study session. The amount of time that you need to plan for your study sessions depends on the type of learner that you are and how quickly you are able to grasp the new content and material. A guideline that you may want to use to begin scheduling your study sessions is to plan 1 hour of study for every 3 hours of class time. So, for example, if your nursing class is scheduled for 3 hours then plan for a 1-hour review of your notes after the class. Then 1 week before the exam, increase the time that you spend in each study session to 2 hours of study for every 3 hours of class time. This is only a guideline to help you think about planning and is not a rigid rule that needs to be strictly followed. Remember that everyone is different when it comes to learning needs, so think about what works best for you and plan accordingly. Chapter 1 provides additional information regarding using your class notes to prepare for an exam.

WILL A STUDY GROUP WORK FOR YOU?

This question is one that only you can answer. If the idea of studying in a group environment has worked for you in the past and you feel comfortable with this type of study arena, by all means continue this way of studying. If you are the type of learner who needs to be alone to study in order to master the content, then a study group will not work. Some combination of alone study time and group study time may also be an option for you. In other words, you can plan to study on your own and once you are comfortable with the content and think that you have mastered it then join a study group to help to reinforce content.

Study groups can be very helpful when preparing for an exam, but the study team needs to be motivated and needs to stay on track with regard to the goal of the group. A study group can easily get off track and waste time discussing "outside of study" issues. If this happens, then the goals of the group may not be met. Be sure to join a study group that has the same goals that you have, and be sure that your study partners have personalities that are compatible with yours so that you can easily work together. This will help with motivating and driving each other to meet group goals.

The size of the study group should be between three and five, and every group member needs to come to the study time prepared to participate. When the study group is initially created, group goals and expectations should be developed. Each study session should have established goals and work to achieve the study goals within the study time. Each group member should accept a task with regard to the contribution or role he or she will take as a member of the group. For example, if the content for a scheduled exam includes the medical-surgical areas of angina, myocardial infarction, and congestive heart failure, then each group member should accept a topic area or a part of it for presentation at the study group session. At the end of each study session the group members should decide when the next study group session will be, what the goals for the session will be, and each member's assignment. Remember that study groups are made of individuals and each individual is a part of the team. If each team member contributes to the study session as planned, then the team will succeed. Chapter 1 provides additional information about study groups.

REFERENCES

National Council of State Boards of Nursing Web site: www.ncsbn.org

Silvestri, L. (2010). *Saunders comprehensive review for the NCLEX-PN® examination* (4th ed.). St. Louis: Saunders.

Silvestri, L. (2008). *Saunders comprehensive review for the NCLEX-RN® examination* (4th ed.). St. Louis: Saunders.

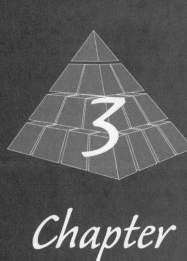

3

Chapter

Reducing Test Anxiety

WHAT IS TEST ANXIETY?

Test anxiety is a psychological condition that can cause a significant amount of stress related to preparing for and taking an examination. Test anxiety is a type of performance anxiety, because the individual is under pressure to do well in order to pass. A person with test anxiety experiences tension and stress before, during, and possibly after finishing an exam. Test anxiety can block the thinking processes and cause poor performance with testing. This chapter provides some tips and strategies to help prevent test anxiety and to reduce the anxiety if it occurs. However, if you feel that your test anxiety is so overwhelming that you are unable to focus or concentrate, seek assistance. As a starting point, you may want to contact your advisor to discuss your test anxiety experiences.

HOW CAN YOU KNOW IF YOU HAVE TEST ANXIETY?

You have attended all your classes, you have done all your reading assignments, you have participated in class discussions, and you followed your study plan. Then the day of the test arrives, and you feel so nervous that you freeze up and are unable to focus, think, or concentrate. It is normal to feel a little nervous and stressed before a test, and actually a little anxiety can keep you sharp and alert during testing. But if the anxiety is overwhelming and you cannot control it, your thinking processes will be blocked, you will have difficulty focusing and concentrating, and you will forget the material that you learned.

Anxiety related to taking an examination can cause various symptoms. Test anxiety can bring on a feeling of "butterflies in the stomach," a stomachache, nausea, vomiting, or diarrhea. Test anxiety also can cause headaches, excessive sweating, a rapid heart rate (feeling like the heart is pounding), and rapid breathing. Some students may describe their physical feelings related to test anxiety as "I feel like throwing up" or "I feel like I might pass out." Test anxiety can also cause overwhelming feelings of helplessness and a sense of feeling out of control of the situation.

WHAT CAUSES TEST ANXIETY?

Taking a test can be stressful because you know that you need to perform well to pass the exam. Physiologically, when you feel stressed your body will release a hormone called *adrenaline,* which prepares you for the stressful situation. This is called the *fight or flight response* and is the same physiological response that occurs when someone encounters a dangerous situation. When the adrenaline is released, the physical symptoms of sweating, the heart pounding, and rapid breathing occur.

Someone who worries about everything or who thinks that he or she needs to achieve a perfect test score is likely to experience test anxiety. This person, who may be termed a *perfectionist,* may find it difficult to obtain anything less than a perfect score and will experience test anxiety because of the great pressure and stress being placed on oneself.

A person with negative thoughts about how he or she will perform promotes test anxiety. Previous experiences, such as poor performance on a previous test, can affect how one might feel about testing. Negative experiences can affect self-confidence and the belief that one can be successful. Focusing on the negative takes a lot of energy and will drain the individual of any energy needed to perform because it causes fatigue and makes the individual feel worse. This pessimistic view of how one might perform will create more intense feelings of anxiety and distracting thoughts, setting the stage for failure on the exam.

Another cause of test anxiety is a lack of preparation for the exam. If you are not prepared for an exam, then you will be worried about passing and this will produce anxiety. Anxiety from lack of preparation occurs as a result of failing to organize and manage your time, poor study habits, not studying enough, or feeling tired because of being up all night and cramming for the test.

WHAT WILL HELP TO PREVENT SOME TEST ANXIETY?

One important way to prevent some test anxiety is to be as prepared as possible for the exam. Time management and a structured study plan will also prevent test anxiety, because you will be planning ahead and working on preparing for a test and other assignments well in advance of the scheduled date. You cannot procrastinate. Procrastinating places unnecessary pressure on you, creating test anxiety or making test anxiety worse. If you study daily rather than cramming at the last minute, you will know the content well enough so that you can recall it even if you are stressed. Preparation will also build your confidence because you will feel more comfortable about knowing the material. Refer to Chapters 1 and 2, because these chapters provide specific tips and strategies on study habits, study skills, and time management that will help you to prepare for an exam. Incorporating these tips and strategies on test preparation into your academic life will help to prevent test anxiety.

WHAT CAN YOU DO WHEN YOU ARE EXPERIENCING TEST ANXIETY?

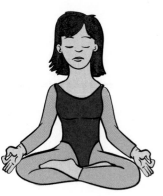

Relaxation techniques can help when you experience test anxiety, because they will relax you and help you gain control. Several types of relaxation techniques that you can use include resting your eyes, muscle relaxation/ tightening exercises, meditation, or breathing exercises. Use whatever technique works for you. Breathing exercises are a commonly used technique that can be done at any time, including during your testing. These exercises will help not only to relax you but also to oxygenate your body. Think about it: you would ask a postoperative client whose pulse oximetry reading is low to take slow, deep breaths. When the client takes the breaths what happens? The pulse oximetry reading rises. This same effect will occur for you if you take slow, deep breaths. Slow, deep breaths will increase oxygenation throughout your body and tissues and help you to relax and control your anxiety. In addition, the slow, deep breaths will give your body and brain an oxygen boost. And wouldn't you want your brain to be as oxygenated as possible when taking the exam?

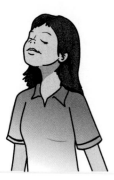

Now how do you effectively take slow, deep breaths? If you become anxious before or during the exam or if you are have difficulty sleeping the night before the exam, sit or lie in a comfortable position, close your eyes, relax, inhale deeply through your nose, hold your breath to a count of 4, exhale slowly through your mouth, and, again, relax. Repeat this breathing exercise several times until you begin to feel relaxed and free from anxiety. During the exam, if you find that you are becoming anxious and distracted and are having difficulty focusing, sit back, close your eyes, and perform your breathing exercises to help relax and get oxygen moving through your body. Remember that the slow, deep-breathing exercises will help you relax and gain control of the moment.

BREATHING EXERCISES

Sit or lie in a comfortable position.
Close your eyes.
Relax.
Inhale deeply through your nose.
Hold your breath to a count of 4.
Exhale slowly through your mouth, and relax.
Repeat until you begin to feel relaxed and free from anxiety.

WHAT IS POSITIVE PAMPERING, AND WHY IS IT IMPORTANT?

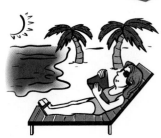

Positive pampering means that you will take care of yourself from a holistic perspective. It will help to maintain an academic and nonacademic balance as you prepare for any examination and will help to alleviate some anxiety. You need to care for yourself by including physical activity, fun and relaxation, and a balanced and healthy diet in your preparation plan. You can implement several measures, identified below, to be sure that you are caring for you. Specific interventions for these measures are described in Chapter 2 under the heading "Top-10 Pyramid Points and Study Habits."

Be sure to read this section to help you incorporate positive pampering strategies into your daily academic life.

POSITIVE PAMPERING

Fun
Relaxation
Physical activity
Balanced and healthy diet

Just as you have developed a schedule for studying, you need a schedule that includes some fun and some form of physical activity. It is your choice—aerobics, running, weight lifting, bowling, a movie, a massage, going to the beach, or whatever makes you feel good about yourself. Time spent away from a hard study schedule and devoted to some form of fun and physical exercise pays its rewards 100-fold. You will feel more energetic and less anxious about your upcoming exam with a schedule that includes these activities.

Establish a balanced diet and healthy eating habits if you have not already done so. Eat lighter and well-balanced meals, and eat more frequently. Include complex carbohydrates and protein in your diet for energy. Avoid caffeine because it will make you jittery and anxious, and avoid eating fatty foods because they will slow you down and make you feel sleepy. If you are having difficulty planning a balanced and healthy diet, another resource is the Food Pyramid Guide, located at www.mypyramid.gov.

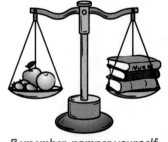

Remember, pamper yourself to maintain balance!

WHAT SHOULD YOU DO THE NIGHT BEFORE THE EXAM?

Remember to avoid cramming the night before the exam, because this will increase your test anxiety. Prepare ahead, and rest your body and your mind. Remember that the mind is like a muscle, and if it is overworked, it has no strength or stamina. Therefore, on the night before the examination, as long as you have prepared well and followed your study plan all along, put your textbook and notes away and get to bed early. At bedtime perform deep-breathing exercises and listen to soothing music to help you relax and fall asleep. Set your alarm clock, and plan to get up 15 to 30 minutes earlier than usual to have some time to wake up and eat a healthy breakfast. Walk to class on the day of the exam to get the circulation and oxygen moving throughout your body. Remember that you have prepared yourself well for the challenge of the day.

HOW CAN YOU CONTROL YOUR TEST ANXIETY BEFORE THE EXAM?

Before the examination you may become anxious and think, "I am not ready!" As a nursing student it is important to remember that it is very difficult to feel 100% prepared for an exam. This feeling is not necessarily caused by inadequate preparation and is usually caused by test anxiety. First, stay away from peers who are experiencing anxiety before the exam. These peers may be discussing content and what might be asked on the test, and this is going to cause confusion and fear about preparing well enough and will cause anxiety. Next, stop whatever you are doing and reflect on all that you have accomplished in your preparation plan. Sit quietly somewhere where you can concentrate on relaxing and tell yourself that you indeed prepared adequately for the test and are ready. Smile, brush those negative feelings away, do your breathing exercises, and keep repeating to yourself, "I am going to do well. I am prepared." Repeating this statement will build the extra confidence that you need, help you to maintain a positive attitude, help you to relax, and help your mind to focus before the exam.

HOW CAN YOU CONTROL YOUR TEST ANXIETY DURING THE EXAM?

During the exam if you begin to experience any anxious feelings, sit back in your chair and perform a relaxation technique, such as breathing exercises. These will help to relax you. The breathing exercises are also helpful if you begin to feel your mind wandering, if you feel distracted, or if you are unable to concentrate on the test question. Oxygenating your body will help you to focus and concentrate on the exam question.

Develop a structured sequence for approaching and taking the exam to help control anxiety, and use this pattern with each exam that you take. What happens if you are presented with a difficult question and have no idea what the answer should be? You become anxious, you feel as if you did not prepare well enough, and your self-confidence diminishes. To avoid this, follow the structured sequence outlined next.

STRUCTURED SEQUENCE FOR TAKING AN EXAM

Place your name on the test and on any other required testing documents.
Read the directions.
Skim through the pages in the test so that you have an idea of how to pace yourself.
If you are allowed to write on the test, jot down data that you needed to memorize and may need as a reference, such as a laboratory value.
Read each question and all options slowly and carefully.
Take your time when answering a question.
Use nursing knowledge and test-taking strategies to help you answer the question.
Skip any questions that are difficult.
Answer all the questions that you know and that are easy for you to answer.
Once you have answered all the easy questions, go back to the questions that were difficult.

✓ **NCLEX® Exam Tip**

On a nursing exam taken while in nursing school, one strategy is to skip questions that are difficult and go back to them once you have answered as many as you can. On the NCLEX exam you need to remember that you will not be able to skip a question and then go back to it. On the NCLEX exam, you must answer the question on the computer screen in front of you or the test will not move. So be prepared for this type of testing when you take the NCLEX exam.

THAT POSITIVE ATTITUDE: HOW CAN YOU MAINTAIN IT?

Maintaining a positive attitude will lead to success. It is natural to be a bit apprehensive about the path before you, especially if you are a beginning nursing student; but it is critical to your continued success that you believe in yourself and your ability to confidently conquer the challenges in your nursing program. Surround yourself with positive thoughts and positive people, and remember that your self-confidence in your ability to succeed is critical to your continued success.

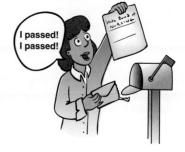

"Yes, I can do this."

When you start to fall into the trap of negative thought, stop! Control the moment, and believe in who you are! Step out of the negative and into the positive, and do not allow anything to stand in your path to success. The one phrase that should become your mantra is "Yes, I can do this." When you open your eyes in the morning and need to face a difficult day, your first thought should be "Yes, I can do this." Use visual reinforcement to help maintain your positive attitude. On a piece of paper write the words "Yes, I can do this" and keep this with you always. When you face a difficult challenge or need to take an exam and have test anxiety, place these written words in front of you so that you can see them. You will constantly be reminded of your self-confidence and ability to be successful.

REFERENCES

Fortinash, K., & Holoday-Worret, P. (2008). *Psychiatric mental health nursing* (4th ed.). St. Louis: Mosby.

Lewis, S., Heitkemper, M., Dirksen, S., & Bucher, L. (2007). *Medical-surgical nursing: Assessment and management of clinical problems* (7th ed.). St. Louis: Mosby.

Silvestri, L. (2010). *Saunders comprehensive review for the NCLEX-PN® examination* (4th ed.). St. Louis: Saunders.

Silvestri, L. (2008). *Saunders comprehensive review for the NCLEX-RN examination* (4th ed.). St. Louis: Saunders.

Varcarolis, E., Carlson, V., & Shoemaker, N. (2006). *Foundations of psychiatric mental health nursing* (5th ed.). Philadelphia: Saunders.

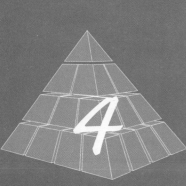

NCLEX® Preparation

WHERE DOES PREPARATION BEGIN?

NCLEX preparation began the moment that you entered your nursing program. Your nursing courses, clinical experiences, reading and other assignments and activities, and any standardized examinations that may have been required to be taken prepared you for the NCLEX exam. In addition, all the practice questions that you reviewed from your course textbooks and NCLEX review book have reinforced content, refined your knowledge base and critical thinking skills, and provided practice with test-taking strategies and how to answer a test question correctly. Now you are an experienced student nurse and are most likely in your final year of nursing school; therefore NCLEX preparation has become your priority focus. Now you need to fine-tune your nursing knowledge base, critical thinking skills, and test-taking skills. You may feel overwhelmed and just not sure where to begin preparing for the NCLEX exam. You may even become more overwhelmed when you look at all the boxes of class notes that you have accumulated and all the textbooks that you have read during nursing school. Now you are saying to yourself, "Where do I start?" Let us look at some points about the NCLEX exam and your plan for preparation!

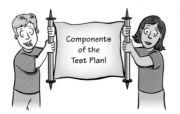

Components of the Test Plan!

THE NCLEX® TEST PLAN: WHY IS IT SO IMPORTANT?

An important strategy for success is to become as familiar as possible with the NCLEX test plan. You can experience a significant amount of anxiety as you face the challenge of this examination. Knowing what the examination is all about will assist in alleviating your fear and anxiety.

The test plan for the NCLEX exam is developed by the National Council of State Boards of Nursing (NCSBN). This test plan is developed based on state laws and regulations, including nursing practice acts, and research studies done with newly licensed nurses to determine the nursing activities that they perform as new nurses. Once this information is identified, the NCSBN formulates the test plan, and the test questions for the NCLEX exam are written. All the information that you will need about the test plan can be located at the NCSBN Web site at www.ncsbn.org. In fact, when you access this Web site you are able to download a copy of the current test plan for your use. The test plan will identify the framework of the NCLEX exam and will list content areas and nursing activities that you will be tested on. This is an extremely valuable resource and can be used as one of your study guides for preparing for the NCLEX exam. See the box below for the NCSBN contact information.

NCSBN CONTACT INFORMATION

National Council of State Boards of Nursing
111 E. Wacker Drive, Suite 2900
Chicago, IL 60601
Web site: www.ncsbn.org

In addition to the test plan, the NCSBN Web site provides much information about the examination process, registering for the NCLEX exam, scheduling a test date, the testing center, and processing results. A tutorial is available to provide you with the experience of answering questions on the NCLEX exam. Multiple-choice questions and alternate item format questions are also available for practice. So take the time to visit the NCSBN Web site and find out everything that you need to know about the test plan and the testing experience. Remember that you want to face this challenge with as much information as possible, and awareness of what the test is all about will help alleviate your anxiety!

WHAT ARE THE STEPS FOR PREPARING?

STEPS FOR PREPARING FOR THE NCLEX® EXAM

Step 1: Your Self-Assessment
Step 2: Your Preparation Plan and Goals
Step 3: Scheduling a Testing Date
Step 4: Implementing Your Preparation Plan
Step 5: Determining Your Readiness for the NCLEX Exam

Step 1: Your Self-Assessment

The first step in preparing for the NCLEX exam is a self-assessment. Your self-assessment is important because it will guide your development of a structured and individualized preparation plan. Open your "My NCLEX Study Guide" binder, and review any notes that you have taken about your strengths or weaknesses. Also review any detailed reports from standardized tests that you have taken, because these reports provide extremely valuable information about your areas of strength and the areas that you need to particularly focus on. If you have not yet set up your binder labeled "My NCLEX Study Guide," you want to do so to begin your preparation for the NCLEX exam. If you do not have copies of standardized test results

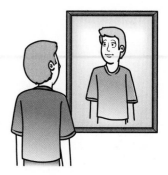

or did not take standardized tests in your nursing program, then use your NCLEX review book to perform a self-assessment. Access the CD in your NCLEX review book to take a 100-question comprehensive exam. Print out the results, and identify your areas of strength and weakness. Place the printout in your "My NCLEX Study Guide" notebook. Then answer the top-10 self-assessment questions listed in the box below in your notebook. Your responses to these questions will assist you in determining your preparation plan and goals.

TOP-10 SELF-ASSESSMENT QUESTIONS

Question 1: What do I feel are my strong and weak areas in nursing content, and what strong and weak areas were identified in standardized testing or other assessment tests that I took?
Question 2: How do I normally study for exams, alone or in groups?
Question 3: Where is my special study place?
Question 4: Am I comfortable using a computer?
Question 5: Do I complete exams within the allotted time?
Question 6: Do I have balance in life; do I exercise, have fun, relax, and eat a balanced and healthy diet?
Question 7: Do I have test anxiety, and how do I control it?
Question 8: Am I able to focus and concentrate during an exam?
Question 9: Am I able to self-discipline and stick to a study plan?
Question 10: Do I have a positive attitude?

Step 2: Your Preparation Plan and Goals

Now that you have answered the self-assessment questions, your next step is to review your answers and develop a plan of preparation and goals. Table 4-1 provides pyramid points ▲ to assist you in determining your preparation plan and goals.

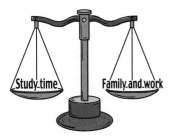

After you graduate from your nursing program, plan to spend at least 2 hours daily preparing for the NCLEX exam. Open your calendar, and mark off days that you have obligations or commitments and will not be able to spend any time on NCLEX preparation. For the remaining days, set a 2-hour time schedule for NCLEX preparation time that will work for you considering your family and personal responsibilities. This is your time and needs to be uninterrupted, so shut off your cell phone and close off the world. This will help you to concentrate and make the most of your preparation time. Remember, though, that you need to maintain balance in your life, so during your off-study hours, exercise, relax, and have fun.

TABLE 4-1 **YOUR PREPARATION PLAN AND GOALS**	
Assessment Question	**Pyramid Points ▲**
Question 1: What do I feel are my strong and weak areas in nursing content, and what strong and weak areas were identified in standardized testing or other assessment tests that I took?	Prioritize your plan of study, listing your weakest to your strongest area(s). You want to plan to begin your NCLEX preparation by reviewing your weakest content areas first; once you have demonstrated improvement in your weak area(s), proceed to review your stronger area(s).

TABLE 4-1 YOUR PREPARATION PLAN AND GOALS—cont'd	
Assessment Question	**Pyramid Points ▲**
Question 2: How do I normally study for exams, alone or in groups?	Study groups are very helpful for some students but not for all students. So you need to think about whether they will help you. You may be the type of learner who requires quiet and alone time to absorb the material, or you may be the type of learner who learns best by reviewing content aloud with others. Continue to do what you have done during your nursing program. If you studied alone, then this is what you should do to prepare for the NCLEX exam. You need to meet your needs, so do not be persuaded to join a study group if it will not work for you. You have been successful thus far, so keep doing what you were doing!
Question 3: Where is my special study place?	Think about how you have normally studied for your nursing exams and where you have studied. If you normally study alone in the early morning, then plan to study at this time. If you have a special study place, then continue to use it. Do not change these study habits, because they have worked for you in the past; otherwise, you would not be at the point that you are, preparing for the NCLEX exam. Do what you normally do, and stick to that special study place that you have been using throughout nursing school!
Question 4: Am I comfortable with using a computer?	If you have been using a computer while in nursing school then you probably are quite comfortable with it. If this is not the case, then you need to begin using a computer so that when you take the NCLEX exam, any anxiety related to testing on a computer is eased. If you do not have a computer, then locate one that you can use, such as at your nursing program, school library, or a public library. Use your CD from your NCLEX review book to begin studying by practicing test questions. In addition, while using the computer, access the NCSBN Web site and do the tutorial and any other NCLEX-related practice sessions provided. This will get you used to testing on a computer.

Continued

TABLE 4-1   YOUR PREPARATION PLAN AND GOALS—cont'd

Assessment Question	Pyramid Points ♠
Question 5: Do I complete exams within the allotted time?	You will have 6 hours to complete the NCLEX-RN, and 5 hours for the NCLEX-PN. The maximum number of questions that need to be answered on the NCLEX-RN is 265, and the maximum number on the NCLEX-PN is 205. Therefore, if each question on the NCLEX exam was individually timed, you would have approximately 1.35 minutes for each question on the NCLEX-RN and approximately 1.46 minutes for each question on the NCLEX-PN. If you did not have a problem completing exams within the allotted time in nursing school, then you will probably not have a problem completing the NCLEX exam within the allotted time. If you had a problem completing exams on time in nursing school, then you need to work on picking up your speed with answering questions without jeopardizing the quality of how you are thinking through the question and answering it. You may ask, "How do I do this?" Practicing is the answer! Use an alarm clock, or set an alarm on your cell phone. Access your CD from your NCLEX review book, and select a 100-question exam. Allow approximately 1.35 minutes or 1.46 minutes for each question depending on which NCLEX exam you are preparing to take. For example, if you are preparing for the NCLEX-RN exam set the alarm to ring in 135 minutes (or 2.25 hours). When the alarm rings, note how many questions you have completed. If you did not complete the 100 questions in the allotted time, note how many were unanswered. Then you need to work on picking up speed. Keep practicing until you are able to complete a 100-question test in the allotted time without jeopardizing the quality of how you are answering the questions.
Question 6: Do I have balance in life; do I exercise, have fun, relax, and eat a	Balance in life is extremely important if you want to be successful. Remember that all work and no play is not healthy. You cannot spend every hour of every day preparing for

TABLE 4-1 YOUR PREPARATION PLAN AND GOALS—cont'd

Assessment Question	Pyramid Points ▲
balanced and healthy diet?	the NCLEX exam. You need to develop a study plan and stick to it, but you also need time to relax, have some fun, and eat healthy, because a healthy diet will build and maintain your energy level and your stamina to meet your set goals. Chapter 2 provides specific strategies related to exercise and eating healthy.
Question 7: Do I have test anxiety, and how do I control it?	Controlling your test anxiety is a must. Some anxiety is useful because it keeps your senses sharp and alert and you definitely want to feel sharp and alert on the day of the NCLEX exam. However, overwhelming anxiety can block your thinking and become an obstacle. So think about what you did when you had to take exams during nursing school, and use these same strategies. Also, be sure to read Chapter 3 for strategies to reduce your test anxiety.
Question 8: Am I able to focus and concentrate during an exam?	If it is difficult to focus and concentrate during an exam, sit back in your chair, close your eyes, and take some slow deep breaths. Breathe in through your nose slowly, hold your breath to a count of 4, and then breathe out through your mouth. Repeat this breathing exercise 4 or 5 times, and then go back to the questions on the exam. These breathing exercises will fill your body and cells, including your brain cells, with oxygen. This will help you to regain control, and you will be better equipped to focus and concentrate.
Question 9: Am I able to self-discipline and stick to a study plan?	Self-discipline is the ability to get yourself to do what you planned, such as adhering to a study plan, regardless of how you feel. It is very easy to get off track with your study plan because "I just do not feel like studying" or because "I would rather be doing something else." If you do not self-discipline, you will not meet your goals. Remember that every successful person works hard and has a great deal of self-discipline. If you want to be successful, self-discipline and stick to your study plan. You will feel great after your study session knowing that you accomplished your goal.

Continued

TABLE 4-1   YOUR PREPARATION PLAN AND GOALS—cont'd

Assessment Question	Pyramid Points ▲
Question 10: Do I have a positive attitude?	A positive attitude will lead to success. You must stay positive about your ability to pass the NCLEX exam. Do not for one moment ever think that you will fail—no negative thoughts! On a large piece of paper write your name in large letters across the top. Now underneath your name, in large letters, write the letters RN or LPN, depending on what your credentials will be when you become licensed. Now doesn't that piece of paper with your name and credentials on it look great? Keep this with you always, especially during your study sessions. This visual will change any negative thoughts that you may have into positive ones!

YOUR PREPARATION PLAN

Do not change your study habits.
Review your weakest areas first.
Plan a 2-hour daily study session.
Practice a *minimum* of 3000 questions.
Review all rationales and test-taking strategies.
Learn ways to control your test anxiety.
Eat healthy and make time to relax, exercise, and have fun.

Step 3: Scheduling a Testing Date

Many nursing graduates ask the question, "How long should I wait to schedule an exam date for the NCLEX exam?" There is no easy or cut-and-dried answer to this question. This is a very individualized decision based on how much preparation that you need to do, your goals, your preparation plan, and your time frame for implementation of your plan. You definitely need to prepare for this exam—this is critical. However, it is also extremely important that you do not wait too long. So, depending on your individual preparation needs, how much preparing you need to do, and how much time you have to prepare, schedule a date within 1½ to 2 months following graduation. Then, after graduation, get working on implementing your preparation plan. So get yourself ready and take that exam!

Step 4: Implementing Your Preparation Plan

Do not for a moment think that the way you will prepare for this exam is to read all your class notes and textbooks cover to cover. This is not the way to prepare for the NCLEX exam, and just the thought of doing this can worsen your already existing overwhelmed feelings. Place your boxes of class notes in a closet out of your sight. The information in them is much too detailed to assist in your preparation. Use your textbooks as a reference to read content areas that you find difficult.

> Practicing answering test questions is a must!

Practicing answering test questions is a must, and the best way to prepare for the NCLEX exam is to practice question after question after question on a computer. Practicing answering test questions yields a twofold reward: (1) you will strengthen your knowledge base of nursing content, and (2) you will become skillful in the use of test-taking strategies. The more you practice, the more prepared you will be for this exam. You should practice answering a *minimum* of 3000 NCLEX-style practice questions before taking the exam. This is very individualized; and to be proficient and skilled with answering exam questions correctly, many graduates need to practice answering between 4000 and 5000 NCLEX-style questions before taking the exam. You also need to score at least an 85% on your practice tests; if you do not obtain this score, then you need to review the content that you are having difficulty with and again answer practice questions in your area of difficulty until you can achieve at least an 85%. It is important to remember here that you also need to read the rationales and test-taking strategies that accompany each practice question, because this will help you refine your nursing knowledge and critical thinking skills. Remember that NCLEX questions will be presented at the cognitive levels of application or analysis or even higher levels. Reading the rationales and test-taking strategies will improve your critical thinking skills for answering future questions.

You may have obtained a comprehensive NCLEX review book during your nursing program, and this book most likely contained both content review and practice questions. You can continue to use this book for NCLEX preparation, but consider selecting a second resource that contains only practice questions. Be selective when deciding on a review book. Also, the preface of this book describes several different NCLEX review products available that will ensure your success on the NCLEX exam.

SELECTING A REVIEW BOOK

Make sure that your resource provides *at least* 3000 practice questions.
Check to see if each question is accompanied by a rationale that provides an explanation for both the correct and incorrect options and a test-taking strategy.
Find out what other information accompanies each question, such as test plan codes and a reference source for the question.
Be sure that a CD accompanies the book.
Check to see what options for content selection are available for the practice questions on the CD.
Note the modes for testing on the CD, and look for a book that provides a study mode, quiz mode, and exam mode.
Be sure that you are given detailed printouts of your performance on quizzes or exams.

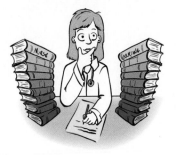

Now that you have your NCLEX resource, start practicing questions. Begin selecting content areas that are your weakest areas, and select the study mode. The study mode will generate all possible available questions on the CD in the content area selected and also provide the correct answer, rationale, and test-taking strategy as soon as you submit your answer. This is an important mode to use when you start your preparation, because you will learn as you go along. When you find that you have difficulty with answering a question, note the problem area in your binder, and after you have completed your study session review this content in your textbooks or your NCLEX review book. Once you feel that you have strengthened your weak area by using the study mode, move to the quiz mode and take a quiz to note your improvement. Normally a quiz mode will provide 10 questions. This mode differs from the study mode in that it provides feedback after you answer all the questions rather than after each question. Continue with this pattern of review, moving from your weak areas to your strong areas.

Step 5: Determining Your Readiness for the NCLEX® Exam

Remember that you are ready to take the NCLEX exam and that you were ready when you completed your nursing program. However, preparation for the NCLEX exam after graduation is a critical piece in becoming successful on this exam. At this point you have implemented your preparation plan and now need to determine your readiness and refine any remaining weak areas while waiting for your scheduled NCLEX date. How will you do this? Using your CD, select the exam mode (100 practice questions) and select all content areas so that you generate an integrated content exam. Review your results, and brush up on any weak areas. Continue to take these 100-question exams and follow this pattern until it is time to take the NCLEX exam. Remember that it is important to maintain momentum and a pattern when getting ready for this exam, so continue to practice questions every day.

It is time to take the NCLEX exam. Are you ready? Of course you are! As long as you followed your preparation plan and worked at strengthening any weak areas, you are ready for the challenge!

REFERENCES

National Council of State Boards of Nursing Web site: www.ncsbn.org

Silvestri, L. (2010). *Saunders comprehensive review for the NCLEX-PN® examination* (4th ed.). St. Louis: Saunders.

Silvestri, L. (2008). *Saunders comprehensive review for the NCLEX-RN® examination* (4th ed.). St. Louis: Saunders.

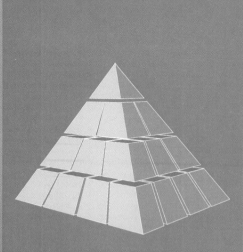

Part II

Strategies for Success

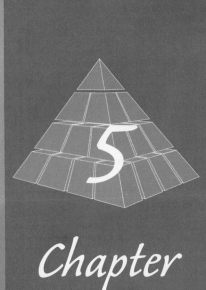

5
Chapter

How to Avoid "Reading Into the Question"

One of the pitfalls that can cause a problem when trying to answer a question correctly is "reading into the question." This means that you are considering issues beyond the information presented in the question. Some strategies that you can use to prevent this from happening when answering a question include the following: identifying the ingredients of a question, reading carefully and looking for strategic words or strategic phrases, identifying the subject of the question and what the question is asking, using the process of elimination, and avoiding the "What if?" syndrome.

▲ INGREDIENTS OF A QUESTION
What Are the Ingredients of a Question?

Each multiple-choice question will contain a case event, a question query, and four options. It is important to identify the ingredients of a question as you read it, because this will help you to sort out the facts and determine what the question is asking.

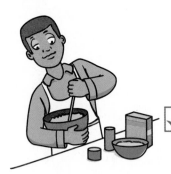

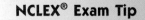

✓ **NCLEX® Exam Tip**

On the NCLEX exam, you will encounter fill-in-the-blank questions and prioritizing (ordered-response) questions.

Fill-in-the-blank questions will contain a case event and a question query but may not contain options. Remember that fill-in-the-blank questions will require you to perform a medication calculation, calculate an intravenous (IV) flow rate, or calculate an intake and output. Because you need to type in the answer for these type of questions, it makes sense that options will not be provided.

In a prioritizing (ordered-response) question, six items will be presented, such as nursing interventions. In this type of question, you will not need to select options; rather, you will be required to list the items presented, such as nursing interventions, in order of priority. On the NCLEX exam you will need to use the computer mouse and drag and drop the options in order of priority. On nursing exams you may be asked to number the options in order of priority. Remember that in a prioritizing (ordered-response) question, all the items listed will be correct.

What Is the Case Event?

The case event is the "heart" of the question. It provides the information that you need to think about to answer the question.

What Is the Question Query?

The question query is a statement that generally follows the case event and asks you something specific about the case event.

What Are the Options?

The options are all the answers presented with the question. A multiple-choice question will have four options, and you must select one. A multiple-response question will have several options, and you must select all options that apply to the case event and the question query.

A figure or illustration question may be presented in a multiple-choice format. For example, you may be given a question with a figure of a rhythm strip, a case event and question query related to the rhythm strip, and four options of which only one will be correct. Or you may be given a question with a figure or illustration, and you will be asked to use the computer mouse to click on the correct option in the figure or illustration. For example, the question may contain a figure of the human body, a case event, and a question query. On the figure you may note small circles, sometimes called "hot spots," and you will be asked to click on the circle that indicates the correct answer to the question.

Examples of the various types of questions that may appear in your nursing exams or on the NCLEX exam and the specific ingredients of the questions are provided in this section. The answers to these example questions and the test-taking strategy also are provided.

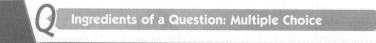

Q Ingredients of a Question: Multiple Choice

Case Event: The nurse is reviewing the laboratory results of a client who is receiving magnesium sulfate by IV infusion and notes that the magnesium level is 3.5 mg/dL.
Question Query: Based on this laboratory result, the nurse would most likely expect to note which of the following in the client?
Options:
1. Tremors
2. Hyperactive reflexes
3. Respiratory depression
4. No specific signs or symptoms because this value is a normal level

Answer: 3
Test-Taking Strategy:
Read each option carefully. Use the process of elimination, and note the strategic words *most likely*. Knowing that the level identified in the question is elevated will assist in eliminating option 4. Next, eliminate options 1 and 2 because they are comparable or alike. Remember to use nursing knowledge, focus on the information in the case event, identify what the question is asking (the subject), note the strategic words, read carefully, and use the process of elimination.

Tip for the Beginning Nursing Student

You need to know that the normal magnesium level is 1.6 to 2.6 mg/dL. Therefore the magnesium level presented in the question is elevated. Next you need to know the signs and symptoms indicative of an elevated magnesium level. Learn this normal level and the signs and symptoms of a magnesium imbalance.

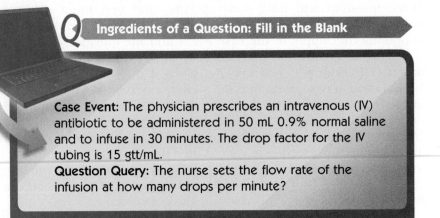

Ingredients of a Question: Fill in the Blank

Case Event: The physician prescribes an intravenous (IV) antibiotic to be administered in 50 mL 0.9% normal saline and to infuse in 30 minutes. The drop factor for the IV tubing is 15 gtt/mL.
Question Query: The nurse sets the flow rate of the infusion at how many drops per minute?

Answer: 25
Test-Taking Strategy:
Note the strategic words *sets the flow rate*. Read the question carefully, focusing on the information in the question and that 50 mL fluid is to infuse in 30 minutes and the drop factor is 15. Use the formula for calculating an IV infusion to answer the question. Always double-check the calculation, and verify your answer. Remember to use nursing knowledge, focus on the information in the case event, identify what the question is asking (the subject), and note the strategic words.

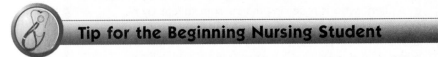

Tip for the Beginning Nursing Student

In this question you need to know the formula for calculating an IV flow rate. The formula and the calculation for this question are as follows:

$$\frac{\text{Total volume to be infused} \times \text{Drop factor}}{\text{Time in minutes}} = \text{Drops per minute}$$

$$\frac{50 \times 15}{30} = 25$$

Use the formula for calculating an IV infusion. Perform the calculation on the note board provided to you, and use the computer on-screen calculator to verify your answer. Read carefully, because in calculation questions you may be asked to round the answer to the nearest whole number or to the nearest tenth.

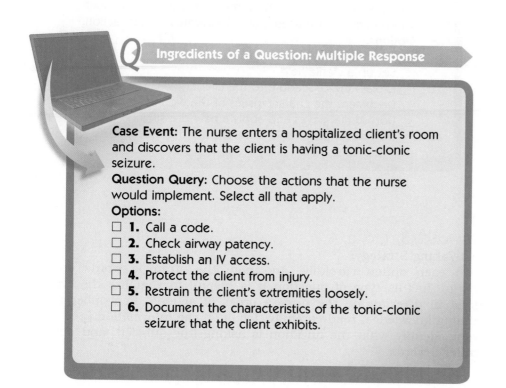

Q Ingredients of a Question: Multiple Response

Case Event: The nurse enters a hospitalized client's room and discovers that the client is having a tonic-clonic seizure.

Question Query: Choose the actions that the nurse would implement. Select all that apply.

Options:
☐ **1.** Call a code.
☐ **2.** Check airway patency.
☐ **3.** Establish an IV access.
☐ **4.** Protect the client from injury.
☐ **5.** Restrain the client's extremities loosely.
☐ **6.** Document the characteristics of the tonic-clonic seizure that the client exhibits.

Answer: 2, 3, 4, 6

Test-Taking Strategy:

Read each option carefully. In this type of question, it is helpful to visualize the event to assist in determining the nurse's actions. Remember that a patent airway and client safety are your priority. Use nursing knowledge, focus on the information in the case event, identify what the question is asking (the subject), note the strategic words, read carefully, and use the process of elimination.

Tip for the Beginning Nursing Student

You need to know that a seizure is an abnormal sudden excessive discharge of electrical activity within the brain. You also need to know what you would do if a client has a seizure. What you need to remember is that a patent airway and client safety are your priority. Learn the nursing interventions for a client experiencing a seizure.

Ingredients of a Question: Prioritizing (Ordered Response)

Case Event: A nurse is preparing to change an abdominal dressing using sterile technique.

Question Query: List in order of priority the actions that the nurse would take to perform this procedure. Number 1 indicates the first action, and 6 indicates the last action.

Options:

___Wash hands.

___Set up a sterile field.

___Explain the procedure to the client.

___Document the characteristics of the wound.

___Don sterile gloves and apply a new dressing.

___Don clean gloves and remove the old dressing.

Answer: 2, 3, 1, 6, 5, 4

Test-Taking Strategy:

Read each option carefully, and note the strategic words *order of priority*. In this type of question it is helpful to visualize the event to assist in determining the nurse's order of actions. Remember to use nursing knowledge, read carefully, focus on the information in the case event, identify what the question is asking (the subject), and note the strategic words.

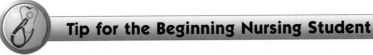

Tip for the Beginning Nursing Student

You need to know the principles that are related to asepsis and the technique for changing a sterile dressing, which you will learn in your fundamentals of nursing class. Learn these principles and techniques, because they are critical in preventing infection in the client.

NCLEX® Exam Tip

For a prioritizing (ordered-response) question on the NCLEX exam, you will need to use the computer mouse to drag and drop the options in order of priority.

Ingredients of a Question: Figure or Illustration

Case Event: The nurse is checking the arterial pulses on an adult client.

Question Query: Mark the area where the nurse would palpate the carotid pulse (see Figure 5-1 on the next page).

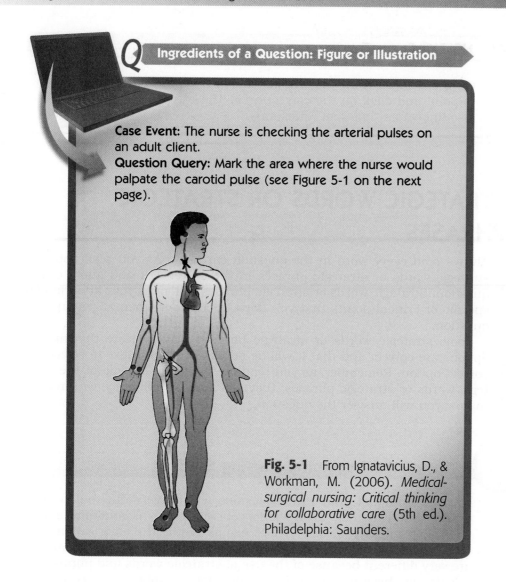

Fig. 5-1 From Ignatavicius, D., & Workman, M. (2006). *Medical-surgical nursing: Critical thinking for collaborative care* (5th ed.). Philadelphia: Saunders.

Answer: answer is indicated by the circle marked with the X

Test-Taking Strategy:

Note the strategic words *carotid pulse.* In this type of question it is helpful to visualize the pulse points for assessment of arterial pulses to identify the correct answer. Remember to use nursing knowledge, read carefully, focus on the information in the case event, identify what the question is asking (the subject), and note the strategic words.

Tip for the Beginning Nursing Student

You need to know where the arterial pulse points are located. Use what you learned in anatomy class to assist in answering this question. You will also learn these pulse points in your fundamentals of nursing class and in your physical assessment class. Be sure to learn these pulse points for assessment of arterial pulses.

✓ **NCLEX® Exam Tip**

On the NCLEX exam you will be asked to use the computer mouse to point and click on the correct area. These types of questions are also known as "hot spot" questions.

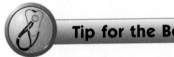

STRATEGIC WORDS OR STRATEGIC PHRASES

Always read every word in the question carefully. As you read, look for strategic words or strategic phrases in the case event and query of the question. Strategic words or strategic phrases will focus your attention on specific or critical points that you need to consider when answering the question.

Some strategic words or strategic phrases may indicate that all the options are correct and that it will be necessary to prioritize to select the correct option. Remember, as you read the question, to look for the strategic words or strategic phrases; they will make a difference with regard to how you will answer the question.

 Tip for the Beginning Nursing Student

You will find that your nursing exams will be very different from exams that you took in previous courses, such as anatomy and physiology or microbiology. Those exams required memorization of facts, which helped you to answer questions correctly. Nursing exams are very different because of the use of strategic words and phrases; the use of these words may indicate that all options are correct. Therefore it is critically important that you learn what these strategic words and phrases are and that you work at using nursing knowledge, critical thinking skills, and test-taking strategies to answer correctly.

What Are the Commonly Used Strategic Words or Strategic Phrases to Look for?

Common Strategic Words or Strategic Phrases That Indicate There Is Only One Correct Option

Some strategic words or strategic phrases used in a question will indicate that *there is only one correct option*. Some of these words and phrases include:

- Early sign
- Late sign
- Understands
- Goal has been achieved

Goals have not yet been fully met
Has not met the outcome criteria
Adequately tolerating
Inadequate
Unable to tolerate
Ineffective
Avoid
Needs additional instructions
Lack of understanding

Common Strategic Words or Strategic Phrases That Indicate the Need to Prioritize

There are also strategic words or strategic phrases that may indicate that all options are correct and that *it will be necessary to prioritize to select the correct option*. Some of these words and phrases include:

Best
First
Initial
Immediately
Most likely or least likely
Most appropriate or least appropriate
Highest or lowest priority
Order of priority
At highest risk
At lowest risk
Best understanding

Common Strategic Words or Strategic Phrases That Indicate a Positive or Negative Event Question/Query

Finally, some strategic words or strategic phrases indicate that the question is a positive or negative event question query. Strategic words or strategic phrases used in these types of questions may indicate that there is only one correct option or may indicate the need to prioritize to select the correct option. (Additional information about positive or negative event queries can be found in Chapter 6.)

Common words or phrases that indicate *a positive event question/query* include:

Early sign
Late sign
Best
First
Initial
Immediately
Most likely
Most appropriate
Highest priority
Order of priority
All nursing interventions that apply
Goal has been achieved
Adequately tolerating

Common words or phrases that indicate *a negative event question/ query* include:

Least likely
Least appropriate
Least priority
Least helpful
At lowest risk
Avoid
Needs additional instructions
Needs additional teaching
Lack of understanding
Goals have not yet been fully met
Has not met the outcome criteria
Ineffective
Inadequate
Unable to tolerate

Use of Strategic Words or Strategic Phrases in a Question

You may be asking yourself: "How are these strategic words or strategic phrases used in a question?" Following are some examples of question queries that contain strategic words:

Select all nursing interventions that apply in the care of the client.
Which statement by a client *indicates an understanding of the instructions*?
What is the *initial* nursing action?
Which of the following is an *early* sign of hypoxia?
List in order of priority the actions that the nurse would take.
Which of the following individuals is *least likely* to develop hypertension?
Which nursing diagnosis is of *least priority*?
The nurse would *avoid* which of the following actions?
The nurse determines that the client *needs additional teaching* if the client stated which of the following?
The nurse determines that the treatment is *ineffective* if which if the following is noted?

▲ THE SUBJECT OF THE QUESTION
What Is the Subject of the Question?

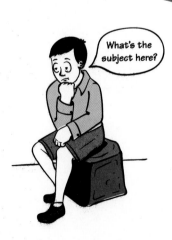

What's the subject here?

The subject of the question is the specific content that the question is asking about. It is important to read every word in the question. As you read and note the strategic words or strategic phrases, determine what the question is asking. Identifying the subject of the question will help you eliminate the incorrect options and direct you to the correct option.

Tip for the Beginning Nursing Student

The questions on nursing exams will cover subjects that you have learned in your nursing course. Focus on these subject areas when preparing for a nursing exam. If your instructor gives you a study guide for the exam, review all subject areas on the study guide.

✓ **NCLEX® Exam Tip**

There are hundreds of subjects that you could be asked about when you take the NCLEX exam. This is understandable, especially when you think about all the information that you needed to learn in nursing school. A test question may ask about any Client Needs area of the NCLEX Test Plan, any content area of nursing, or anything that has to do with the role and responsibilities of the nurse. Therefore the list of subjects that could be tested is never-ending. It is extremely helpful to obtain a copy of the detailed NCLEX Test Plan, which is published by the National Council of State Boards of Nursing (NCSBN). This Test Plan, which identifies some of the content that will be tested on the NCLEX exam, can be obtained at no fee at the NCSBN Web site (www.ncsbn.org). Be sure to download the detailed Test Plan.

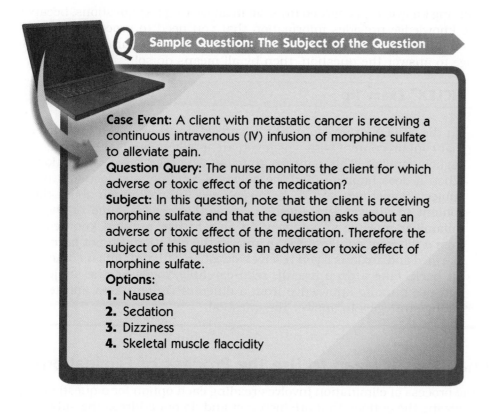

Q Sample Question: The Subject of the Question

Case Event: A client with metastatic cancer is receiving a continuous intravenous (IV) infusion of morphine sulfate to alleviate pain.

Question Query: The nurse monitors the client for which adverse or toxic effect of the medication?

Subject: In this question, note that the client is receiving morphine sulfate and that the question asks about an adverse or toxic effect of the medication. Therefore the subject of this question is an adverse or toxic effect of morphine sulfate.

Options:

1. Nausea
2. Sedation
3. Dizziness
4. Skeletal muscle flaccidity

Answer: 4

Test-Taking Strategy:
Read every word in the question, and specifically determine what the question is asking. The question is asking about the adverse or toxic effect of morphine sulfate. Dizziness, sedation, and nausea are side effects of morphine sulfate that the client may experience, but they are not adverse or toxic effects. Remember to focus on the information in the question and what the question is asking!

Tip for the Beginning Nursing Student

You need to know that morphine sulfate is an opioid analgesic and that it causes depression of the central nervous system. Next noting that the question is asking about an adverse or toxic effect will assist in answering correctly. You will learn about morphine sulfate in your nursing courses, and it is important that you are very familiar with the side effects and adverse and toxic effects of the medication. In addition to skeletal muscle flaccidity, a major concern is that the medication causes respiratory depression. Learn the side effects and adverse effects of this medication.

USING NURSING KNOWLEDGE AND THE PROCESS OF ELIMINATION
Why Is Nursing Knowledge So Important?

Nursing knowledge is needed to assist in answering test questions, because the knowledge provides information that you need to process and think about critically to answer the question. If you can use your nursing knowledge to answer the question, then by all means do so!

✓ NCLEX® Exam Tip

On the NCLEX exam, do not be surprised if you are given questions that contain content with which you are totally unfamiliar or are only vaguely familiar. This happens to many who take this examination. When it does happen, read the question carefully and focus on the subject. Sometimes you do not even need to know much about the content to answer the question. In addition, with some of these unfamiliar questions, you may be able to use nursing knowledge from a different content area to answer the question. Do not become alarmed and anxious if you receive a question with unfamiliar content. Sit back, take a deep breath, read carefully, focus on the subject, and use nursing knowledge from a different content area and test-taking strategies to answer the question.

What Does It Mean to Use the Process of Elimination?

The process of elimination involves reading each option for a question and removing the options that are incorrect and do not address the subject of the question. Using the process of elimination is extremely important when you are reading the options to a question and trying to determine the correct answer. Do not hastily select an option because it sounds good. Always read every option carefully before selecting an answer.

Some students will read a question, and before looking at the options they will determine a correct answer. This is a helpful strategy for answering a test question, because you are using nursing knowledge to help answer the question correctly. The problem with this strategy is that you may have an answer to the question in mind, but when you look at the options your answer is not there. This can be very frustrating and anxiety provoking. Let's look at the example on the next page.

Sample Question: The Process of Elimination

Case Event: A client who has type 1 diabetes mellitus describes shakiness and hunger 2 hours after receiving a dose of regular insulin.

Question Query: The nurse determines that the client is having a hypoglycemic reaction and prepares to give the client which best item from the dietary kitchen to treat the reaction?

After you read this question, you will immediately think, "Orange juice! Yes, orange juice is the best item! I know the answer to this question." Then you look at the options and find the following:

Options:

1. Milk
2. Diet soda
3. Sugar-free gelatin
4. Sugar-free cookies

Answer: 1

Test-Taking Strategy:

Your answer, orange juice, is not there! So now what do you do? You need to use your nursing knowledge and think about what thought processes led you to identify orange juice as the answer to the question. Remember that a food item that contains 10 to 15 g carbohydrate is used to treat a hypoglycemic reaction. Now look at your options and use the process of elimination. In this question you can eliminate options 2, 3, and 4 because these items do not contain carbohydrates.

Tip for the Beginning Nursing Student

You need to know that diabetes mellitus is a chronic disorder of impaired carbohydrate, protein, and lipid metabolism that is caused by a deficiency of effective insulin. You also need to know that hypoglycemia is a complication of diabetes mellitus, and you need to know the signs of hypoglycemia. You will learn a great deal about diabetes mellitus during your nursing courses because it is a major health disorder. In this question you can use medical terminology skills to determine that *hypoglycemia* means a low blood glucose level. When the blood glucose is low then we need to provide glucose to the client. The only item in the options that will provide a form of glucose is milk. Learn about diabetes mellitus, the signs of hypoglycemia, and its treatment.

What Do You Do if You Eliminate Two Options and Are Unsure of the Final Two?

As you use the process of elimination to rule out the incorrect options, it is likely that you will be able to easily eliminate two of the four options in a multiple-choice question. Now what do you do with the last two options, and how do you proceed to select the correct one? Follow these helpful steps when you are trying to decide which of the last two options is correct.

1. Read the question again.
2. Identify the case event from the query of the question.
3. Look for the strategic words or strategic phrases.
4. Identify the subject of the question.
5. Ask yourself, "What is the question asking?"
6. Read the options again.
7. Make your final choice by focusing on what the question is asking, using nursing knowledge, and implementing test-taking strategies.

What Is the "What If?" Syndrome?

The "What if?" syndrome occurs when you read a test question and, instead of simply focusing on the information in the question, you start asking yourself, "Well, what if?" You need to avoid asking yourself this question, because this leads you right into the dreaded pitfall of "reading into the question." Read the question carefully, identify strategic words or strategic phrases, and focus on the subject of the question. You may need to think critically to answer the question, but stay on track! Asking yourself "What if?" moves you off track with regard to what the question is asking. Let's look at two questions and then examine the ways to avoid reading into them.

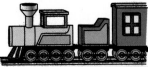

STAY ON TRACK!

Q Sample Question 1

Case Event: A nurse is changing the tapes on a tracheostomy tube. The client coughs, and the tube is dislodged.

Question Query: The *initial* nursing action is to:

1. Call the physician to reinsert the tube
2. Grasp the retention sutures to spread the opening
3. Call the respiratory therapy department to reinsert the tube
4. Cover the tracheostomy site with a sterile dressing to prevent infection

Now you may immediately think, "The tube is dislodged, and I need the physician!" Read the question carefully. Note the strategic word *initial,* and focus on the subject—the client's tube is dislodged. The question is asking you for a nursing action, so that is what you need to look for. This will direct you to option 2. Use nursing knowledge and test-taking strategies to assist in answering the question.

Answer: 2

Test-Taking Strategy:
Use the process of elimination, and focus on the subject. Eliminate options 1 and 3 first because they are comparable or alike and will delay the immediate intervention needed. Eliminate option 4 because this action will block the airway. If the tube is accidentally dislodged, the initial nursing action is to grasp the retention sutures and spread the opening. In addition, use of the ABCs—airway, breathing, and circulation—will direct you to the correct option.

Tip for the Beginning Nursing Student

A tracheostomy is an opening into the trachea that is created surgically for the purpose of establishing an airway. You will learn about the care of a client with a tracheostomy tube when you learn about nursing care for a client with a respiratory condition; but the important thing to remember for any client, is that maintaining a patent airway is the nurse's priority. In this question the only nursing action that will open the airway is the action identified in option 2. Learn about tracheostomy care and the nurse's responsibilities in the care of the client.

Q Sample Question 2

Case Event: A nurse is caring for a hospitalized client with a diagnosis of heart failure who suddenly reports shortness of breath and dyspnea.

Question Query: The nurse takes which *immediate* action?

1. Calls the physician
2. Administers oxygen to the client
3. Elevates the head of the client's bed
4. Prepares to administer furosemide (Lasix)

Now you may immediately think that the client has developed pulmonary edema, a complication of heart failure, and needs a diuretic. Although pulmonary edema is a complication of heart failure, there is no information in the question indicating the presence of pulmonary edema. The question simply states that the client suddenly reports shortness of breath and dyspnea. Read the question carefully. Note the strategic word *immediate,* and focus on the subject—the client's symptoms. The question is asking you for a nursing action, so that is what you need to look for. This will direct you to option 3. Use nursing knowledge and test-taking strategies to assist in answering the question.

Answer: 3

Test-Taking Strategy:

Use the process of elimination, and focus on the information in the question and on the subject. Note the strategic word *immediate*. Think about the client's symptoms, and look for the *immediate* nursing action. Although the physician may need to be notified, this is not the immediate action. A physician's order is needed to administer oxygen. Furosemide is a diuretic and may or may not be prescribed for the client. Because no data in the question indicate the presence of pulmonary edema, option 3 is correct.

Tip for the Beginning Nursing Student

Heart failure is an inability of the heart to maintain adequate circulation to meet the metabolic needs of the body because of an impaired pumping ability. Pulmonary edema is a serious complication of heart failure in which fluid accumulates in the pulmonary system as a result of the impaired pumping ability of the heart. You will learn about heart failure and pulmonary edema when you learn about cardiac disorders. One thing to remember is that with all clients, airway is the priority and that as the nurse you need to take an immediate action that will assist the client to breathe easily. In many questions that ask for an immediate action, the action that identifies a client position is usually the immediate action, as long as the position is a correct one. For clients with respiratory or cardiac problems, elevation of the client's head will assist with breathing. Learn about heart failure and pulmonary edema, the signs and symptoms, and immediate nursing actions to take.

REFERENCES

Hodgson, B., & Kizior, R. (2008). *Saunders nursing drug handbook 2008.* Philadelphia: Saunders.

Lewis, S., Heitkemper, M., Dirksen, S., O'Brien, P., & Bucher, L. (2007). *Medical-surgical nursing: Assessment and management of clinical problems* (7th ed.). St. Louis: Mosby.

National Council of State Boards of Nursing Web site: www.ncsbn.org

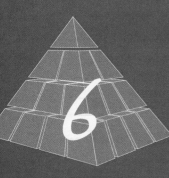

6
Chapter

Positive and Negative Event Queries

The questions presented on the National Council Licensure Examination (NCLEX), including multiple-choice, fill-in-the-blank, multiple-response, figure or illustration, and prioritizing (ordered-response) questions, will be written to include either a positive or a negative event query. The questions primarily will be written as positive event queries; however, you need to be prepared for either type.

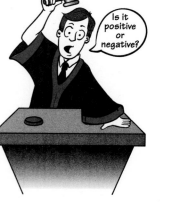

POSITIVE EVENT QUERIES

What Is a Positive Event Query?

A positive event query asks you to make a decision and select the option that is accurate or correct with regard to the data presented in the question. How will you know that the question includes a positive event query? Read the question carefully, and focus on the query of the question. The query of the question will contain strategic words or strategic phrases that will indicate that the question includes a positive event query.

> **POSITIVE EVENT QUERY**
>
> Select an option that is positive or correct!

What Strategic Words and Strategic Phrases Are Commonly Used in Positive Event Queries?

Remember to read the question carefully and focus on the query of the question, because the query of the question will contain strategic words or strategic phrases that will indicate that the question includes a positive event query. Several examples of question queries and sample questions that indicate that the question includes a positive event query are listed below.

POSITIVE EVENT QUERIES: STRATEGIC WORDS AND STRATEGIC PHRASES

Early	Initial	Select all that apply
Late	First	Understands
Most likely	Immediately	Has been achieved
Highest	Most appropriate	Adequately tolerating
Best	Order of priority	

Positive Event Queries: Examples of Queries

What is the earliest sign of a change in level of consciousness?

Which of the following is a late sign of shock?

The nurse would most likely expect to note:

Which of the following individuals is at the greatest risk for committing suicide?

The nurse plans to administer how many milliliters of medication?

What best action will the nurse implement?

Which action will the nurse do first?

What is the initial nursing action?

Based on these findings, the nurse immediately:

Which nursing action is most appropriate?

List in order of priority the actions that the nurse takes.

The most appropriate response to the client is:

Which intervention would be of highest priority in the preoperative teaching plan?

Select all nursing interventions that apply in the care of the client.

Which statement made by the client indicates the best understanding of how to prevent transmission of the disease?

Which of the following outcomes would indicate that the most important goal has been achieved for this client?

The nurse determines that the client is adequately tolerating the procedure if which of the following observations is made?

Positive Event Queries: Sample Questions

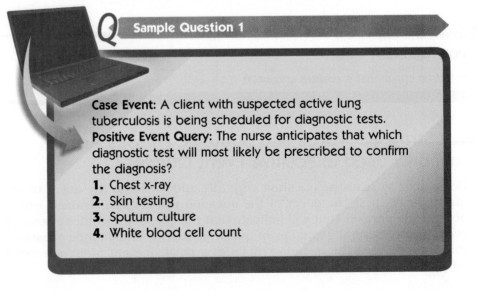

Sample Question 1

Case Event: A client with suspected active lung tuberculosis is being scheduled for diagnostic tests.
Positive Event Query: The nurse anticipates that which diagnostic test will most likely be prescribed to confirm the diagnosis?
1. Chest x-ray
2. Skin testing
3. Sputum culture
4. White blood cell count

Answer: 3
Test-Taking Strategy:
This question identifies an example of a positive event query. Note the strategic words *most likely.* Additional strategic words are *active* and *confirm.* Focus on the diagnosis presented in the question and the associated pathophysiology to assist in directing you to option 3. Remember that tuberculosis is an infectious disease caused by *Mycobacterium tuberculosis*, and the demonstration of tubercle bacilli using bacteriology is essential for establishing a diagnosis. It is not possible to make a diagnosis solely on the basis of a chest x-ray, and a positive reaction to a skin test indicates the presence of tuberculosis infection but does not show whether the infection is active or dormant. A white blood cell count may be increased, but it is not specifically related to the presence of tuberculosis. Remember to focus on the strategic words!

Tip for the Beginning Nursing Student

Tuberculosis is an infectious disease of the lung caused by the acid-fast bacillus *Mycobacterium tuberculosis*. It is generally transmitted by the inhalation or ingestion of infected droplets and usually affects the lungs, although infection of multiple organ systems can occur. It is a major public health concern because of its infectious nature. Because of the presence of the acid-fast bacillus in the lung, the way that the infection is confirmed is by its presence in the sputum. You may have already learned about this disease during your microbiology course but will learn more about it when you study the respiratory system and infectious diseases. Be sure to learn about this infectious disease.

Q Sample Question 2

Case Event: The nurse is preparing to administer digoxin (Lanoxin) 0.25 mg orally. The label on the medication bottle reads "digoxin (Lanoxin) 0.125 mg per tablet."
Positive Event Query: How many tablets will the nurse plan to administer to the client?

Answer: 2
Test-Taking Strategy:
Note the strategic words *plan to administer.* Focus on the information in the question and that a dose of 0.25 mg is prescribed. Use the formula for calculating a medication dose to answer the question. Always double-check the calculation, and verify your answer. Remember to use nursing knowledge, focus on the information in the case event, identify what the question is asking (the subject), and note the strategic words.

Tip for the Beginning Nursing Student

In this question you need to know the formula for calculating a medication dose. The formula and the calculation for this question are as follows:

$$\frac{\text{Desired}}{\text{Available}} \times \text{Quantity} = \text{Number of tablet(s)}$$

$$\frac{0.25 \text{ mg}}{0.125 \text{ mg}} \times 1 \text{ tablet} = 2 \text{ tablets}$$

✓ NCLEX® Exam Tip

Use the formula for calculating a medication dose. Perform the calculation on the note board provided to you, and use the computer on-screen calculator to verify your answer. Read carefully because in calculation questions you may be asked to round the answer to the nearest whole number or to the nearest tenth.

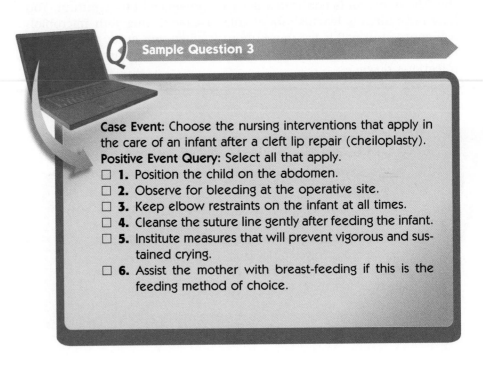

Q Sample Question 3

Case Event: Choose the nursing interventions that apply in the care of an infant after a cleft lip repair (cheiloplasty).
Positive Event Query: Select all that apply.
☐ **1.** Position the child on the abdomen.
☐ **2.** Observe for bleeding at the operative site.
☐ **3.** Keep elbow restraints on the infant at all times.
☐ **4.** Cleanse the suture line gently after feeding the infant.
☐ **5.** Institute measures that will prevent vigorous and sustained crying.
☐ **6.** Assist the mother with breast-feeding if this is the feeding method of choice.

Answer: 2, 4, 5, 6
Test-Taking Strategy:
Note the strategic words *select all that apply*, and focus on the surgical procedure: a cleft lip repair. Visualize each intervention, and think about its effect on the surgical repair to assist in selecting the correct interventions. Remember to focus on the strategic words and the surgical procedure!

Tip for the Beginning Nursing Student

A cleft lip is a craniofacial malformation that results from the incomplete fusion of the embryonic structures surrounding the primitive oral cavity. It may be unilateral or bilateral. Closure of the lip defect is usually done between 6 and 12 weeks of age as long as the infant is free of any oral, respiratory, or systemic infection. Interventions in the postoperative period are directed toward protecting the operative site, preventing infection, and maintaining nutrition. Keeping these goals of care in mind will assist in answering the question correctly. You will learn about disorders of the newborn and infant in your newborn care and pediatric nursing courses. Learn about cleft lip repair and the important nursing interventions.

✓ NCLEX® Exam Tip

Focus on the strategic words and the surgical procedure. Think about the goals of care in the care of an infant with cleft lip repair. Remember that interventions in the postoperative period are directed toward protecting the operative site, preventing infection, and maintaining nutrition. Keeping these goals of care in mind will assist in answering questions regarding this content area correctly.

Q Sample Question 4

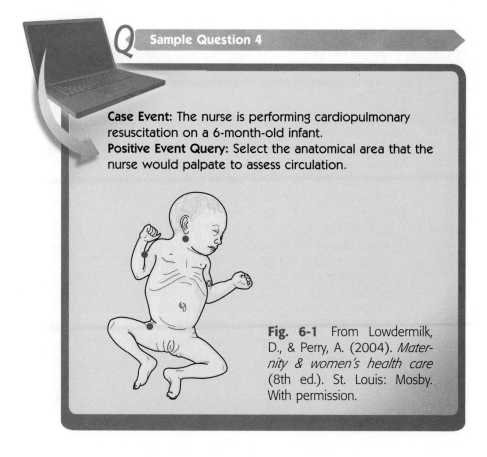

Case Event: The nurse is performing cardiopulmonary resuscitation on a 6-month-old infant.
Positive Event Query: Select the anatomical area that the nurse would palpate to assess circulation.

Fig. 6-1 From Lowdermilk, D., & Perry, A. (2004). *Maternity & women's health care* (8th ed.). St. Louis: Mosby. With permission.

Answer: Answer is indicated by the circle marked with the X

Test-Taking Strategy:

Focus on the strategic words *6-month-old infant* and *assess circulation.* Visualize the body structure of a 6-month-old infant, and recall that the very short and fat neck of the infant makes the carotid pulse difficult to palpate. In an infant younger than 12 months, the brachial pulse is used to assess circulation. Remember to focus on the strategic words!

Tip for the Beginning Nursing Student

You need to know where the arterial pulse points are located, but you need to note that this question focuses on the 6-month-old infant. Use what you learned in anatomy class, fundamentals of nursing class, and physical assessment class. You will also learn more about the infant in your newborn care and pediatric nursing courses. Think about the anatomical structure of the 6-month-old infant, and remember that in an infant younger than 12 months, the brachial pulse is used to assess circulation.

NCLEX® Exam Tip

On the NCLEX exam, you will be asked to use the computer mouse to point and click on the correct area. These types of questions are also known as "hot spot" questions.

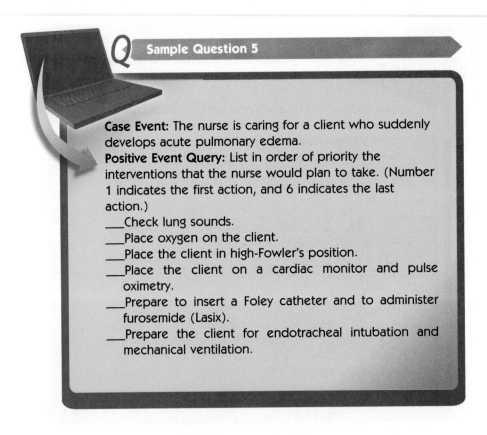

Q Sample Question 5

Case Event: The nurse is caring for a client who suddenly develops acute pulmonary edema.

Positive Event Query: List in order of priority the interventions that the nurse would plan to take. (Number 1 indicates the first action, and 6 indicates the last action.)

___Check lung sounds.

___Place oxygen on the client.

___Place the client in high-Fowler's position.

___Place the client on a cardiac monitor and pulse oximetry.

___Prepare to insert a Foley catheter and to administer furosemide (Lasix).

___Prepare the client for endotracheal intubation and mechanical ventilation.

Answer: 4, 2, 1, 3, 5, 6
Test-Taking Strategy:
Focus on the strategic words *order of priority.* Think about the pathophysiology associated with acute pulmonary edema. This will assist in determining that positioning the client in high-Fowler's position would be the first action so that breathing will be easier for the client. Next, use the ABCs—airway, breathing, and circulation—to guide your selections. This will assist in determining that administering oxygen to the client would be the next action, followed by placing the client on a cardiac monitor and pulse oximetry. Next check the lung sounds because this is an assessment or data collection procedure, and you would want to evaluate the status of lung sounds so that you will be able to determine the response to furosemide when it is administered. The Foley catheter is also inserted so the urine output can be assessed as a response to the furosemide. If there is no response to the treatment, then finally the client may need intubation and mechanical ventilation. Remember to focus on the strategic words!

Tip for the Beginning Nursing Student

Pulmonary edema is a life-threatening event that can result from severe heart failure. In pulmonary edema the left ventricle of the heart fails to eject sufficient blood, and pressure increases in the lungs because of the accumulated fluid. The client has severe dyspnea and struggles for air. Therefore interventions are aimed at alleviating this severe dyspnea and removing the excess fluid from the body. You will learn about pulmonary edema in your medical-surgical nursing course when you study cardiovascular disorders. Be sure to learn the signs and symptoms of heart failure and pulmonary edema and the associated interventions.

✓ NCLEX® Exam Tip

Positive event queries are primarily used in questions on the NCLEX exam.

◆ NEGATIVE EVENT QUERIES

What Is a Negative Event Query?

A negative event query asks you to make a decision and select the option that is inaccurate or incorrect with regard to the data presented in the question. How will you know that the question includes a negative event query? Read the question carefully, and focus on the query of the question. The query of the question will contain strategic words or strategic phrases that will indicate that the question includes a negative event query.

Generally, negative event queries are used in evaluation-type questions and evaluate the effectiveness of a treatment, procedure, medication, or teaching.

> ✓ **NCLEX® Exam Tip**
>
> Negative event queries are used less frequently on the NCLEX exam than positive event queries, but you need to be alert in noting these types of questions. It is unlikely that negative event queries will be presented in alternate item formats. You will most likely note negative event queries presented in a multiple-choice format.

> **NEGATIVE EVENT QUERY**
>
> Select an option that is incorrect or inaccurate with regard to the data in the question!

What Strategic Words and Strategic Phrases Are Commonly Used in Negative Event Queries?

Remember to read the question carefully and focus on the query of the question, because the query of the question will contain strategic words or strategic phrases that will indicate that the question includes a negative event query. Examples of strategic words and strategic phrases are listed in the following box. In addition, examples of negative event queries and sample questions that indicate that the question includes a negative event query are listed below.

> **NEGATIVE EVENT QUERIES: STRATEGIC WORDS AND STRATEGIC PHRASES**
>
> | | |
> |---|---|
> | Least likely | Needs additional discharge instructions |
> | Least priority | Have not yet been fully met |
> | Least helpful | Needs additional medication administration instructions |
> | Avoid | Has not met the outcome criteria |
> | Ineffective | |

Negative Event Queries: Examples of Queries

Which of the following individuals is least likely to develop coronary artery disease?

Which nursing diagnosis is of least priority?

Which of the following approaches by the nurse would be least helpful in assisting this client?

The nurse would avoid which of the following actions?

The nurse determines that the family needs additional discharge instructions if the nurse observed which of the following being done by the family?

Which of the following outcomes indicates to the nurse that the goals have not yet been fully met?

The nurse determines that the medication is ineffective if the client continues to experience which symptom?

The nurse determines that the client needs additional medication administration instructions if the client makes which of the following statements?

The nurse determines that the client has not met the outcome criteria by discharge if the client:

Negative Event Queries: Sample Questions

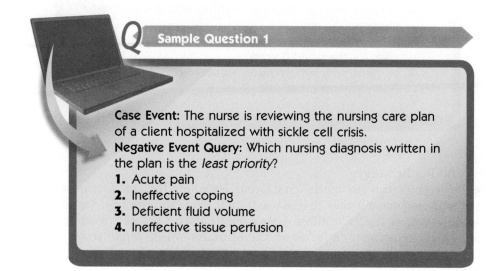

Q **Sample Question 1**

Case Event: The nurse is reviewing the nursing care plan of a client hospitalized with sickle cell crisis.
Negative Event Query: Which nursing diagnosis written in the plan is the *least priority*?
1. Acute pain
2. Ineffective coping
3. Deficient fluid volume
4. Ineffective tissue perfusion

Answer: 2

Test-Taking Strategy:
Focus on the strategic words *least priority.* According to Maslow's Hierarchy of Needs theory, physiological needs are the priority, followed by safety needs, and then psychosocial needs. Using Maslow's theory will direct you to option 2 because this is the only option that addresses a psychosocial need. Remember to focus on the strategic words *least priority!*

Tip for the Beginning Nursing Student

Sickle cell disease is a genetic disorder that results in chronic anemia, pain, organ damage, and disability. The client also has an increased risk of infection. In sickle cell disease the hemoglobin contains an abnormal beta chain known as hemoglobin S. The hemoglobin S is sensitive to oxygen changes occurring on the red blood cells; when decreased oxygen states occur, the abnormal cells pile together distorting its shape, and these cells form a sickle shape, become rigid, and block blood flow. The client with sickle cell disease can have episodes of crises that occur in response to conditions that cause hypoxemia. This causes acute pain. The primary treatment for crisis consists of hydration, comfort measures with analgesics, and oxygen administration. You will learn about sickle cell disease when you study hematological problems. Be sure to learn about the causes of crisis and its treatment measures.

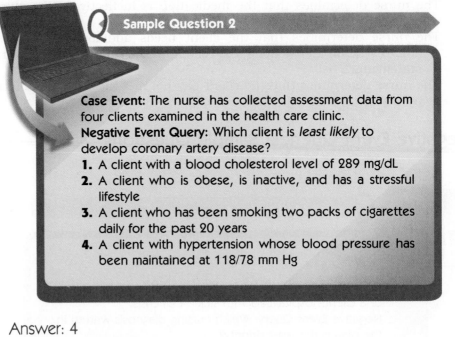

Sample Question 2

Case Event: The nurse has collected assessment data from four clients examined in the health care clinic.
Negative Event Query: Which client is *least likely* to develop coronary artery disease?
1. A client with a blood cholesterol level of 289 mg/dL
2. A client who is obese, is inactive, and has a stressful lifestyle
3. A client who has been smoking two packs of cigarettes daily for the past 20 years
4. A client with hypertension whose blood pressure has been maintained at 118/78 mm Hg

Answer: 4
Test-Taking Strategy:
Focus on the strategic words *least likely*. Recalling the risk factors associated with coronary artery disease will direct you to option 4. Option 4 is the only option that identifies a risk factor that has been modified and controlled. Remember to focus on the strategic words *least likely!*

Tip for the Beginning Nursing Student

Coronary artery disease affects the arteries that supply blood to the myocardium. When blood flow to the myocardium is partially or completely blocked, ischemia or infarction of the myocardium can occur and the client suffers a heart attack. Coronary artery disease is a major concern because it is a life-threatening disease and that is why there is great emphasis on reducing or eliminating the modifiable risk factors, such as obesity, high blood pressure, stress, smoking, and high cholesterol. You will learn about coronary artery disease when you study the cardiovascular system in medical-surgical nursing. Be sure to learn the associated risk factors and measures to reduce or eliminate them.

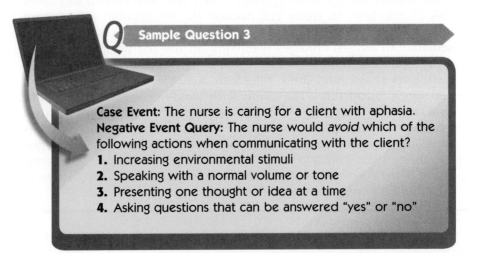

Sample Question 3

Case Event: The nurse is caring for a client with aphasia.
Negative Event Query: The nurse would *avoid* which of the following actions when communicating with the client?
1. Increasing environmental stimuli
2. Speaking with a normal volume or tone
3. Presenting one thought or idea at a time
4. Asking questions that can be answered "yes" or "no"

Answer: 1
Test-Taking Strategy:
Focus on the strategic word *avoid*. Recalling that the client with aphasia may need extra time to comprehend and respond to communication will direct you to option 1. Increased environmental stimuli may be distracting and disrupting to communication efforts. Remember to focus on the strategic word *avoid*!

Tip for the Beginning Nursing Student

Aphasia is an abnormal neurological condition in which language function is disordered or absent because of injury to certain areas of the cerebral cortex. This condition is most often seen in a client with a brain attack (stroke). The aphasic client needs repetitive directions to understand and complete a task, and each task needs to be broken down into parts, with directions given one step at a time. The client needs time to process the information. This is why increased environmental stimuli can be disruptive to the communication process. You will learn about aphasia when you study the neurological system in your medical-surgical nursing course. Be sure to learn about the nursing interventions for a client with aphasia.

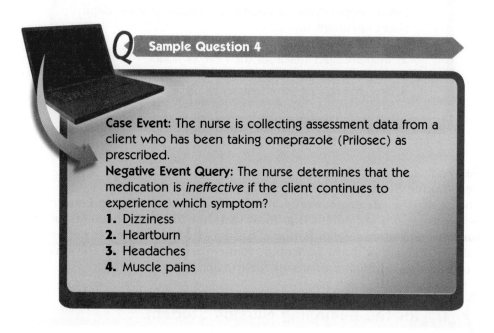

Sample Question 4

Case Event: The nurse is collecting assessment data from a client who has been taking omeprazole (Prilosec) as prescribed.
Negative Event Query: The nurse determines that the medication is *ineffective* if the client continues to experience which symptom?
1. Dizziness
2. Heartburn
3. Headaches
4. Muscle pains

Answer: 2
Test-Taking Strategy:
Focus on the strategic word *ineffective*. Recalling that omeprazole is a gastric acid pump inhibitor (most medication names that end with the letters *-zole* are gastric acid pump inhibitors) will direct you to option 2. Remember to focus on the strategic word *ineffective*!

Tip for the Beginning Nursing Student

Omeprazole (Prilosec) is a gastric acid pump inhibitor that is most often used to treat gastrointestinal disorders, such as esophagitis, gastroesophageal reflux disease, and certain stomach ulcers. Therefore this medication will assist in relieving heartburn. You will learn about this medication when you study pharmacology and when you study gastrointestinal disorders in your medical-surgical nursing course. Be sure to learn the action, intended effect, and client teaching points for this medication.

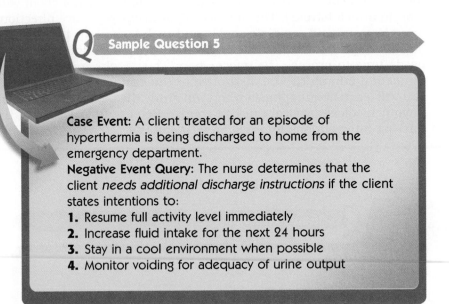

Sample Question 5

Case Event: A client treated for an episode of hyperthermia is being discharged to home from the emergency department.
Negative Event Query: The nurse determines that the client *needs additional discharge instructions* if the client states intentions to:
1. Resume full activity level immediately
2. Increase fluid intake for the next 24 hours
3. Stay in a cool environment when possible
4. Monitor voiding for adequacy of urine output

Answer: 1
Test-Taking Strategy:
Focus on the strategic words *needs additional discharge instructions*. Select the client statement that indicates that the nurse needs to provide further instructions. Resumption of full activity immediately is not helpful; rather, rest periods are indicated. Remember to focus on the strategic words *needs additional discharge instructions*!

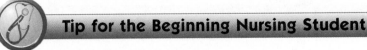

Tip for the Beginning Nursing Student

Hyperthermia is a condition in which the client's body temperature is elevated above his or her normal range. It can be caused by various factors, such as a hot environment, vigorous activity, medications or anesthesia, increased metabolic rate, illness or trauma, dehydration, or the inability to perspire. Treatment involves lowering the body temperature and treating and eliminating its cause. You will learn about hyperthermia during your nursing program in many of your courses. Be sure to focus on the causes of the hyperthermia and its treatment.

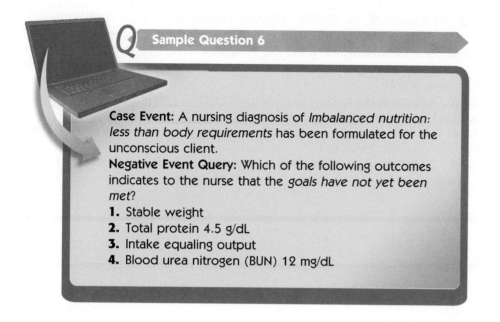

Sample Question 6

Case Event: A nursing diagnosis of *Imbalanced nutrition: less than body requirements* has been formulated for the unconscious client.

Negative Event Query: Which of the following outcomes indicates to the nurse that the *goals have not yet been met*?

1. Stable weight
2. Total protein 4.5 g/dL
3. Intake equaling output
4. Blood urea nitrogen (BUN) 12 mg/dL

Answer: 2

Test-Taking Strategy:
Focus on the strategic words *goals have not yet been met*. Because stable weight and equal intake and output are satisfactory indicators and the BUN is a normal value, option 2 is the answer to the question. Remember to focus on the strategic words *goals have not yet been met*!

Tip for the Beginning Nursing Student

A nursing diagnosis is a statement of a client's problem. This problem can be treated by a nurse using nursing interventions. The nursing diagnosis of *Imbalanced nutrition: less than body requirements* indicates that the client's intake of nutrients is insufficient to meet the client's metabolic needs. This can be due to various causes, such as, but not limited to, disease, injury, malabsorption, social factors, or cultural factors. Nursing interventions focus on addressing the nutritional deficits. You will learn about nursing diagnoses in your fundamentals of nursing course and will formulate nursing diagnoses when you care for clients in the clinical area.

REFERENCES

Ackley, B., & Ladwig, G. (2008). *Nursing diagnosis handbook: An evidence-based guide to planning care* (8th ed.). St. Louis: Mosby.

Chernecky, C., & Berger, B. (2008). *Laboratory tests and diagnostic procedures* (5th ed.). Philadelphia: Saunders.

Hockenberry, M., & Wilson, D. (2007). *Nursing care of infants and children* (8th ed.). St. Louis: Mosby.

Hodgson, B., & Kizior, R. (2008). *Saunders nursing drug handbook 2008*. Philadelphia: Saunders.

Ignatavicius, D., & Workman, M. (2006). *Medical-surgical nursing: Critical thinking for collaborative care* (5th ed.). Philadelphia: Saunders.

Kee, J., & Marshall, S. (2009). *Clinical calculations: With applications to general and specialty areas* (6th ed.). Philadelphia: Saunders.

Monahan, F., Sands, J., Marek, J., Neighbors, M., & Green, C. (2007). *Phipps' medical-surgical nursing: Health and illness perspectives* (8th ed.). St. Louis: Mosby.

National Council of State Boards of Nursing (eds.). (2007). *2007 NCLEX-RN® Detailed Test Plan.* Chicago: Author.

National Council of State Boards of Nursing (eds.). (2008). *2008 Detailed Test Plan for the NCLEX-RN® Examination.* Chicago: Author.

Perry, A., & Potter, P. (2009). *Clinical nursing skills & techniques* (7th ed.). St. Louis: Mosby.

Chapter 7

Chapter

Questions Requiring Prioritization

Be prepared! Many test questions in the National Council Licensure Examination (NCLEX) will require you to use the skill of prioritizing nursing actions. Most prioritizing questions will be presented in the multiple-choice format; however, you may be presented with a question in the prioritizing (ordered-response) format. Prioritizing questions will address content in any nursing area. These types of questions can be difficult, because when a question requires prioritization, all options may be correct, but you need to determine the correct order of action. Some test-taking strategies that you can use to assist in answering these questions correctly include noting the strategic words or strategic phrases that indicate the need to prioritize; the ABCs—airway, breathing, and circulation; Maslow's Hierarchy of Needs theory; and the steps of the nursing process. Let's review the definition of prioritizing and these test-taking strategies.

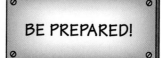

BE PREPARED!

GUIDES FOR PRIORITIZING

Strategic words or phrases
The ABCs
Maslow's Hierarchy of Needs theory
The steps of the nursing process (clinical problem-solving process)

◆ PRIORITIZING
What Does Prioritizing Mean?

Prioritizing means that you need to rank the client's problems in order of importance. It is important to read a question carefully and focus on the information in the question, because the order of importance may vary depending on the subject of the question, the clinical setting, the client's condition, and the client's needs. It also is important to consider what the client deems a priority, which may be quite different from what the nurse thinks is most important. Remember to always consider what the client believes is the priority when planning care.

When you prioritize, you are deciding which client needs or problems require immediate action and which ones could be delayed until a later time because they are not urgent. As you read a question and are trying

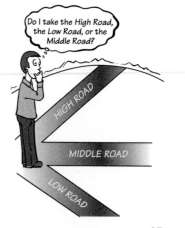

Do I take the High Road, the Low Road, or the Middle Road?

HIGH ROAD
MIDDLE ROAD
LOW ROAD

to determine which option identifies the nurse's priority, use the priority classification system to rank nursing actions as a high, intermediate (middle), or low priority. The description of these three types of classifications is listed below.

PRIORITY CLASSIFICATION SYSTEM

High Priority: a client need that is life threatening or if untreated could result in harm to the client

Intermediate (Middle) Priority: a nonemergency and non–life-threatening client need that does not require immediate attention

Low Priority: a client need that is not directly related to the client's illness or prognosis, is not urgent, and does not require immediate attention

When Is It a Priority to Select the Option "Call the Physician"?

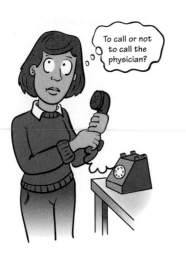

To call or not to call the physician?

An important point to remember is that the NCLEX exam tests your competence and ability to care for a client and to implement necessary measures in a particular situation. It is critically important to read the question carefully, note the information in the question, and read all available options. If the question describes a client situation that is not life threatening and there is an option that directly relates to a nursing action relevant to the situation, then it is best to select that option and not the option that indicates to "call the physician." Remember that there is usually an action that the nurse would take in a non–life-threatening situation before calling the physician. *NOTE:* For those nursing students who are studying to become licensed practical/vocational nurses rather than registered nurses, it is very important to report any changes in a client's condition immediately to the registered nurse.

If the question presents a client situation that is life threatening, then the correct option *may* be to call the physician. Unfortunately, this is not always clear-cut and can present a dilemma in your efforts to answer a question correctly. That is why it is so important to carefully read the question and all the options. Let us review some sample questions that illustrate when to and when not to select the option "call the physician."

Q **When *TO* Select the Option "Call the Physician" as the Priority Action**

Case Event: A nurse is caring for a client who just returned from the recovery room after a tonsillectomy and adenoidectomy. The client is restless, and the pulse rate is increased. The nurse prepares to continue assessing the client, but the client begins to vomit large amounts of bright red blood.

Question Query: The *immediate* nursing action is to:

1. Call the surgeon
2. Obtain a flashlight and gauze
3. Check the client's blood pressure
4. Continue assessing the client

Answer: 1

Test-Taking Strategy:
Read the question carefully, noting the strategic words and the subject of the question. Several strategic words in this question that you need to note include *restless, pulse rate is increased, large amounts, bright red blood,* and *immediate.* The subject of the question is that the client is actively bleeding and is exhibiting signs of shock (restlessness and increased pulse rate). Remember to always read each option carefully. In this situation and from the options provided, the nurse would contact the surgeon. Options 2, 3, and 4 would delay necessary interventions needed in this life-threatening situation.

Tip for the Beginning Nursing Student

Whenever you note that a client is bleeding and the amount is large and bright red, you would become concerned because this indicates active bleeding. Active bleeding is a concern after any type of surgery, including a tonsillectomy and adenoidectomy. You will learn about postoperative complications in your fundamentals of nursing course, and you will learn specifically about tonsillectomy and adenoidectomy in your pediatrics nursing course. Be sure to learn the postoperative complications and the immediate nursing interventions.

Q When *NOT TO* Select the Option "Call the Physician" as the Priority Action

Case Event: The nurse enters a client's room and finds the client slumped over in bed. The nurse quickly assesses the client and discovers that the client is not breathing.
Question Query: The nurse *immediately:*
1. Calls the physician
2. Sits the client upright in bed
3. Begins cardiopulmonary resuscitation (CPR)
4. Places oxygen via a nasal cannula on the client

Answer: 3

Test-Taking Strategy:
Read the question carefully, note the strategic word *immediately*, and focus on the subject—the client is not breathing. Although the information in the question indicates a life-threatening situation, you need to read all options carefully. In this situation and based on the options provided, the nurse needs to intervene *immediately*. Although the physician needs to be called, the *immediate* nursing action would be to administer CPR and provide breaths to the client. This option also represents the use of the ABCs—airway, breathing, and circulation—as a strategy to answer the question. Options 2 and 4 are incorrect, because neither of these options will assist this client.

Tip for the Beginning Nursing Student

It is important to read all the information in the question and focus on every word. Note that the client is not breathing. Therefore you need to begin CPR. You were most likely required to obtain health care certification in basic life support and CPR before entering nursing school. Be sure to review these procedures, especially because you will begin clinical experiences in your nursing program.

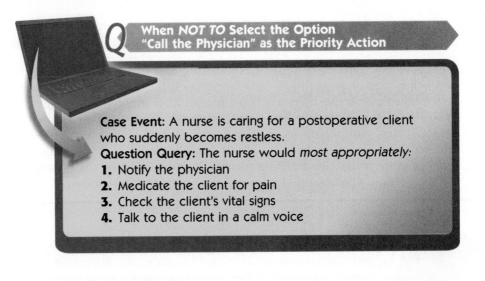

**Q   When *NOT TO* Select the Option
"Call the Physician" as the Priority Action**

Case Event: A nurse is caring for a postoperative client who suddenly becomes restless.
Question Query: The nurse would *most appropriately*:
1. Notify the physician
2. Medicate the client for pain
3. Check the client's vital signs
4. Talk to the client in a calm voice

Answer: 3

Test-Taking Strategy:
Read the question carefully, note the strategic words *most appropriately*, and focus on the subject—a postoperative client who becomes restless. No data in the question indicate that the client has pain; therefore eliminate option 2. Because option 4 is a psychosocial action rather than a physiological one (physiological needs are the priority), eliminate that option. Recall that restlessness can be an early sign of shock. However, no data in the question indicate a life-threatening condition. Therefore the nurse would gather more data about the client's condition and would *most appropriately* check the client's vital signs.

Tip for the Beginning Nursing Student

One complication following surgery is the development of shock, which is usually due to bleeding or an excessive loss of blood during the surgical procedure. The nurse always monitors the postoperative client for signs of shock. One of the earliest signs of shock is restlessness. If restlessness is noted, the nurse would check the client's vital signs next. In shock the nurse would note that the blood pressure decreases and the pulse rate increases. You will learn about shock as a postoperative complication in your fundamentals of nursing course. Be sure to focus on the signs of shock and the immediate nursing interventions.

STRATEGIC WORDS OR STRATEGIC PHRASES

What Strategic Words or Strategic Phrases Indicate the Need to Prioritize Nursing Actions?

Remember that when a question requires prioritization, all options may be correct; therefore you will need to determine the correct order of nursing action. Read the question carefully, and look for the strategic words or strategic phrases in the question that indicate the need to prioritize. Some common strategic words or strategic phrases that indicate the need to prioritize are listed below and are followed by sample questions to illustrate how some of these words or phrases are used in a question.

Strategic Words!

Note the strategic words that indicate the need to prioritize!

Common Strategic Words That Indicate the Need to Prioritize

Common strategic words that indicate *the need to prioritize* include:
Best
Essential
First
Highest priority
Immediately
Initial
Most appropriate
Most effective
Most important
Most likely
Next
Order of priority
Priority
Primary
Vital

✓ NCLEX® Exam Tip

Remember that many if not most questions on the NCLEX exam will require you to prioritize. This means that you can expect that the options presented for the question will all be correct options and that you will need to use prioritizing skills to answer correctly. Remember to look for the strategic words in the event query to assist in answering correctly!

Sample Question: Prioritizing and Strategic Words

Case Event: A nurse is caring for a client with angina pectoris who begins to experience chest pain. The nurse administers a sublingual nitroglycerin (Nitrostat) tablet as prescribed, but the pain is unrelieved.
Question Query: Which action would the nurse take *next*?
1. Reposition the client
2. Contact the physician
3. Call the client's family
4. Administer another nitroglycerin tablet

Answer: 4

Test-Taking Strategy:
Note the strategic word *next,* and focus on the subject—the client is experiencing chest pain. Recalling that the nurse would administer three nitroglycerin tablets 5 minutes apart from each other to relieve chest pain will assist in directing you to option 4. Repositioning the client will not alleviate pain associated with angina pectoris. The nurse would call the physician if three nitroglycerin tablets administered 5 minutes apart from each other did not alleviate the pain. There is no useful reason to call the client's family at this time.

Tip for the Beginning Nursing Student

Angina pectoris refers to chest pain that is most often caused by a lack of oxygen to myocardial tissue and occurs as a result of atherosclerosis (clogged blood vessels) or spasm of the coronary arteries. The pain may be relieved by rest and vasodilation of the coronary arteries by medication, such as nitroglycerin. The usual protocol for administering nitroglycerin is to administer a total of three tablets, 5 minutes apart each, to relieve the chest pain. In other words, a nitroglycerin tablet is administered and if the pain is not relieved in 5 minutes another is administered. This is repeated in 5 minutes, one more time, if the pain is not relieved by the second nitroglycerin tablet. After administering three nitroglycerin tablets, if the pain is still unrelieved, the physician is called. It is also important for the nurse to monitor the client's blood pressure, because nitroglycerin will cause a drop in the blood pressure. You will learn about angina pectoris and nitroglycerin during your medical-surgical nursing course. Because this is a major, life-threatening disorder, it is critical that you learn about its signs and symptoms and immediate treatment.

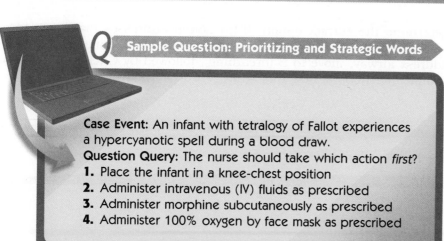

Sample Question: Prioritizing and Strategic Words

Case Event: An infant with tetralogy of Fallot experiences a hypercyanotic spell during a blood draw.
Question Query: The nurse should take which action *first*?
1. Place the infant in a knee-chest position
2. Administer intravenous (IV) fluids as prescribed
3. Administer morphine subcutaneously as prescribed
4. Administer 100% oxygen by face mask as prescribed

Answer: 1

Test-Taking Strategy:
Note the strategic word *first*, and focus on the subject of the question—a hypercyanotic spell. In questions that require you to determine the first nursing action, if one of the options indicates client positioning, that option may be the correct one. Positioning a client can relieve a symptom and is an intervention that takes only seconds to implement. Placing the infant in the knee-chest position reduces the venous return from the legs (which is desaturated) and increases systemic vascular resistance, which diverts more blood flow into the pulmonary artery. Note that the remaining options all require a physician's order. Your next action would be to administer oxygen to the infant. Remembering that morphine sulfate reduces spasm that occurs with these spells and that IV fluids are not always needed to treat these spells will assist in determining the order of priority for the remaining two interventions.

Tip for the Beginning Nursing Student

Tetralogy of Fallot is a congenital cardiac anomaly that consists of four defects in the heart: pulmonary stenosis, ventricular septal defect, malposition of the aorta so that it arises from the septal defect or the right ventricle, and right ventricular hypertrophy. The treatment consists primarily of supportive measures and palliative surgical procedures until the child is old enough to tolerate total corrective surgery. It would be helpful to review the anatomy and physiology of the heart. In addition, you will learn about tetralogy of Fallot when you take your pediatrics nursing course.

THE ABCs
What Are the ABCs, and How Will They Help Answer a Prioritizing Question?

The ABCs—airway, breathing, and circulation—direct the order of priority of nursing actions. Airway is always the first priority in caring for any client. When a question requires prioritization, use the ABCs to help determine the correct option. If an option addresses maintenance of a patent airway, that will be the correct option. If none of the options address airway, move to B (breathing), followed by C (circulation). Some sample questions of how this strategy works are provided below.

Use the ABCs to prioritize!

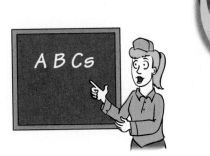

Q Sample Question: The ABCs

Case Event: A client with a diagnosis of cancer is receiving morphine sulfate 10 mg subcutaneously every 3 to 4 hours for pain.
Question Query: When preparing the plan of care for the client, the nurse includes which priority action?
1. Monitor stools
2. Encourage fluid intake
3. Monitor urine output
4. Encourage the client to cough and deep breathe

Answer: 4

Test-Taking Strategy:
Note the strategic word *priority,* and focus on the subject—morphine sulfate. Use the ABCs as a guide to direct you to the correct option. Recall that morphine sulfate suppresses the cough reflex and the respiratory reflex. Although options 1, 2, and 3 are components of the plan of care, the correct option addresses airway. Remember to use the ABCs to prioritize.

Tip for the Beginning Nursing Student

Morphine sulfate is an opioid analgesic that is used to alleviate pain. One of the primary concerns when a client receives morphine sulfate is that the medication depresses the respiratory and cough reflex. Therefore the nurse focuses primarily on the client's respiratory status when administering morphine sulfate. You will learn about morphine sulfate in your medical-surgical nursing courses and in your pharmacology course.

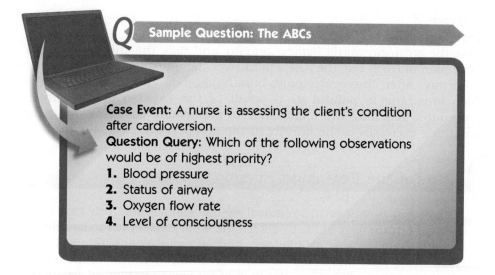

Sample Question: The ABCs

Case Event: A nurse is assessing the client's condition after cardioversion.

Question Query: Which of the following observations would be of highest priority?

1. Blood pressure
2. Status of airway
3. Oxygen flow rate
4. Level of consciousness

Answer: 2

Test-Taking Strategy:

Note the strategic words *highest priority,* and focus on the subject—assessment after cardioversion. Nursing responsibilities after cardioversion include maintenance of a patent airway, oxygen administration, assessment of vital signs and level of consciousness, and dysrhythmia detection. Airway, however, is always the highest priority. Use the ABCs to direct you to option 2.

Tip for the Beginning Nursing Student

Cardioversion is a procedure in which an electrical shock is delivered to the heart with the use of a defibrillator. Cardioversion is used to slow the heart or to restore the heart to a normal sinus rhythm when medication therapy is ineffective. You will learn about cardioversion when you study cardiac disorders and dysrhythmias in your medical-surgical nursing course.

Sample Question: The ABCs

Case Event: The nurse is providing preoperative teaching to a client scheduled for a cholecystectomy.

Question Query: Which intervention would be of highest priority in the preoperative teaching plan?

1. Teaching leg exercises
2. Instructions regarding fluid restrictions
3. Teaching coughing and deep-breathing exercises
4. Assessing the client's understanding of the surgical procedure

Answer: 3

Test-Taking Strategy:

Note the strategic words *highest priority*, and note the subject—preoperative plan of care. Use the ABCs to answer the question. Option 3 relates to airway. After cholecystectomy, breathing tends to be shallow because deep breathing is painful as a result of the location of the surgical procedure. Teaching the importance of performing coughing and deep-breathing exercises is the priority in the preoperative plan of care.

Tip for the Beginning Nursing Student

A cholecystectomy is the removal of the gallbladder. You can use medical terminology skills to determine what cholecystectomy refers to: *cholecyst-* means gallbladder, and *-ectomy* means removal of. Next, using your knowledge of anatomy, think about the anatomical location of the gallbladder. Because of its close anatomical location to the diaphragm, it makes sense that the client would have difficulty coughing and deep breathing after surgery.

MASLOW'S HIERARCHY OF NEEDS THEORY
What Is Maslow's Hierarchy of Needs Theory, and How Will It Help Answer Prioritizing Questions?

Abraham Maslow theorized that human needs are satisfied in a particular order, and he arranged human needs in a pyramid or hierarchy. According to Maslow, basic physiological needs, such as airway, breathing, circulation, water, food, and elimination needs, are the priority. These basic physiological needs are followed by safety and then the psychosocial needs, including security needs, love and belonging needs, self-esteem needs, and self-actualization needs, in that order.

Maslow's Hierarchy of Needs theory is a helpful guide when prioritizing client needs. When you are answering a question that requires you to prioritize, select an option that relates to a physiological need, remembering that physiological needs are the first priority.

If a physiological need is not addressed in the question or noted in one of the options, then continue to use Maslow's Hierarchy of Needs theory as a guide and look for the option that addresses safety. If neither physiological nor safety needs are addressed, then look for the option that addresses the client's psychosocial need. Figure 7-1 illustrates Maslow's Hierarchy of Needs theory. The sample questions that follow point out how Maslow's theory can be used as a guide when answering questions that require prioritizing.

Use Maslow's Hierarchy of Needs theory to prioritize!

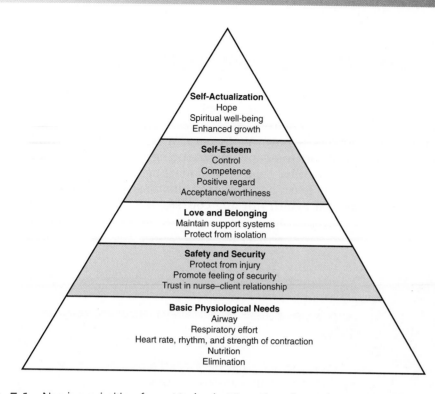

Fig. 7-1 Nursing priorities from Maslow's Hierarchy of Needs. (From Harkreader, H., Hogan, M.A., & Thobaben, M. [2007]. *Fundamentals of nursing: Caring and clinical judgment* [3rd ed.]. Philadelphia: Saunders.)

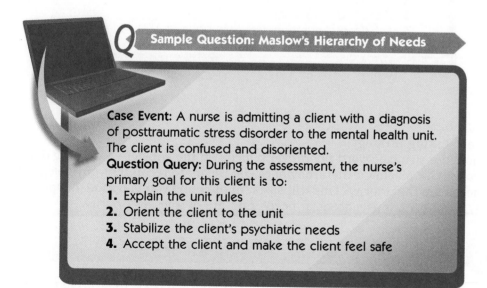

Case Event: A nurse is admitting a client with a diagnosis of posttraumatic stress disorder to the mental health unit. The client is confused and disoriented.

Question Query: During the assessment, the nurse's primary goal for this client is to:

1. Explain the unit rules

2. Orient the client to the unit

3. Stabilize the client's psychiatric needs

4. Accept the client and make the client feel safe

Answer: 4

Test-Taking Strategy:

Note the strategic word *primary*, and focus on the subject—a client being admitted to the mental health unit. Using Maslow's Hierarchy of Needs theory, remember that when a physiological need does not exist, then safety needs take precedence. It is important to accept a client and make a confused and disoriented client feel safe. Stabilizing psychiatric needs is a long-term goal. Orientation and explaining the unit rules are part of any admission process and are not specific to this client.

Tip for the Beginning Nursing Student

Posttraumatic stress disorder is a mental health disorder that is characterized by an acute emotional response to a traumatic event that involved severe environmental stress. This event could include situations such as a natural disaster, a terrorist attack, military combat, physical torture, rape, experiencing or witnessing an automobile accident or other type of accident, or witnessing a shooting or murder. You will learn about posttraumatic stress disorder in your psychiatric/mental health nursing course.

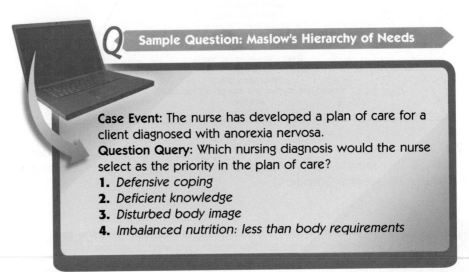

Sample Question: Maslow's Hierarchy of Needs

Case Event: The nurse has developed a plan of care for a client diagnosed with anorexia nervosa.
Question Query: Which nursing diagnosis would the nurse select as the priority in the plan of care?
1. *Defensive coping*
2. *Deficient knowledge*
3. *Disturbed body image*
4. *Imbalanced nutrition: less than body requirements*

Answer: 4
Test-Taking Strategy:
Note the strategic word *priority*, and focus on the subject—a nursing diagnosis. Use Maslow's Hierarchy of Needs theory to recall that physiological needs are the priority. This will assist in directing you to option 4. Options 1, 2, and 3 are psychosocial needs and are of a lesser priority.

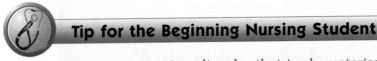

Tip for the Beginning Nursing Student

Anorexia nervosa is a disorder that is characterized by a prolonged refusal to eat. The client believes that he or she is obese, although the body weight is well below the individual's normal expected weight. It results in emaciation, amenorrhea, an emotional disturbance concerning body image, and the fear of becoming obese. The condition is primarily seen in adolescent girls and is usually associated with emotional stress or conflict such as anger, fear, or anxiety. Treatment includes measures to improve nutritional status and therapy to overcome the emotional conflicts associated with the disorder. You will learn about anorexia nervosa in your psychiatric/mental health nursing course.

Sample Question: Maslow's Hierarchy of Needs

Case Event: A nurse is preparing to teach a client how to use crutches. Before initiating the lesson, the nurse performs an assessment on the client.

Question Query: The priority nursing assessment should include which of the following?

1. The client's feelings about the restricted mobility
2. The client's fear related to the use of the crutches
3. The client's muscle strength and previous activity level
4. The client's understanding of the need for increased mobility

Answer: 3

Test-Taking Strategy:

Note the strategic word *priority*, and focus on the subject—teaching a client how to use crutches. Using Maslow's Hierarchy of Needs theory, remember that physiological needs take precedence over psychosocial needs. This should direct you to option 3. Assessing muscle strength will help determine whether the client has enough strength for crutch walking and if muscle-strengthening exercises are necessary. Previous activity level will provide information related to the tolerance of activity. Options 1, 2, and 4 are also components of the assessment but relate to psychosocial needs.

Tip for the Beginning Nursing Student

Crutches are devices that are usually made of wood or metal and that aid a person in walking. Crutches require the use of some upper and lower body muscle strength; otherwise, injury, such as a fall, can occur. It is also important for the nurse to determine the client's previous activity level in order to determine if crutches would be an appropriate assistive device. If the client's previous activity level was minimal and muscle strength was poor, crutches would not be an appropriate ambulatory device and the client would be at risk for injury with their use. It is also important for the crutches to be fitted properly and for the individual to be taught how to safely walk using them to achieve a stable gait. You will learn about the use of crutches and other assistive devices for ambulation in your fundamentals of nursing course.

▲ NURSING PROCESS (CLINICAL PROBLEM-SOLVING PROCESS)

How Will the Nursing Process (Clinical Problem-Solving Process) Help Answer Prioritizing Questions?

The Test Plan for the NCLEX exam identifies the nursing process (clinical problem-solving process) as an Integrated Process. The nursing process provides a systematic method for providing care to a client. For the student studying to become a registered nurse, these steps include assessment, analysis, planning, implementation, and evaluation. For the student studying to become a licensed practical/vocational nurse, these steps include data collection, planning, implementation, and evaluation. These steps are usually followed in sequence, with assessment/data collection being the first step and evaluation being the last step. However, once the nursing process begins, it becomes a cyclical process. The steps of the nursing process can be used as a guide to help you when answering questions that require prioritization. Remember that it is always important to read the question carefully to determine what the question is asking. When a question asks for the first or initial nursing action, use these steps and look for an assessment/data collection action in one of the options. If an assessment/data collection action is not addressed in one of the options, then continue to use the nursing process in a systematic order. Figure 7-2 illustrates the steps of the nursing process for the student studying to become a registered nurse, and Figure 7-3 illustrates the steps of the nursing process (clinical problem-solving process) for the student studying to become a licensed practical/vocational nurse. A description for each step follows.

> Use the steps of the nursing process (clinical problem-solving process) to prioritize!

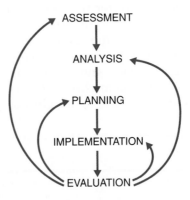

Fig. 7-2   Steps of the nursing process—RN nursing student. (From Ignatavicius, D., & Workman, M. [2006]. *Medical-surgical nursing: Critical thinking for collaborative care* [5th ed.]. Philadelphia: Saunders.)

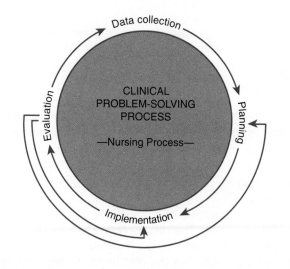

Fig. 7-3 Steps of the nursing process—PN nursing student.

Assessment/Data Collection

Assessment/data collection questions address the process of gathering subjective and objective data relative to the client, confirming that data, and communicating and documenting the data.

Remember that assessment/data collection is the first step in the nursing process. When you are asked to select your first and initial nursing action, look for an option that addresses assessment/data collection. If an option contains the concept of assessment or the collection of client data, it is best to select that option. Some strategic words to look for in the options that indicate an assessment/data collection action, are listed below. A sample question follows.

Strategic Words in Options That Indicate Assessment/Data Collection

Strategic words that indicate *assessment/data collection* include:
  Ascertain
  Assess
  Check
  Collect
  Determine
  Find out
  Identify
  Monitor
  Observe
  Obtain information
  Recognize

If an assessment/data collection action is not noted in one of the options, follow the steps of the nursing process (clinical problem-solving process) as your guide in selecting your initial or first action. ***Possible exception to this guideline for prioritizing:*** If the question presents an emergency situation, read carefully; in an emergency situation, an intervention may be the priority!

Q Sample Question: Assessment/Data Collection

Case Event: A nurse is teaching a client with coronary artery disease about dietary measures that should be followed.

Question Query: During the session the client expresses frustration in learning the dietary regimen. The nurse would initially:

1. Notify the physician
2. Continue with the dietary teaching
3. Identify the cause of the frustration
4. Tell the client that the diet needs to be followed

Answer: 3

Test-Taking Strategy:
Note the strategic word *initially,* and focus on the subject—a nursing action. Use the steps of the nursing process. Of the four options presented, the only assessment/data collection action is option 3. Options 1, 2, and 4 identify the implementation step of the nursing process. The initial action is to identify the cause of the frustration. Remember that assessment/data collection is the first step of the nursing process.

Tip for the Beginning Nursing Student

Coronary artery disease affects the arteries that supply blood to the myocardium. When blood flow to the myocardium is partially or completely blocked, ischemia or infarction of the myocardium can occur and the client experiences a heart attack. Because coronary artery disease is a life-threatening disease, great emphasis is placed on reducing or eliminating the modifiable risk factors, such as obesity, high blood pressure, stress, smoking, and high cholesterol. Dietary measures include limiting foods high in cholesterol. High-fat foods, such as fried foods, are high in cholesterol. Because cholesterol is also found in foods of animal origin, meats such as organ meats, beef, bacon, and sausage are high in cholesterol. You will learn about coronary artery disease when you study the cardiovascular system in medical-surgical nursing, and you will learn about the foods high in cholesterol when you study nutrition related to cardiovascular disorders. Be sure to learn about these foods that are high in cholesterol, because you will need to teach your client with cardiovascular disease about limiting them in the diet.

Analysis

Beware! For the student studying to become a *registered nurse*, analysis questions are the most difficult, because they require understanding of the principles of physiological responses and require interpretation of the data on the basis of assessment. Analysis questions also require critical thinking and determining the rationale for therapeutic interventions that may be addressed in the question; therefore many questions on the NCLEX-RN exam will be analysis type of questions. Questions that address this step of the nursing process may also address the formulation of a nursing diagnosis and the communication and documentation of the results of the process of analysis. Remember to read the question carefully, identify the strategic words and the subject, and use the process of elimination to select the correct option. An example of an analysis-type question is provided below.

> **Sample Question: Analysis**
>
> **Case Event:** A nurse is reviewing the laboratory results of an infant suspected of having pyloric stenosis.
> **Question Query:** Which of the following laboratory findings would the nurse most likely expect to note in this infant?
> **1.** A blood pH of 7.50
> **2.** A blood pH of 7.30
> **3.** A blood bicarbonate of 22 mEq/L
> **4.** A blood bicarbonate of 19 mEq/L

Answer: 1

Test-Taking Strategy:
Note the strategic words *most likely*, and focus on the subject—laboratory results. It is necessary to understand the physiology associated with pyloric stenosis and that metabolic alkalosis is likely to occur as a result of vomiting. Next, it is necessary to know which laboratory findings would be noted in this acid-base condition. The normal pH ranges from 7.35 to 7.45. In an alkalotic condition the pH is elevated. Analysis of these data will direct you to the correct option.

Tip for the Beginning Nursing Student

Pyloric stenosis is a condition in which a narrowing of the pyloric sphincter at the outlet of the stomach occurs. This results in an obstruction that blocks the flow of food into the small intestine. The condition primarily occurs as a congenital defect in newborns. The infant experiences forceful projectile vomiting, causing the loss of hydrochloric acid, which results in metabolic alkalosis in the infant. The condition is treated by surgical correction. You will learn about acid-base disorders in your fundamentals of nursing course and in your medical-surgical nursing course. You will also learn about pyloric stenosis in your maternity and newborn course and in your pediatrics nursing course.

Planning

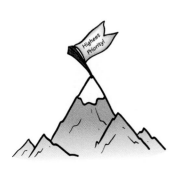

Planning questions frequently address nursing diagnoses. These questions require prioritizing nursing diagnoses, determining goals and outcome criteria for goals of care, developing the plan of care, and communicating and documenting the plan of care. With regard to questions that address the planning step of the nursing process, keep two important points in mind. First, remember that this is a nursing examination and the answer to the question most likely involves something related to the nursing plan rather than to the medical plan, unless the question asks what you anticipate the physician will prescribe. The second point to remember relates to questions that contain options listing nursing diagnoses and require you to prioritize them or to select the nursing diagnosis of highest priority. In these questions it is important to remember that actual client problems rather than potential or at-risk client problems will most likely be the priority. Read the information in the question carefully; this information will guide you to select the correct option in this type of question. An example of a planning type of question is provided below.

Sample Question: Planning

Case Event: A nurse is reviewing the plan of care for a client with a diagnosis of sickle cell anemia.
Question Query: Which nursing diagnosis, if stated on the plan of care, would the nurse select as receiving the highest priority?
1. *Anxiety*
2. *Ineffective coping*
3. *Disturbed body image*
4. *Deficient fluid volume*

Answer: 4
Test-Taking Strategy:
Note the strategic words *highest priority,* and focus on the subject—a nursing diagnosis in the plan of care. To correctly answer this question, use Maslow's Hierarchy of Needs theory to prioritize, remembering that physiological needs come first. Using this guideline will direct you to option 4. *Deficient fluid volume* is a physiological need and is the priority nursing diagnosis. Options 1, 2, and 3 are psychosocial needs and may or may not be a concern for the client, but remember that physiological needs are the priority.

Tip for the Beginning Nursing Student

Sickle cell anemia is a severe and chronic incurable anemic condition in which the abnormal hemoglobin called hemoglobin S (Hb S) results in distortion and fragility of the erythrocytes. It is characterized by crises in which the sickled cells clump and cause obstruction of the blood vessels. Joint pain, thrombosis, fever, lethargy, weakness, and splenomegaly occur. You may have learned about sickle cell anemia in your anatomy and physiology course. You will also learn more about this type of anemia in your medical-surgical nursing course and pediatrics course. Sickle cell anemia may also be discussed in your maternity nursing course because this type of anemia in a pregnant client places the client at risk for complications during the pregnancy.

Implementation

Implementation questions address the process of organizing and managing care, counseling and teaching, providing care to achieve established goals, supervising and coordinating care, and communicating and documenting nursing interventions. Because the NCLEX exam tests your competence and ability to function as a professional nurse, many questions on the examination will be implementation-type questions.

When you are presented with a question that requires you to determine what the nurse will do, there are two important points to keep in mind. The first point is that the only client that you need to be concerned about is the client in the question; remember that the client in the question is your only assigned client. This is an important point to bear in mind as you are trying to select the correct option.

> You have only one client to be concerned about!

The second important point to keep in mind when you are answering NCLEX questions is that you need to answer the question from an ideal and textbook perspective, not a reality perspective; you also need to answer the question as if the nurse has all the time available to care for the client and all the needed resources available at the client's bedside.

> Answer the question from an ideal and textbook perspective!

> Answer the question as if the nurse had all the time available to care for the client and all the resources needed at the client's bedside!

To illustrate these important points, let us look at the following sample questions.

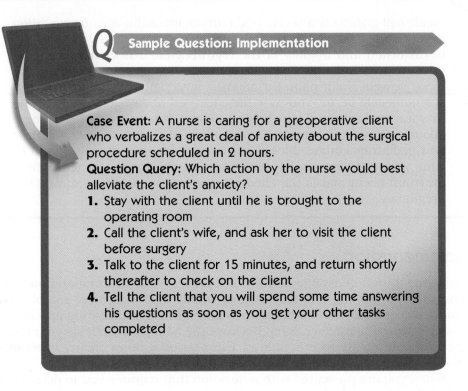

Sample Question: Implementation

Case Event: A nurse is caring for a preoperative client who verbalizes a great deal of anxiety about the surgical procedure scheduled in 2 hours.

Question Query: Which action by the nurse would best alleviate the client's anxiety?

1. Stay with the client until he is brought to the operating room
2. Call the client's wife, and ask her to visit the client before surgery
3. Talk to the client for 15 minutes, and return shortly thereafter to check on the client
4. Tell the client that you will spend some time answering his questions as soon as you get your other tasks completed

Answer: 1

Test-Taking Strategy:

Note the strategic word *best,* and focus on the subject—alleviating the client's anxiety. As you are reading the options, you may hesitate to select option 1 and may say to yourself, "I could never stay with a client for 2 hours. I would never get any of my other clients taken care of." Stop right there and remember that on the NCLEX exam, the only client that you are caring for is the client in the question. Therefore option 1 is the *best* of the four options.

Tip for the Beginning Nursing Student

A preoperative client is a client who is either preparing for surgery or is waiting to be transferred to the operating room. Many times these clients are anxious about the surgery and the nurse is responsible for alleviating the anxiety. You will learn about the many ways to alleviate a client's anxiety, but one way is to be present and available for the client to answer questions if necessary and to provide comfort. Many times just the nurse's presence provides comfort to a client. You will learn about caring for the client having surgery in your fundamentals of nursing course, and you will also learn about the many measures that you can implement to alleviate a client's anxiety.

Sample Question: Implementation

Case Event: A nurse is caring for a client after a cardiac catheterization. The client suddenly reports a feeling of wetness in the groin at the catheter insertion site.

Question Query: The nurse checks the site, notes that the client is actively bleeding, and takes which best action?

1. Contacts the physician
2. Checks the client's peripheral pulse in the affected extremity
3. Dons a sterile glove and places pressure on the insertion site using sterile gauze
4. Dons a clean glove and places pressure on the insertion site with the gloved hand

Answer: 3

Test-Taking Strategy:

Note the strategic word *best*, and focus on the subject—a nursing action. Active bleeding indicates the need for intervention and the application of pressure at the site of bleeding. This directs you to options 3 and 4 as the possible correct options. You may hesitate to select option 3 because you may say to yourself, "I would not use the sterile gloves or gauze, because by the time I went to the treatment room, obtained these sterile items, and returned to the room, the client would have lost a critically large amount of blood." Stop right there, and remember that on the NCLEX exam, you have all the resources needed and readily available at the client's bedside. Because the catheter insertion site is an open area, the best option is to don a sterile glove and place pressure on the insertion site using sterile gauze.

Tip for the Beginning Nursing Student

A cardiac catheterization is a diagnostic procedure in which a catheter is introduced through an incision into a large blood vessel and threaded through the circulatory system of the heart. This procedure is primarily done to assess the status of the coronary arteries in the heart and to determine if any blockage is present and, if so, the extent of the blockage. Following the procedure the client is at risk for bleeding, infection, thrombophlebitis, and dysrhythmias (irregular heart beat patterns). You will learn about this important cardiac diagnostic procedure when you study cardiovascular disorders in your medical-surgical nursing course.

Evaluation

Evaluation questions focus on comparing the actual outcomes of care with the expected outcomes and focus on how the nurse should monitor or make a judgment concerning a client's response to therapy or to a nursing action. These questions also address evaluating the client's ability to implement self-care, health care team members' ability to implement care, and the process of communicating and documenting evaluation findings.

In an evaluation question, it is important to note if the question includes a negative event query. Look for the words or phrases that indicate a negative event query, because they may be used in evaluation type of questions and ask for inaccurate information related to the subject of the question. (Strategic words or strategic phrases used in a negative event query are listed in Chapter 6.) Following is an example of an evaluation type of question.

Sample Question: Evaluation

Case Event: A client recovering from an exacerbation of left-sided heart failure has a nursing diagnosis of *Activity intolerance.*

Question Query: The nurse determines that the client best tolerates mild exercise if the client exhibits which of the following changes in vital signs during activity?
1. Pulse rate increased from 80 to 104 beats/min
2. Oxygen saturation decreased from 96% to 91%
3. Respiratory rate increased from 16 to 19 breaths/min
4. Blood pressure decreased from 140/86 to 110/68 mm Hg

Answer: 3

Test-Taking Strategy:
Note the strategic word *best*, and focus on the subject—the client's ability to tolerate exercise. Use the process of elimination and nursing knowledge regarding normal vital sign values. Options 1 and 2 are incorrect, because they represent changes from normal to abnormal values. Blood pressure decreases by more than 10 mm Hg could indicate an orthostatic hypotensive change and that the client is not tolerating the exercise. The only option that identifies values that remain within the normal range is option 3.

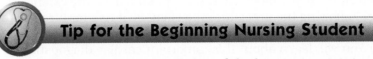

Tip for the Beginning Nursing Student

Heart failure is an inability of the heart to maintain adequate circulation to meet the metabolic needs of the body because of an impaired pumping ability. Because of the imbalance of the oxygen supply and demand that occurs in this disorder, *Activity intolerance* can be a problem for the client. In the case of a client with heart failure, *Activity intolerance* refers to an insufficient amount of physiological energy necessary to tolerate or complete the desired activity or exercise. You will learn about heart failure when you learn about cardiac disorders. One important thing to remember is that with all clients, airway is the priority.

REFERENCES

Ackley, B., & Ladwig, G. (2006). *Nursing diagnosis handbook: A guide for planning care* (7th ed.). St. Louis: Mosby.

Christen, B., & Kockrow, E. (2006). *Adult health nursing* (5th ed.). St. Louis: Mosby.

Fortinash, K., & Holoday-Worret, P. (2008). *Psychiatric mental health nursing* (4th ed.). St. Louis: Mosby.

Harkreader, H., Hogan, M.A., & Thobaben, M. (2007). *Fundamentals of nursing: Caring and clinical judgment* (3rd ed.). Philadelphia: Saunders.

Hockenberry, M., & Wilson, D. (2007). *Nursing care of infants and children* (8th ed.). St. Louis: Mosby.

Hodgson, B., & Kizior, R. (2008). *Saunders nursing drug handbook 2008*. Philadelphia: Saunders.

Ignatavicius, D., & Workman, M. (2006). *Medical-surgical nursing: Critical thinking for collaborative care* (5th ed.). Philadelphia: Saunders.

Leifer, G. (2007). *Introduction to maternity and pediatric nursing* (5th ed.). Philadelphia: Saunders.

Linton, A., & Maebius, N. (2007). *Introduction to medical-surgical nursing* (4th ed.). Philadelphia: Saunders.

Monahan, F., Sands, J., Marek, J., Neighbors, M., & Green, C. (2007). *Phipps' medical-surgical nursing: Health and illness perspectives* (8th ed.). St. Louis: Mosby.

Potter, P., & Perry, A. (2009) *Fundamentals of nursing* (7th ed.). St. Louis: Mosby.

Price, D., & Gwin, J. (2008). *Pediatric nursing: An introductory text* (10th ed.). Philadelphia: Saunders.

Varcarolis, E., Carlson, V., & Shoemaker, N. (2006). *Foundations of psychiatric mental health nursing* (5th ed.). Philadelphia: Saunders.

Wong, D., Perry, S., Hockenberry, M., Lowdermilk, D., & Wilson, D. (2006). *Maternal-child nursing care* (3rd ed.). St. Louis: Mosby.

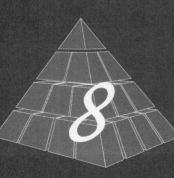
Leading and Managing, Delegating, and Assignment-Making Questions

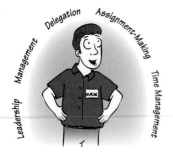

The nurse is both a leader and a manager. As a leader and a manager, the nurse needs to assume many roles and responsibilities. Some of these roles include managing, organizing, and prioritizing care; making client care or related task assignments and delegating care; supervising care delivered by other health care providers; and managing time efficiently. The National Council Licensure Examination (NCLEX) Test Plan, developed by the National Council of State Boards of Nursing (NCSBN), which can be obtained at the NCSBN Web site at www.ncsbn.org, identifies the content related to these roles and responsibilities in the Safe and Effective Care Environment Client Needs category. It is important to review the information related to this content area to ensure that you are well prepared for questions regarding the roles and responsibilities of the nurse as a leader and a manager. This chapter reviews the roles and responsibilities of the nurse and other health care providers, such as the licensed practical or vocational nurse and the nursing assistant. This chapter also reviews the guidelines and principles related to delegating and assignment making, which are two important roles of the nurse. In addition, this chapter identifies guidelines for time management, because managing time efficiently is a key factor for completing activities and tasks within a definite time period.

✓ NCLEX® Exam Tip

Many test questions on the NCLEX exam in the Safe and Effective Care Environment Client Needs category relate to the nurse's responsibilities regarding delegating care and assignment making and the supervisory role of these responsibilities. You may also be presented with questions that require you to determine the priority of care for a group of clients. These questions most likely will be in the multiple-choice format; however, you may be presented with questions that address these responsibilities in the multiple-response or the prioritizing (ordered-response) format.

DELEGATION AND ASSIGNMENT MAKING
What Is Delegation?

Delegation is the process of transferring a selected nursing task in a client situation to an individual who is competent to perform that specific task. It involves sharing activities and achieving outcomes with other individuals who have the competency to accomplish the task. The nurse practice act and any other practice limitations, such as agency policies and procedures, define the aspects of care that can be delegated and the tasks and activities that need to be performed by the registered nurse, those that can be performed by the licensed practical nurse or licensed vocational nurse, and those that can be performed by an unlicensed individual, such as a nursing assistant. When delegating an activity, the nurse needs to determine the degree of supervision that the delegatee may require and provide supervision as appropriate.

> **Delegation:** Transferring a nursing task to an individual who is competent to perform the task

What Is Assignment Making?

Assignment making is a specific activity that involves planning care activities for a client or a group of clients and determining specifically who will provide the care or perform certain activities. As with delegating, the nurse practice act and any other practice limitations, such as agency policies and procedures, that define the aspects of care need to be used as a guide when planning assignments for activities and client care. Supervision of performance of the activity as appropriate also is important.

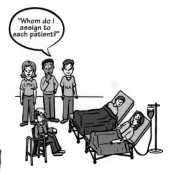

> **Assignment Making:** Planning care activities for a client or a group of clients and determining who will provide the care or perform certain activities

What Are the Important Points to Keep in Mind When Delegating or Making Assignments?

When you are answering questions related to either delegating or assignment making, keep two important points in mind. First, even though a task or activity may be delegated to someone, the nurse who delegates the task or activity maintains accountability for the overall nursing care of the client. Remember that only the task, not the ultimate accountability, may be delegated to another.

The second point to keep in mind is that this examination is a national examination. Therefore use general guidelines, such as the nurse practice act, regarding what a health care provider can competently and legally perform to answer the question correctly. Avoid using agency policies and procedures and agency position descriptions to answer the question,

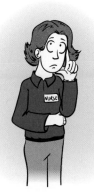

unless the question provides information to do so, because they are specific to the agency.

Let us review two sample questions: one that illustrates the use of general guidelines related to delegating and assignment making and one that relates to specific agency policies and procedures.

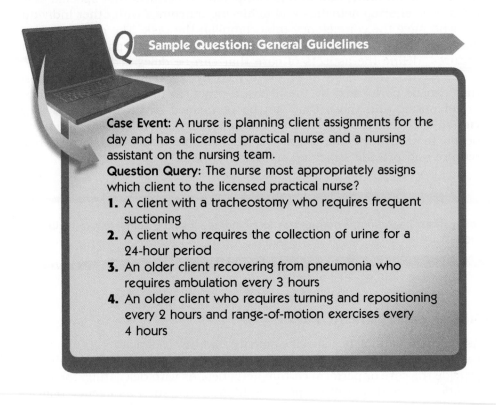

Sample Question: General Guidelines

Case Event: A nurse is planning client assignments for the day and has a licensed practical nurse and a nursing assistant on the nursing team.
Question Query: The nurse most appropriately assigns which client to the licensed practical nurse?
1. A client with a tracheostomy who requires frequent suctioning
2. A client who requires the collection of urine for a 24-hour period
3. An older client recovering from pneumonia who requires ambulation every 3 hours
4. An older client who requires turning and repositioning every 2 hours and range-of-motion exercises every 4 hours

Answer: 1
Test-Taking Strategy:
This question requires that you determine which client should most appropriately be assigned to the licensed practical nurse. No information in the question indicates the need to use agency policies, procedures, or position descriptions to determine the most appropriate assignment; therefore use general guidelines, such as the nurse practice act. As you read each option, think about and visualize the client's needs. The client described in option 1 has needs that cannot be met by the nursing assistant. Remember that the health care provider needs to be competent and skilled to perform the assigned task or client activity.

Tip for the Beginning Nursing Student

You will learn about the specific roles and responsibilities of various health care providers in your fundamentals of nursing course. You will also learn more specific content about these roles and responsibilities when you begin your leadership and management course. The important thing to remember is that the registered nurse is educationally prepared to assume the highest level of responsibilities. The licensed practical or vocational nurse can assume some responsibilities that are invasive, and the nursing assistant can assume responsibilities that are noninvasive. A tracheostomy is a surgically created opening into the neck that provides an airway for a client who is unable to breathe through the upper airway. A client with a tracheostomy requires suctioning, which involves, as needed, the insertion of a tube that provides suction to remove secretions to maintain a clear airway. This is an invasive procedure, and thus a licensed nurse needs to be assigned to this client. The collection of urine, ambulating a client, and turning and repositioning and range-of-motion exercises are noninvasive procedures and thus can be assigned to a nursing assistant.

Q Sample Question: Specific Agency Policies and Procedures

Case Event: A licensed nurse employed in a hospital is assigning client care activities to a nursing assistant. The nursing assistant is a first-semester senior nursing student and works at the hospital as a nursing assistant part-time on weekends. The hospital position description for a nursing student who is employed as a nursing assistant indicates that he or she may perform basic procedures learned in nursing school if supervised by a licensed nurse.

Question Query: Based on the hospital's position description, the licensed nurse assigns which most appropriate activity to the nursing assistant?

1. Change a sterile abdominal dressing
2. Hang a unit of red blood cells on a client
3. Insert an intravenous (IV) catheter into an infant
4. Administer digoxin (Lanoxin) by IV push

Answer: 1

Test-Taking Strategy:
In this question, information is provided that directs you to use the hospital's position description to determine the most appropriate activity to assign to the nursing assistant. The strategic words in the question are *most appropriate.* Based on the data provided in the question and in the options, it is best to select the least invasive activity. Also, recall that blood administration and medication administration must be performed by a licensed health care provider. Inserting an IV catheter into an infant is an invasive procedure that needs to be performed by a health care provider specially trained to perform it. Remember that the health care provider needs to be competent and skilled to perform the assigned task or client activity.

Tip for the Beginning Nursing Student

You will learn about the specific roles and responsibilities of various health care providers in your fundamentals of nursing course and your leadership and management course. When answering these types of questions, remember to focus on the subject of who the task is being assigned to and to select the least invasive task if the health care provider is not licensed. Hanging red blood cells means that the client will receive blood by the IV route, and this is a highly invasive procedure. Inserting an IV catheter and administering digoxin (a cardiac medication) intravenously are also highly invasive procedures that need to be performed by licensed personnel. Although changing a sterile dressing is invasive to some degree and requires education in its performance to maintain sterility, it is the least invasive of the procedures provided in the options.

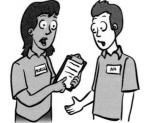

This is what you need to do and how you need to do it.

What Principles and Guidelines Can Be Used to Delegate and Make Assignments?

If you are presented with a question on an examination that requires you to delegate or plan assignments for a group of clients, certain principles and guidelines can be used to assist in answering the question correctly. As you are using the process of elimination to determine the correct option, keep these principles and guidelines in mind. Also, read each option carefully. Think about and visualize the client's needs to determine which health care provider could best meet the client's needs. Following is a review of the principles and guidelines for delegating and assignment making.

Principles and Guidelines for Delegating and Assignment Making

1. Always ensure client safety—never select an option that could potentially harm the client.
2. Focus on the subject of the question and what the question is asking; for example, is the question asking you to delegate to another registered nurse, a licensed practical or vocational nurse, or a nursing assistant?
3. Determine which tasks or client care activities can be delegated and to whom and match the task to the delegatee on the basis of the nurse practice act, agency policies and procedures, or position descriptions as appropriate; that is, think about the activities that the delegatee can safely and legally perform.
4. Think about individual variations in work abilities, and determine the degree of supervision that may be required; for example, if the question asks you to delegate or assign a client care activity to a new graduate, then you must think about the need for providing adequate supervision and the need to teach the new graduate about the assigned activity.
5. Always provide directions to the delegatee that are clear, concise, accurate, and complete and that validate the person's understanding of the directions and expectations; that is, ask the delegatee to verbalize the procedure for performing the task or activity that was delegated.
6. Communicate a feeling of confidence to the delegatee, and provide feedback promptly after the task or activity is performed regarding his or her performance; ensure that the delegatee completed the task, and evaluate the outcome of the care provided.

7. Provide the delegatee with a timeline for completion of the task or activity; for example, if a client is scheduled for a diagnostic test and an activity or task needs to be completed before the test, it is important to identify this timeline to the delegatee.

8. Maintain continuity of care as much as possible when assigning client care; for example, it is best for the client to be cared for by a nurse with whom the client has developed a therapeutic relationship. However, it is also important to remember that in some client situations, maintaining continuity of care would be unfavorable with regard to ensuring a safe environment for a health care provider, such as with the client with an infectious disease or the client with a radiation implant.

Sample Question: Assignment Making

Case Event: A nurse is planning the client assignments for the day and is reviewing client data and the needs of the clients on the nursing team.

Question Query: To maintain continuity of care, the nurse would ensure that which client is cared for by the nurse who cared for the client on the previous day?

1. A client with active tuberculosis
2. A client with herpes zoster (chickenpox)
3. A client with a cervical radiation implant
4. A client recently diagnosed with inoperable cancer

Answer: 4

Test-Taking Strategy:
Focus on the subject of the question—to maintain continuity of care. Read each option carefully, keeping two points in mind: the client's needs and ensuring a safe environment for the health care provider. The clients described in options 1, 2, and 3 can potentially present a risk to the health care provider. The client in option 4 will likely have psychosocial needs that can best be met if the client is cared for by a health care provider with whom the client has developed a therapeutic relationship.

Tip for the Beginning Nursing Student

Tuberculosis is an infection caused by an acid-fast bacillus known as *Mycobacterium tuberculosis* and usually affects the lungs, although infection of multiple organ systems can occur. In its active stage it is highly contagious and is transmitted by the inhalation of infected droplets. Herpes zoster (chickenpox) is an acute and highly contagious viral disease caused by the varicella zoster virus. This disease is transmitted by direct contact with skin lesions or by droplet spread from the respiratory tract of an infected person. A radiation implant is a device that is placed internally into a client to treat cancer. This type of therapy is also known as brachytherapy. When a radiation implant is in place, the client is strictly isolated because the implant emits radiation and can affect and be harmful to other individuals. Cancer, also known as a neoplasm, is a growth. It is characterized by the uncontrolled growth of cells that invades surrounding tissue and spreads (metastasizes) to other parts of the body. Cancer is not a contagious disorder. You will learn about the spread of infectious diseases in your fundamentals of nursing course. You will also learn about tuberculosis and radiation implants in your medical-surgical nursing course and about herpes zoster (chickenpox) in your pediatrics course.

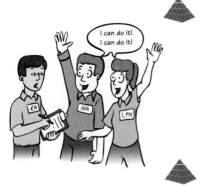

Who Can Do What?

There are some general guidelines to follow when answering a question that requires determining what tasks and client care activities should be assigned to which health care provider. Remember that these are general guidelines, and the general guidelines are the ones that you need to follow when taking a national examination. These guidelines (listed below) are followed by sample questions in both multiple-choice and multiple-response formats.

Unlicensed Personnel, Such as a Nursing Assistant

Generally, noninvasive tasks and basic client care activities can be assigned to an unlicensed individual, such as a nursing assistant. Some of these tasks and activities include:

Ambulation
Bathing
Client transport
Grooming
Hygiene measures
Positioning
Range-of-motion exercises
Skin care
Some specimen collections, such as urine or stool

Licensed Practical or Vocational Nurse

In addition to the tasks that the unlicensed personnel (nursing assistant) can perform, a licensed practical or vocational nurse can perform certain invasive tasks and client care activities. Some of these additional tasks include:

Administering oral medications
Administering intramuscular injections
Administering subcutaneous injections
Administering intradermal medications
Administering medications by the rectal, vaginal, eye, ear, nose, or topical routes
Administering medications by a gastrointestinal tube
Administering some IV piggyback medications

Changing dressings

Irrigating wounds

Monitoring an IV flow rate

Suctioning

Teaching about basic hygienic and nutritional measures

Urinary catheterization

Using the nursing process (clinical problem-solving process): data collection, planning, implementing, and evaluating

Registered Nurse

The registered nurse is competent to perform many tasks and client care activities. In addition to the tasks and client care activities that a licensed practical or vocational nurse can perform, the registered nurse can perform numerous other procedures. To assist you in differentiating the role of the registered nurse and the licensed practical or vocational nurse, some tasks and client care activities that only the registered nurse can perform are:

Administering IV medications by continuous IV, by piggyback, and by IV push

Initiating client teaching

Using the nursing process: assessment, analyzing data, planning, implementing, and evaluating

---

Q | Sample Question: Multiple Response

Case Event: A nurse is planning the client assignments for the day and has a registered nurse, a licensed practical nurse, and a nursing assistant on the nursing team.

Question Query: Choose all clients that could be safely assigned to the licensed practical nurse. Select all that apply.

☐ **1.** A client scheduled for an ultrasound of the heart

☐ **2.** A client with an open abdominal wound who requires wound irrigations every 3 hours

☐ **3.** A client newly diagnosed with diabetes mellitus who requires teaching about insulin administration

☐ **4.** A client with a spinal cord injury who requires intermittent urinary catheterization every 4 hours

☐ **5.** A client with pulmonary edema who was admitted to the hospital 2 hours ago and requires frequent respiratory assessments

☐ **6.** A client with a central IV line who is receiving parenteral nutrition and lipids and has a physician's order to receive 2 units of packed red blood cells

Answer: 1, 2, 4

Test-Taking Strategy:

Focus on the subject of the question—a client assignment to a licensed practical nurse. Use general principles and guidelines to assist in answering the question correctly. Think about and visualize the client's needs, and determine whether the licensed practical nurse can competently and legally perform activities to meet these needs. Initial teaching about insulin administration needs to be done by a registered nurse. Client assessment is done by the registered nurse; however, the licensed practical nurse can collect data. A client with a central IV line who needs to receive blood transfusions needs to be cared for initially by a registered nurse. In addition, this client has complex needs with regard to the central IV line, because the client is also receiving parenteral nutrition and lipids. Remember that the health care provider needs to be competent and skilled to perform the assigned task or client activity.

Tip for the Beginning Nursing Student

An ultrasound of the heart is a noninvasive procedure in which the heart chambers and valves are visualized and examined for abnormalities. There is no client preparation for the procedure, and the procedure is painless for the client. Wound irrigations may be prescribed for certain clients who have wound infections or are at risk for a wound infection. This procedure requires sterile technique and cleansing of the wound with a sterile solution, such as normal saline, or another type of solution as prescribed by the physician. Diabetes mellitus is a disorder of carbohydrate, fat, and protein metabolism that occurs primarily as a result of a deficiency or complete lack of insulin secretion by the beta cells of the pancreas or resistance to insulin. Many clients with diabetes mellitus require insulin (although some may be controlled with oral medications). Insulin needs to be administered by subcutaneous injection, and these clients need to learn how to properly administer the insulin. In addition to insulin, diet and exercise are important components of management of the disease. A spinal cord injury occurs as a result of a traumatic disruption of the spinal cord, such as from a car or other type of accident or from some sort of violent impact. Such trauma can cause varying degrees of paralysis; depending on the level of injury in the spinal cord, some individuals lose the ability to urinate on their own. As a result these individuals require urinary catheterization (insertion of a tube to drain the bladder), an invasive procedure. Heart failure is an inability of the heart to maintain adequate circulation to meet the metabolic needs of the body because of an impaired pumping ability. Pulmonary edema is a serious complication of heart failure in which fluid accumulates in the pulmonary system as a result of the impaired pumping ability of the heart. A client with pulmonary edema requires frequent respiratory assessments. The registered nurse is the health care provider who is responsible for client assessment. A central IV line is one that is inserted into a central vein, usually the subclavian vein. Clients with this type of IV line can receive solutions such as parenteral nutrition (a solution containing a high concentration of nutrients and glucose) and lipids (fat emulsion to prevent fatty acid deficiency) through the line. Red blood cells, usually administered to a client with anemia, can also be administered through a central IV line, and a registered nurse is responsible for administering the blood transfusion. You will learn about these client conditions in your fundamentals of nursing course and in your medical-surgical nursing course.

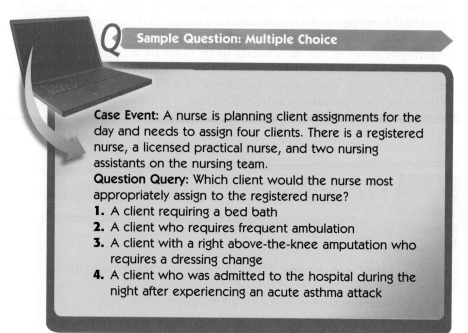

Case Event: A nurse is planning client assignments for the day and needs to assign four clients. There is a registered nurse, a licensed practical nurse, and two nursing assistants on the nursing team.

Question Query: Which client would the nurse most appropriately assign to the registered nurse?

1. A client requiring a bed bath
2. A client who requires frequent ambulation
3. A client with a right above-the-knee amputation who requires a dressing change
4. A client who was admitted to the hospital during the night after experiencing an acute asthma attack

Answer: 4

Test-Taking Strategy:

Note the strategic words *most appropriately,* and focus on the subject of the question—a client assignment to a registered nurse. Use general principles and guidelines to assist in answering the question correctly. Think about and visualize the client's needs. The client who was admitted to the hospital during the night after experiencing an acute asthma attack would most appropriately be assigned to the registered nurse, because this client would require frequent respiratory assessments. The nursing assistant can most appropriately give a bed bath and ambulate a client. The licensed practical nurse can perform dressing changes. Remember that the health care provider needs to be competent and skilled to perform the assigned task or client activity.

Tip for the Beginning Nursing Student

You will learn about the procedure for giving a client a bed bath (bathing a client while the client is in bed) and will learn about the safe procedure for ambulating a client during your fundamentals of nursing course. These are noninvasive procedures and can therefore be assigned to a nursing assistant, because these health care providers are trained to perform these procedures safely. A right above-the-knee amputation means that the client underwent a surgical procedure in which the right limb to the level above the knee was surgically removed. This client requires dressing changes, which are an invasive procedure that requires sterile technique. The licensed practical or vocational nurse is trained to perform sterile dressing changes. You will also learn about the procedure for changing sterile dressings in your fundamentals of nursing course and in your medical-surgical nursing course. Asthma is a respiratory disorder that is characterized by recurring episodes of dyspnea, wheezing, constriction of the bronchi, coughing, and the production of mucoid bronchial secretions. Acute attacks can occur that require aggressive treatment to maintain a patent airway. These clients require frequent respiratory assessment that needs to be done by a registered nurse. You will learn about asthma in your medical-surgical nursing course when you study respiratory problems. You will also learn about asthma in your pediatrics nursing course.

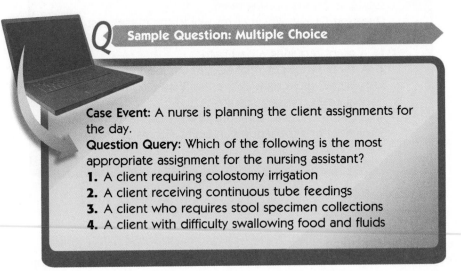

Sample Question: Multiple Choice

Case Event: A nurse is planning the client assignments for the day.
Question Query: Which of the following is the most appropriate assignment for the nursing assistant?
1. A client requiring colostomy irrigation
2. A client receiving continuous tube feedings
3. A client who requires stool specimen collections
4. A client with difficulty swallowing food and fluids

Answer: 3
Test-Taking Strategy:
Note the strategic words *most appropriate,* and focus on the subject of the question—a client assignment to a nursing assistant. Use general principles and guidelines to assist in answering the question correctly. Think about and visualize the client's needs, and determine whether the nursing assistant can competently and legally perform activities to meet these needs. In this situation the most appropriate assignment for a nursing assistant would be to care for the client who requires stool specimen collections. The client with difficulty swallowing food and fluids is at risk for aspiration. Colostomy irrigations and tube feedings are not performed by unlicensed personnel. Remember that the health care provider needs to be competent and skilled to perform the assigned task or client activity.

Tip for the Beginning Nursing Student

A colostomy is the surgical creation of a stoma (an artificial anus) on the abdominal wall that allows for the elimination of feces (bowel contents). This is created for the client with a bowel tumor who is experiencing bowel obstruction or for the client with a tumor or other disorder who requires removal of part of the colon. The colostomy may require irrigations to empty the content of the colon. This is an invasive procedure that can be performed by the licensed practical or vocational nurse or the registered nurse. Tube feedings involve the administration of liquid food to a client through a tube placed in the client's stomach or other area of the client's gastrointestinal tract. Because this procedure places that client at risk for aspiration (breathing in fluid or food into the lungs resulting in a blocked airway), a licensed nurse needs to perform this procedure. Likewise, a client having difficulty swallowing food and fluids is at risk for aspiration and requires care from a licensed nurse. The collection of stool specimens is a noninvasive procedure, and therefore a nursing assistant can perform this procedure. You will learn about caring for these types of clients in your fundamentals of nursing course and in your medical-surgical nursing course.

TIME MANAGEMENT
What Is Time Management, and Why Is It Important?

Time management is a technique used by the nurse to assist in completing tasks within a definite period. It involves learning how, when, and where to use one's time and involves establishing personal goals and time frames. Time management requires an ability to anticipate the day's activities, to combine activities when possible, and to avoid being interrupted by nonessential activities. It also involves efficiency in completing tasks quickly and thoroughly and effectiveness in deciding on the most important task to do and doing it correctly. The ability to manage time efficiently is important to complete tasks and client care activities within a reasonable time frame. In many client care situations, time management requires prioritizing. The nurse needs to be skilled in planning time resourcefully and needs to assist other health care providers with time management. Some principles and guidelines to use to assist in managing time efficiently are listed below.

> **Time Management:** The ability to manage time efficiently in order to complete tasks and client care activities within a reasonable time frame

Principles and Guidelines of Time Management

Following is a list of the principles and guidelines of time management:
1. Identify tasks, obligations, and client care activities and write them down.
2. Organize the workday; identify which tasks and client care activities must be completed in specified time frames.
3. Prioritize client needs.
4. Anticipate the needs of the day, and provide time for unexpected and unplanned tasks or client care activities that may arise.

5. Focus on beginning the daily tasks by working on the most important first, while keeping goals in mind; look at the final goal for the day, which will help to break down tasks into manageable parts.

6. Begin client rounds at the beginning of the shift, assessing/collecting data on each assigned client.

7. Delegate tasks when appropriate.

8. Keep a daily hour-by-hour log to assist in providing structure to the tasks that must be accomplished, and cross tasks off the list as they are accomplished.

9. Use hospital and agency resources efficiently, anticipating resource needs and gathering the necessary supplies before beginning the task.

10. Organize paperwork, and continuously document task completion and necessary client data throughout the day.

11. At the end of the day, evaluate the effectiveness of time management.

TIME MANAGEMENT

Think!
Organize!
Plan!
Prioritize!

Q Sample Question: Prioritizing and Time Management

Case Event: A nurse on the day shift is assigned to care for four clients.

Question Query: Following report from the night shift, which client will the nurse plan to assess/collect data from first?

1. Client scheduled for a cardiac catheterization at 10:00 AM

2. Client scheduled to have an electrocardiogram (ECG) at 9:00 AM

3. Client with pulmonary edema who was treated with furosemide (Lasix) at 5:00 AM

4. Client newly diagnosed with diabetes mellitus who is scheduled for discharge to home

Answer: 3

Test-Taking Strategy:
Note the strategic word *first,* and focus on the subject—which client the nurse plans to assess/collect data from first. This question describes a situation in which the nurse needs to prioritize and manage his or her

time with regard to the assigned clients. Use the ABCs—airway, breathing, and circulation—to answer the question. Airway is always a high priority; therefore the nurse would assess and collect data from the client with pulmonary edema who was treated with furosemide (Lasix) at 5:00 AM first. The nurse would next assess/collect data from the client scheduled for the cardiac catheterization, because this client will require preprocedural preparation. The client scheduled for discharge would be attended to next because there may be discharge needs that require attention. The client scheduled for an ECG can be checked last.

Tip for the Beginning Nursing Student

Heart failure is an inability of the heart to maintain adequate circulation to meet the metabolic needs of the body because of an impaired pumping ability. Pulmonary edema is a serious complication of heart failure in which fluid accumulates in the pulmonary system as a result of the impaired pumping ability of the heart. The client is treated with a diuretic, which is a medication that will result in an increased urine output, thus ridding the body of the excess fluid that accumulated in the pulmonary system. Furosemide (Lasix) is a diuretic. A major concern for the client with pulmonary edema is airway and breathing, so this is the reason why assessing/collecting data from this client is the priority. A cardiac catheterization is a diagnostic procedure in which a catheter is introduced through an incision into a large blood vessel and threaded through the circulatory system of the heart. This procedure is primarily done to assess the status of the coronary arteries in the heart and to determine if any blockage is present and if so, the extent of the blockage. The client requires some preprocedural preparation, such as ensuring informed consent has been obtained, checking for client allergies, obtaining height and weight and vital signs and noting the quality and presence of peripheral pulses, ensuring that an IV line is inserted, client teaching, and administering prescribed medications. Because this procedure is scheduled for 10:00 AM, this client can be assessed second. Diabetes mellitus is a disorder of carbohydrate, fat, and protein metabolism that occurs primarily as a result of a deficiency or complete lack of insulin secretion by the beta cells of the pancreas or resistance to insulin. Insulin therapy or oral medications, diet therapy, and an exercise regimen are important components for management of the disease to prevent complications, and the nurse needs to ensure that the client has been taught about management and understands the treatment prescribed for the disorder. Because the client is scheduled for discharge it is important that the nurse ensure that the client's needs are met and that the client understands the prescribed treatment. Therefore in this situation this client is the nurse's third priority. An ECG is a diagnostic test that is performed using a device that records the electrical activity of the myocardium and detects the transmission of the cardiac impulse through the tissues of the heart muscle. This test can diagnose specific abnormalities of the heart. It is a noninvasive test that requires no specific preparation except for explaining the procedure to the client. Therefore in this situation this client would be the nurse's last priority.

REFERENCES

Christen, B., & Kockrow, E. (2006). *Adult health nursing* (5th ed.). St. Louis: Mosby.

Fortinash, K., & Holoday-Worret, P. (2008). *Psychiatric mental health nursing* (4th ed.). St. Louis: Mosby.

Harkreader, H., Hogan, M.A., & Thobaben, M. (2007). *Fundamentals of nursing: Caring and clinical judgment* (3rd ed.). Philadelphia: Saunders.

Hockenberry, M., & Wilson, D. (2007). *Nursing care of infants and children* (8th ed.). St. Louis: Mosby.

Hodgson, B., & Kizior, R. (2008). *Saunders nursing drug handbook 2008.* Philadelphia: Saunders.

Ignatavicius, D., & Workman, M. (2006). *Medical-surgical nursing: Critical thinking for collaborative care* (5th ed.). Philadelphia: Saunders.

Linton, A., & Maebius, N. (2007). *Introduction to medical-surgical nursing* (4th ed.). Philadelphia: Saunders.

Monahan, F., Sands, J., Marek, J., Neighbors, M., & Green, C. (2007). *Phipps' medical-surgical nursing: Health and illness perspectives* (8th ed.). St. Louis: Mosby.

National Council of State Boards of Nursing (Eds.) (2008). *2008 NCLEX-PN® detailed test plan, National Council of State Boards of Nursing.* Chicago: Author.

National Council of State Boards of Nursing (Eds.) (2007). *2007 NCLEX-RN® Detailed Test Plan.* Chicago: Author.

National Council of State Boards of Nursing Web site: www.ncsbn.org

Potter, P., & Perry, A. (2009). *Fundamentals of nursing* (7th ed.). St. Louis: Mosby.

Price, D., & Gwin, J. (2008). *Pediatric nursing: An introductory text* (10th ed.). Philadelphia: Saunders.

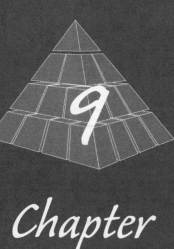

9 Chapter

Communication Questions

Communication is a process in which information is exchanged, either verbally or nonverbally, between two or more individuals (Figure 9-1). According to the National Council of State Boards of Nursing (NCSBN), an Integrated Process of the Test Plan is a process that is fundamental to the practice of nursing and is incorporated throughout the Client Needs categories of the Test Plan. In the National Council Licensure Examination (NCLEX) Test Plan, the NCSBN identifies the concept of communication as a component of one of the Integrated Processes. In addition, in the Psychosocial Integrity category of Client Needs, therapeutic communication and cultural considerations are listed as content that is tested on the NCLEX exam. Therefore it is likely that you will be presented with questions related to the communication process. This chapter reviews the guidelines to follow when answering communication questions and identifies various cultural considerations to consider when communicating and caring for clients. Several sample questions are included to illustrate how these guidelines are used.

HOW ARE COMMUNICATION CONCEPTS TESTED IN A QUESTION?

Communication is an important characteristic of the nurse–client relationship. Therefore test questions that refer to the concept of communication may address a client situation in any clinical setting and any nursing care area. That is, communication questions may address client situations in the adult health area, the maternity area, the pediatric area, or the mental health area in settings such as the hospital, clinic, physician's office, or other health care setting.

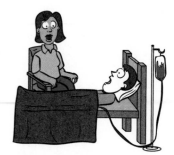

When we think about communication concepts and the nurse–client relationship, we usually visualize an interaction between the nurse and the client. Although this is an accurate visualization, it is important to broaden our thinking with regard to the communication process and the concepts that will be tested on the examination. Test questions not only will address the communication process between the nurse and the client,

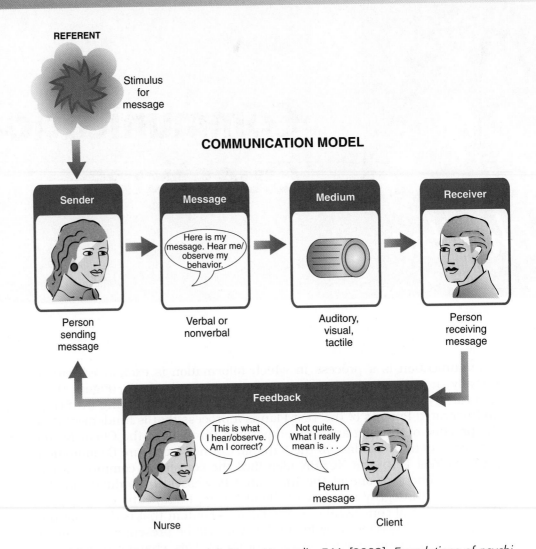

Fig. 9-1 Communication model. (From Varcarolis, E.M. [2002]. *Foundations of psychiatric mental health nursing* [4th ed.]. Philadelphia: Saunders.)

but also will address the process between the nurse and a client's family member or significant other, or the nurse and another member of the health care team, such as another nurse, a nursing assistant, or a physician. For example, you may be asked about how you would respond to a staff member who makes an inappropriate statement or how you would respond to a physician who is demanding. Most questions that test the concept of communication will be in the multiple-choice format and will relate to how the nurse would respond to the person with whom he or she is communicating.

✓ **NCLEX® Exam Tip**

Remember that communication questions may address client situations in the adult health area, the maternity area, the pediatric area, or the mental health area in settings such as the hospital, clinic, physician's office, or other health care setting. In addition, these questions may identify a client from a culture different from your own, and you will need to consider cultural differences in order to answer the question correctly.

WHAT GUIDELINES CAN BE USED TO ANSWER COMMUNICATION QUESTIONS?

The four primary guidelines to use when answering communication questions are as follows:

1. Use therapeutic communication techniques to answer communication questions because of their effectiveness in the communication process. As you read the question and each option, find the option that indicates the use of a therapeutic communication technique.

2. Nontherapeutic communication techniques are ineffective and should be avoided when responding to a client, a client's family member or significant other, or another member of the health care team. As you read the question and each option, eliminate the options that indicate the use of a nontherapeutic communication technique.

3. Focus on feelings, concerns, anxieties, or fears. As you read the question and each option, look for the option that indicates the use of a therapeutic communication technique and focuses on the feelings, concerns, anxieties, or fears of the client, the client's family member or significant other, or the health care team member.

4. Consider cultural differences as you answer the question. If you note that a question contains information that identifies a specific cultural group, think about specific cultural characteristics to answer the question correctly. Remember that each culture is unique with regard to characteristics related to the process of communication.

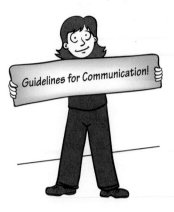
Guidelines for Communication!

> **GUIDELINES FOR COMMUNICATION**
>
> Use therapeutic communication techniques.
> Avoid nontherapeutic communication techniques.
> Focus on the client's feelings, concerns, anxieties, or fears.
> Consider cultural differences.

COMMUNICATION TECHNIQUES
What Are the Therapeutic Communication Techniques?

Using therapeutic communication techniques encourages the client, or other individual with whom the nurse is communicating, to express his or her thoughts and feelings. Many therapeutic communication techniques can be used to promote verbalization. If you are not familiar with these techniques, you will learn them in your first nursing course in nursing school. Table 9-1 provides a brief review of these techniques.

Tip for the Beginning Nursing Student

You will learn about therapeutic and nontherapeutic communication techniques in your first nursing course. These techniques are very important, because they provide a foundation for your interaction with your client or others in any clinical setting. So be sure to read your assigned reading in your textbook carefully, because you will use these techniques throughout nursing school and your profession.

TABLE 9-1 THERAPEUTIC COMMUNICATION TECHNIQUES

Technique	Description
Active listening	Carefully noting what the client is saying and observing the client's nonverbal behavior
Broad openings	Encouraging the client to select topics for discussion
Clarifying	Providing a means for making the message clearer, to correct any misunderstandings, and to promote mutual understanding
Focusing	Directing the conversation on the topic being discussed
Informing	Giving information to the client
Offering self to help	Includes staying with the client or talking to the client for consideration
Open-ended questions	Encouraging conversation because these questions require more than one-word answers
Paraphrasing	Restating in different words what the client said
Reflecting	Directing the client's question or statement back to the client for consideration
Restating	Repeating what the client has said and directing the statement back to the client to provide the client the opportunity to agree or disagree or to clarify the message further
Silence	Allowing time for formulating thoughts
Summarizing	Stating briefly what was discussed during the conversation
Validating	Verifying that both the nurse and the client are interpreting the topic or message in the same way

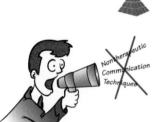

What Are the Nontherapeutic Communication Techniques?

Nontherapeutic communication techniques impair or block the flow of a conversation. They are also known as the barriers to an effective communication process. The many nontherapeutic communication techniques need to be avoided when communicating because of their ineffectiveness. Table 9-2 briefly reviews some nontherapeutic communication techniques.

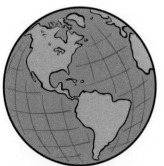

WHY ARE CULTURAL CONSIDERATIONS IMPORTANT?

The nurse needs to be aware of certain cultural characteristics that relate to the communication process and other aspects of care that may differ from his or her own cultural uniqueness. Questions on the NCLEX exam may address the concept of communication with a client from a specific cultural group. If you note that a question contains information identifying a specific cultural group, think about specific cultural characteristics to answer the question correctly.

TABLE 9-2 NONTHERAPEUTIC COMMUNICATION TECHNIQUES

Technique	Description
Approval	Implying that the client is thinking or doing the right thing and is not thinking or doing what is wrong; this may direct the client to focus on thinking or behavior that pleases the nurse
Asking excessive questions	Demanding information from the client without respect for the client's willingness or readiness to respond
Changing the subject	Avoiding addressing the client's thoughts, feelings, or concerns; implying that the client's statement is not important
Close-ended questions	Questions that ask for specific information such as a "yes" or "no" answer and therefore inhibit communication
Disagreeing	Opposing the client's thinking or opinions, implying that the client is wrong
Disapproving	Indicating a negative value judgment about the client's behavior or thoughts
False reassurance	Making a statement that implies that the client has no reason to be worried or concerned; belittling a client's concerns
Giving advice	Assuming that the client cannot think for himself or herself, which inhibits problem solving and fosters dependence
Minimizing the client's feelings	Making a statement that implies that the client's feelings are not important
Parroting	Repeating the client's words before determining what the client has said
Placing the client's feelings on hold	Avoiding addressing the client's thoughts, feelings, or concerns; making a statement that places the responsibility of addressing the client's thoughts, feelings, or concerns elsewhere or on another person
Value judgments	Making a comment that addresses the client's morals; this can make the client feel angry or guilty or as though he or she is not being supported
"Why?" questions	Cause the client to feel defensive because many times he or she does not know the reason "why"; these types of questions also often imply criticism

Communication involves three cultural characteristics: communication style, use of eye contact, and the meaning of touch. Review the characteristics associated with specific cultures and become familiar with them before taking the NCLEX exam. The box below identifies the three characteristics of specific cultural groups that you need to consider. Appendix B also identifies other important aspects of care for clients in specific cultural groups. This appendix includes the dietary preferences of various cultural groups and various religions, beliefs and practices of the Amish society, and religion and end-of life care practices. If you are unfamiliar with content related to the characteristics of various cultures, refer to this appendix and *Saunders Comprehensive Review for the NCLEX®-RN Examination* or *Saunders Comprehensive Review for the NCLEX®-PN Examination*. This product contains information about cultural characteristics and a specific chapter, entitled "Cultural Diversity," that describes many features related to cultural differences for various cultural groups.

CULTURAL COMMUNICATION POINTS TO CONSIDER!

Communication style
Use of eye contact
Meaning of touch

Communication Style

The following sections provide some background information to consider when developing your communication style with specific cultural groups.

African Americans

Personal questions asked on initial contact with the client may be viewed as intrusive.
Head nodding by the client does not necessarily mean agreement.

Asian Americans

Asian cultures may believe that feelings and emotions are private, and an open expression of emotions is regarded as a weakness.
Silence is valued by the client.
Criticism or disagreement is not expressed verbally by the client.
Head nodding by the client does not necessarily mean agreement.
The client may interpret the word "no" as disrespect for others.
The client does not use hand gestures.

European (White) Americans

Silence can be used by the client to show respect or disrespect for another, depending on the situation.

French and Italian Americans

The client may use expressive hand gestures and animated facial expressions during conversation.

German and British Americans

The client may show little facial emotion, because these clients highly value the concept of self-control.

Hispanic Americans

The client may use dramatic body language, such as gestures or facial expressions, to express emotion or pain.
The client may tend to be verbally expressive, yet confidentiality is important.
Hispanic Americans may believe that direct confrontation is disrespectful and the expression of negative feelings is impolite.

Native Americans

To Native Americans, silence indicates respect for the speaker.
Many of these clients speak in a low tone of voice and expect others to be attentive.
Body language is important.
Obtaining input from members of the extended family is important.

Use of Eye Contact

The following sections provide information regarding how clients of specific cultural groups view the use of eye contact.

African Americans

Direct eye contact may be interpreted as rude or aggressive behavior.

Asian Americans

Eye contact is limited and may be considered inappropriate or disrespectful.

European (White) Americans

Eye contact may be viewed as indicating trustworthiness.

Native Americans

Eye contact may be viewed as a sign of disrespect.
The nurse needs to understand that the client may be attentive even when eye contact is absent.

Hispanic Americans

Some Hispanic Americans believe that avoiding eye contact with a person in authority indicates respect and attentiveness.

Meaning of Touch

The following sections discuss how specific cultural groups view touch.

African Americans

African Americans may feel comfortable with close personal space when they are interacting with family and friends.

Asian Americans

Asian Americans prefer a formal personal space except with family and close friends.
They usually do not touch others during conversation.
Touching is unacceptable with members of the opposite gender; if possible, a female client prefers a female health care provider.
The head is considered to be sacred; therefore touching someone on the head may be considered disrespectful.
The nurse would avoid physical closeness and excessive touching and would only touch a client's head when necessary, informing the client before doing so.

European (White) Americans

European Americans tend to avoid close physical contact.
The nurse needs to respect the client's personal space.

Native Americans

Personal space is very important to Native Americans.
Native American clients may lightly touch another person's hand during greetings.
In this culture, massage is used for the newborn infant to promote bonding between the infant and mother.
Touching a dead body may be prohibited in some tribes.

Hispanic Americans

Hispanic Americans are comfortable with close proximity with family, friends, and acquaintances and value the physical presence of others.
The nurse needs to protect the client's privacy.
Hispanic Americans are very tactile and use embraces and handshakes.
The nurse needs to ask if it would be all right to touch a child before examining him or her.

SAMPLE COMMUNICATION QUESTIONS

Following are sample communication questions that illustrate the use of therapeutic and nontherapeutic communication techniques.

Tip for the Beginning Nursing Student

Remember to use the following communication guidelines:
1. Use therapeutic communication techniques.
2. Avoid the use of nontherapeutic communication techniques.
3. Focus on the client's feelings, concerns, anxieties, or fears.
4. Consider cultural differences.

Q Sample Question 1

Case Event: A mother says to the nurse in the physician's office, "I am afraid that my child might have another seizure."

Question Query: Which response by the nurse is most therapeutic?
1. "Tell me what frightens you the most about seizures."
2. "Why worry about something that you cannot control?"
3. "Most children will never experience a second seizure."
4. "Phenytoin (Dilantin) can prevent another seizure from occurring."

Answer: 1

Test Taking Strategy:

Note the strategic words *most therapeutic.* Option 1 is the only option that addresses the client's fears. Option 2 is a nontherapeutic response, because it states that the mother should not worry. Options 3 and 4 are incorrect, because the nurse is giving false reassurance to the mother that a seizure will not recur or can be prevented in this child.

Tip for the Beginning Nursing Student

A seizure is a hyperexcitation of the neurons in the brain leading to a sudden, violent involuntary series of contractions of a group of muscles. There are different types of seizures. The most important nursing measures when a client experiences a seizure are to maintain a patent airway and to ensure safety for the client. You will learn about caring for a client with seizures when you study neurological disorders in your medical-surgical nursing class. To answer this question correctly, remember to use therapeutic communication techniques and focus on the client's feelings, concerns, anxieties, and fears!

Sample Question 2

Case Event: A client examined in the health care clinic has been diagnosed with hypertension and has been taking a prescribed antihypertensive medication. On a follow-up visit, the client says to the nurse, "I don't understand why I have to take this medication. It makes me feel awful."

Question Query: The most appropriate nursing response is which of the following?

1. "You will need to ask your doctor about that."
2. "Everyone who takes that medication says the same thing."
3. "You have to take this medication if you want to prevent a stroke."
4. "Describe what you mean when you say that the medication makes you feel awful."

Answer: 4

Test-Taking Strategy:

Note the strategic words *most appropriate.* Option 1 avoids the client's concern and places the client's feelings on hold. Option 2 minimizes the client's feelings and implies that the client's complaint is not important. In option 3 the nurse gives advice and also provides false reassurance that the medication will prevent a stroke. In this option the nurse also avoids the client's complaint, is somewhat threatening, and may induce fear in the client. In option 4 the nurse uses the therapeutic communication technique of restating. In this technique the nurse explores by repeating what the client has said and directing the statement back to the client to provide the client the opportunity to clarify the message further.

Tip for the Beginning Nursing Student

Hypertension is a condition characterized by an elevated blood pressure above the normal value and is a known cardiovascular risk factor. Many times clients with hypertension do not even know that they are experiencing the disorder and are without signs and symptoms. This is why the disorder is sometimes called a "silent disease" and may not be discovered until a routine physical exam is performed. Antihypertensive medications are prescribed to lower the blood pressure, but unpleasant side effects of the medication can occur. This is why noncompliance can be a concern for clients with hypertension taking antihypertensive medications. You will learn about hypertension in your medical-surgical nursing course. For this sample question, remember to use therapeutic communication techniques and focus on the client's feelings, concerns, anxieties, and fears!

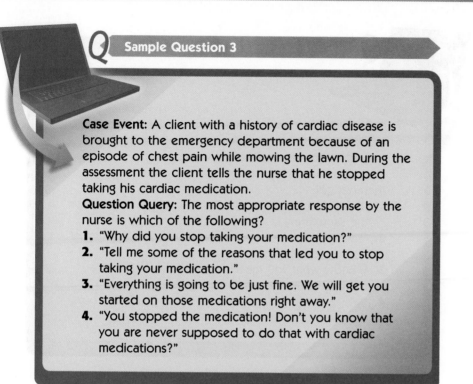

Sample Question 3

Case Event: A client with a history of cardiac disease is brought to the emergency department because of an episode of chest pain while mowing the lawn. During the assessment the client tells the nurse that he stopped taking his cardiac medication.

Question Query: The most appropriate response by the nurse is which of the following?

1. "Why did you stop taking your medication?"
2. "Tell me some of the reasons that led you to stop taking your medication."
3. "Everything is going to be just fine. We will get you started on those medications right away."
4. "You stopped the medication! Don't you know that you are never supposed to do that with cardiac medications?"

Answer: 2

Test-Taking Strategy:

Note the strategic words *most appropriate.* Option 2 is an open-ended and broad opening question that will promote and encourage the client to communicate. The statement in option 1 uses the word *why.* Use of this word implies criticism and often makes the client feel defensive; in addition, many times the client does not know why he or she stopped the medication. In option 3 the nurse provides false reassurance by telling the client that everything is going to be fine. Also, the nurse avoids exploring the reason(s) that led the client to stop the medication. In option 4 the nurse demoralizes, belittles, and lectures the client, which is nontherapeutic.

 Tip for the Beginning Nursing Student

Cardiac disease can result from a variety of causes, including but not limited to angina pectoris (chest pain), myocardial infarction (heart attack), heart failure, or valvular disorders. If a client experiences chest pain this could result from a lack of oxygen to the myocardial tissue and needs to be attended to immediately to prevent myocardial tissue death. You will learn about cardiac disease during your medical-surgical nursing course; because heart disease is a major health concern, focus on the ways to teach a client to prevent it. For this question, remember to use therapeutic communication techniques and focus on the client's feelings, concerns, anxieties, and fears!

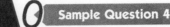

Sample Question 4

Case Event: A client recently diagnosed with ovarian cancer says to the nurse, "I cannot believe this has happened to me. I wish that I were dead!"

Question Query: Which nursing response is most therapeutic?

1. "Every client diagnosed with this type of cancer says the same thing."
2. "You must be feeling very upset. Are you thinking of hurting yourself?"
3. "I know what you mean, but there are a lot of treatments available for ovarian cancer."
4. "Why are you talking that way? Your children would not want to hear you say that, would they?"

Answer: 2

Test-Taking Strategy:

Note the strategic words *most therapeutic.* In option 2 the nurse focuses on the client's statement and addresses the client's feelings in the response. In options 1 and 3 the nurse minimizes the client's feelings. In addition, option 3 provides false reassurances. In option 4 the nurse uses the word *why,* which implies criticism and often makes the client feel defensive. In addition, option 4 focuses on the client's children and their feelings rather than on the client's feelings.

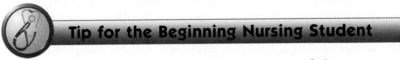

Tip for the Beginning Nursing Student

Ovarian cancer is a malignant tumor of the ovary or ovaries. It is rarely detected in its early stages and is usually far advanced when diagnosed. Regular yearly pelvic examinations contribute significantly to early diagnosis; thus it is important to teach clients about the importance of these pelvic examinations. You will learn about ovarian cancer and other types of cancer in your medical-surgical nursing course. For this sample question, remember to use therapeutic communication techniques and focus on the client's feelings, concerns, anxieties, and fears!

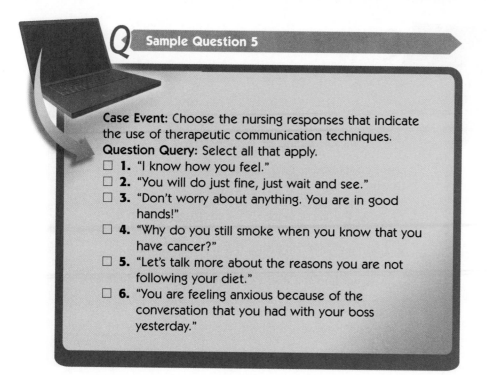

Case Event: Choose the nursing responses that indicate the use of therapeutic communication techniques.
Question Query: Select all that apply.
- ☐ **1.** "I know how you feel."
- ☐ **2.** "You will do just fine, just wait and see."
- ☐ **3.** "Don't worry about anything. You are in good hands!"
- ☐ **4.** "Why do you still smoke when you know that you have cancer?"
- ☐ **5.** "Let's talk more about the reasons you are not following your diet."
- ☐ **6.** "You are feeling anxious because of the conversation that you had with your boss yesterday."

Answer: 5, 6

Test-Taking Strategy:
Focus on the subject—therapeutic communication techniques. Review the following nursing responses:

1. "I know how you feel."—nontherapeutic and minimizes the client's feelings
2. "You will do just fine, just wait and see."—nontherapeutic and minimizes and avoids the client's feelings
3. "Don't worry about anything. You are in good hands!" —nontherapeutic; avoids the client's feelings and provides false reassurance
4. "Why do you still smoke when you know that you have cancer?"—nontherapeutic; demoralizes the client and also can make the client feel guilty, angry, anxious, or unsupported
5. "Let's talk more about why you are not following your diet."—therapeutic and uses the technique of focusing
6. "You are feeling anxious because of the conversation that you had with your boss yesterday."—therapeutic and indicates the use of reflection

 Tip for the Beginning Nursing Student

This question asks you to select the statements that reflect the use of therapeutic communication techniques. So think about these techniques when selecting the correct statements. You will learn about these therapeutic and nontherapeutic techniques in your fundamentals of nursing course. Remember to use therapeutic communication techniques and focus on the client's feelings, concerns, anxieties, and fears when answering communication questions!

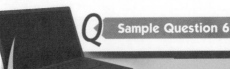

Sample Question 6

Case Event: A nurse is providing instructions to an Asian client regarding obtaining a stool specimen for testing for occult blood. As the nurse explains the instructions, the client continuously turns away.

Question Query: Which nursing action is most appropriate?

1. Stress the importance of the instructions with the client.
2. Continue with the instructions, verifying client understanding.
3. Walk around the client so that the nurse continuously faces the client.
4. Give the client the list of instructions and return later to continue with the instructions.

Answer: 2

Test-Taking Strategy:

In this question you need to consider the characteristics of the Asian culture. Note the strategic words *most appropriate.* If the client turns away from the nurse during a conversation, the most appropriate action is to continue with the conversation. Telling the client about the importance of the instructions may be viewed as degrading. Walking around the client so that the nurse faces the client is in direct conflict with the cultural practice. The client may view returning later to continue with the explanation as a rude gesture.

Tip for the Beginning Nursing Student

When a question addresses a specific culture, consider the cultural characteristics of the specific group to answer the question. Many Asian clients maintain a formal distance with others, which is a form of respect. Also, many Asian clients are uncomfortable with face-to-face communications, especially when there is direct eye contact. So if the client turns away from the nurse during a conversation, the most appropriate action is to continue with the conversation. You will learn about the cultural characteristics of various cultural groups in your fundamentals of nursing course and other nursing courses. Remember that if the question identifies a specific cultural group, you need to consider the characteristics of the culture to answer the question!

Sample Question 7

Case Event: A nurse in an ambulatory care clinic is performing an admission assessment on an African-American client scheduled for a laparoscopic cholecystectomy.

Question Query: Which of the following questions would be inappropriate for the nurse to ask on initial assessment?

1. "Do you ever experience chest pain?"

2. "Do you have any difficulty breathing?"

3. "Do you have a close family relationship?"

4. "Do you frequently have episodes of abdominal pain?"

Answer: 3

Test-Taking Strategy:

Note the strategic words *inappropriate* and *initial assessment*. In this question you need to consider the characteristics of the African-American culture. In the African-American culture it is considered intrusive to ask personal questions on the initial contact. African Americans are highly verbal and express feelings openly to family or friends, but what transpires within the family is viewed as private. Options 1, 2, and 4 are appropriate to ask the client on initial assessment. In addition, use Maslow's Hierarchy of Needs theory: options 1, 2, and 4 include cardiovascular, respiratory, and gastrointestinal assessments; physiological assessments are the priority assessments.

 Tip for the Beginning Nursing Student

A laparoscopic cholecystectomy is the surgical excision of the gallbladder through small incisions made in the abdominal wall done with the client under general anesthesia. You will learn more about this type of surgery when you study gastrointestinal disorders in your medical-surgical nursing course. For this question, focus on the cultural characteristics of the African-American culture, and remember that in the African-American culture it is considered intrusive to ask personal questions at the initial meeting. Remember that if the question identifies a specific cultural group, you need to consider the characteristics of the culture to answer the question!

REFERENCES

Giger, J., & Davidhizar, R. (2008). *Transcultural nursing assessment & intervention* (5th ed.). St. Louis: Mosby.

Grodner, M., Long, S., & Walkinshaw, B. (2007). *Foundations and clinical applications of nutrition: A nursing approach* (4th ed.). Philadelphia: Mosby.

Harkreader, H., Hogan, M.A., & Thobaben, M. (2007). *Fundamentals of nursing: Caring and clinical judgment* (3rd ed.). St. Louis: Saunders.

Jarvis, C. (2008). *Physical examination & health assessment* (5th ed.). Philadelphia: Saunders.

Linton, A., & Maebius, N. (2007). *Introduction to medical-surgical nursing* (4th ed.). Philadelphia: Saunders.

National Council of State Boards of Nursing Web site: www.ncsbn.org

Nix, S. (2005). *Williams' basic nutrition and diet therapy* (12th ed.). St. Louis: Mosby.

Schlenker, E., & Long, S. (2007). *Williams' essentials of nutrition & diet therapy* (9th ed.). St. Louis: Mosby.

Skidmore-Roth, L. (2006). *Mosby's handbook of herbs & natural supplements* (3rd ed.). St. Louis: Mosby.

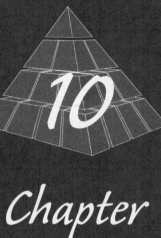

10 Chapter

Pharmacology Questions

Pharmacology is one of the most difficult nursing content areas to master. One reason why it is so difficult is because of the enormous number of medications available. Another reason is that there is a vast amount of information to know about each medication. The National Council Licensure Examination (NCLEX) Test Plan addresses pharmacological and parenteral therapies in the Physiological Integrity category. The registered nurse (RN) Test Plan identifies 13% to 19% as the percentage of this type of test question that will possibly appear on the examination, and the licensed practical/vocational (LPN/LVN) Test Plan identifies 9% to 15% as the percentage of this type of test question that will possibly appear on the examination. This means that if you took a 100-question examination, 13 to 19 of the questions (RN Test Plan) or 9 to 15 of the questions (LPN/LVN Test Plan) would relate to pharmacology and parenteral therapies. Therefore it is important to spend ample time reviewing pharmacology in preparation for the NCLEX exam, and it is best to do your review from a question-and-answer perspective.

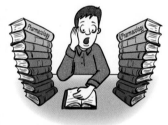

✓ NCLEX® Exam Tip

When a pharmacology question appears on the exam, note the name of the medication and remember that the question will identify both the generic name and the trade name. Focus on the client's diagnosis, and use medical terminology skills to break the name of the medication down into parts to determine the medication and its intended use. Also, use other pharmacology strategies and guidelines to answer the question.

This chapter provides the strategies for preparing to answer pharmacology questions and also various general guidelines to use when attempting to answer the questions correctly. The pharmacology strategies are listed in the box below. In addition, remember to read the question carefully, noting the strategic words and the subject of the question, and always use the process of elimination to select the correct option. As with any

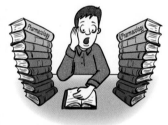

type of question, it is best to use your nursing knowledge to answer the question. However, a question may appear on your examination that contains a medication name with which you are unfamiliar. When this occurs, the guidelines and the strategies to answer a pharmacology question correctly will be valuable. After you read this chapter, practice as many pharmacology questions as you can. Several resources are available that contain hundreds of pharmacology practice questions. For the RN nursing student, these resources include *Saunders Comprehensive Review for the NCLEX-RN® Examination, Saunders Q&A Review for the NCLEX-RN® Examination, Saunders Q&A Review Cards for the NCLEX-RN® Examination,* and *Saunders Online Review Course for the NCLEX-RN® Examination.* For the LPN/LVN student, these resources include *Saunders Comprehensive Review for the NCLEX-PN® Examination, Saunders Q&A Review for the NCLEX-PN® Examination,* and *Saunders Review Cards for the NCLEX-PN® Examination.* These products can be obtained at the Elsevier Web site (www.elsevierhealth.com).

PHARMACOLOGY STRATEGIES

Read the question carefully.
Note the strategic words.
Note the subject.
Use the process of elimination.
Use nursing knowledge.
Use general and other pharmacology guidelines.
Use test-taking strategies.

▲ PHARMACOLOGY: GENERAL GUIDELINES TO FOLLOW

Some general guidelines to keep in mind as you are trying to select the correct option are given in the following list. These guidelines are also located in Appendix C.

1. Medication absorption, distribution, metabolism, and excretion are affected by age and physiological processes; the older client and the neonate and infant are at greater risk for toxicity than an adult.
2. Many medications are contraindicated in pregnancy and during breast-feeding.
3. Antacids are not usually administered with medication, because the antacid will affect the absorption of the medication.
4. Grapefruit juice is not usually administered with medication because it contains a substance that will interact with the absorption of the medication.
5. Enteric-coated and sustained-release tablets should not be crushed; also, capsules should not be opened.
6. Nursing interventions always include monitoring for intended effects, side effects, adverse effects, or toxic effects of the medication.
7. Nursing interventions always include client education.

8. The nurse or client should never adjust or change a medication dose, abruptly stop taking a medication, or discontinue a medication.

9. The nurse may withhold a medication if he or she suspects that the client is experiencing an adverse or toxic effect of a medication; the nurse must immediately contact the physician if either of these effects occurs.

10. The client needs to avoid taking any over-the-counter medications or any other medications, such as herbal preparations, unless they are approved for use by the health care provider.

11. The client needs to know how to correctly administer the medication.

12. The client needs to be aware of the side effects and adverse effects of medications and how to check his or her own temperature, pulse, and blood pressure.

13. The client needs to take the prescribed dose for the prescribed length of therapy and understand the necessity of compliance.

14. The client needs to avoid consuming alcohol and to avoid smoking.

15. The client should wear a Medic-Alert bracelet if he or she is taking medications such as, but not limited to, anticoagulants, oral hypoglycemics or insulin, certain cardiac medications, corticosteroids and glucocorticoids, antimyasthenic medications, anticonvulsants, and monoamine oxidase inhibitors.

16. The client needs to follow up with a health care provider as prescribed.

The following sample pharmacology question illustrates how these general pharmacology guidelines may be helpful.

Q Sample Question: General Pharmacology Guidelines

Case Event: A client taking amitriptyline hydrochloride (Elavil) calls the nurse at the physician's office and reports that he has an upset stomach whenever he takes the medication.

Question Query: The nurse most appropriately tells the client to:

1. Take the medication with food.
2. Take the medication with an antacid.
3. Take the medication on an empty stomach.
4. Stop the medication for 2 days and then resume the prescribed medication schedule.

Answer: 1

Test-Taking Strategy:
Remember to read the question carefully, noting the subject of the question and the strategic words. In this question the strategic words are *most appropriately*, and the subject is the client's complaint of an upset stomach. Recalling that antacids are not usually administered with medication and that the nurse would not tell a client to discontinue a medication will

assist in eliminating options 2 and 4. From the remaining options, focusing on the subject will assist in eliminating option 3.

Tip for the Beginning Nursing Student

Amitriptyline hydrochloride (Elavil) is a medication that is called a tricyclic antidepressant. It affects chemicals in the brain that may become unbalanced and is used to treat symptoms of depression. You will learn about this medication in your pharmacology nursing course and in your mental health nursing course.

PHARMACOLOGY: ASSESSMENT/DATA COLLECTION GUIDELINES
What Are the Pharmacology Assessment/Data Collection Guidelines, and How Will They Help in Answering a Pharmacology Question?

There are some specific assessment/data collection guidelines to follow when you administer medication to a client. In addition to using the six rights when administering medications, these guidelines include client assessment and assessment of other factors related to the medication, such as checking certain laboratory values or vital signs; checking for potential interactions or contraindications related to the medication; client teaching; monitoring for intended effects, side effects, adverse effects, or toxic effects; and evaluating the client's response to the medication therapy. When you are presented with a pharmacology question and are trying to select the correct option, using the pharmacology assessment/data collection guidelines will assist you in eliminating incorrect options. Some of these guidelines are listed in the following box.

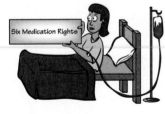

SIX MEDICATION RIGHTS

Right client
Right medication
Right dose
Right time and frequency
Right route
Right documentation

PHARMACOLOGY: ASSESSMENT/DATA COLLECTION GUIDELINES TO FOLLOW

The following list gives pharmacology assessment/data collection guidelines to follow when administering medication to a client:
1. Always assess for client allergies or hypersensitivity to a medication.
2. Always assess the client for existing medical disorders that are contraindicated with the administration of a prescribed medication.

3. Always assess for potential interactions related to the medication.
4. Always check pertinent laboratory results.
5. Always check the client's vital signs, particularly if medications such as antihypertensive or cardiac medications are being administered.
6. Always assess the client for intended effects, side effects, adverse effects, or toxic effects of the medication.
7. Always assess the client's response to the medication.

These guidelines will be particularly helpful if the question asks for the priority nursing action when administering a medication. Below is a sample pharmacology question illustrating how these assessment/data collection guidelines may be helpful.

Sample Question: Pharmacology

Case Event: The nurse notes that a physician has prescribed sulfamethoxazole and trimethoprim (Bactrim) for a client with a urinary tract infection.

Question Query: Which priority action will the nurse take before administering this medication?

1. Call the pharmacy to order the medication.
2. Ask the client about an allergy to sulfonamides.
3. Inform the client about the need to increase fluid intake.
4. Check the medication supply room to find out whether the medication needs to be ordered.

Answer: 2

Test-Taking Strategy:
Remember to read the question carefully, noting the subject of the question and the strategic words. In this question the strategic word is *priority*, and the subject is the action that the nurse will take. Also note that the client has a urinary tract infection. Using the pharmacology assessment/data collection guidelines will direct you to option 2. In addition, use of the steps of the nursing process will direct you to the correct option, because option 2 is the only option that addresses client assessment/data collection.

Tip for the Beginning Nursing Student

Bactrim contains a combination of sulfamethoxazole and trimethoprim and is an antibiotic that treats different types of infection caused by bacteria. It is used to treat ear infections, urinary tract infections, bronchitis, *Pneumocystis jiroveci* pneumonia, and other types of infection. You will learn about this medication in your pharmacology nursing course and in your medical-surgical nursing course when you study the immune system.

◢ MEDICATION EFFECTS
What Are the Differences Among an Intended Effect, a Side Effect, an Adverse Effect, and a Toxic Effect of a Medication?

It is important to understand these differences; understanding them will assist in eliminating the incorrect options in a pharmacology question that asks about one of these effects. When you are presented with a question on the examination that asks about an effect of a medication, note the specific subject—is the subject of the question an intended effect, a side effect, an adverse effect, or a toxic effect? The differences are described in the following sections, and each section has a sample question related to the specific effect discussed in that section.

Intended Effect

An intended effect is the desired and expected effect of a medication. For example, the intended effect of morphine sulfate is pain relief. A sample question that asks about an intended effect is provided.

> **INTENDED EFFECT**
>
> A desired effect

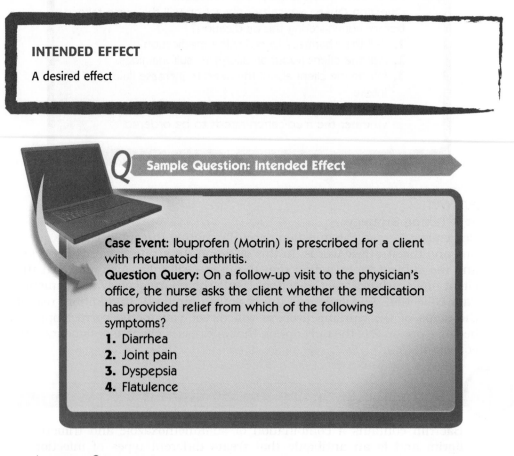

Sample Question: Intended Effect

Case Event: Ibuprofen (Motrin) is prescribed for a client with rheumatoid arthritis.
Question Query: On a follow-up visit to the physician's office, the nurse asks the client whether the medication has provided relief from which of the following symptoms?
1. Diarrhea
2. Joint pain
3. Dyspepsia
4. Flatulence

Answer: 2

Test-Taking Strategy:
Read the question carefully, noting the subject of the question and the strategic words. In this question the strategic words are *provided relief from*, and the subject is an intended effect of the medication. Note that the question provides the client's diagnosis. Recalling the pathophysiology

related to rheumatoid arthritis will assist in directing you to option 2. Also note that options 1, 3, and 4 are comparable or alike in that they all address gastrointestinal symptoms. When options are comparable or alike, it is best to eliminate those options because they are unlikely to be correct. In addition, options 1, 3, and 4 are side effects of ibuprofen, not intended effects.

Tip for the Beginning Nursing Student

Ibuprofen (Motrin) is in a group of medications called nonsteroidal anti-inflammatory drugs (NSAIDs). It works by reducing hormones that cause inflammation and pain in the body. It is used to reduce fever and treat pain or inflammation caused by many conditions, such as headache, toothache, back pain, arthritis, menstrual cramps, or minor injury. You will learn about this medication in your pharmacology course and in your medical-surgical nursing course.

Side Effect

A side effect is a physiological effect of a medication that is unrelated to the intended medication effects. For example, a side effect of an antihistamine medication is drowsiness. A side effect of a medication is not usually life threatening, and normally there are measures that will either eliminate the side effect or alleviate the discomfort associated with it. A sample question that asks about a side effect is provided.

SIDE EFFECT

Not a desired effect
Not usually life threatening
Can usually be alleviated with specific measures

Sample Question: Side Effect

Case Event: Erythromycin (E-Mycin) has been prescribed for a client with a respiratory infection.
Question Query: The nurse tells the client that which frequent side effect can occur from this medication?
1. Severe diarrhea
2. Yellow-colored skin
3. Abdominal cramping
4. Yellow discoloration to the white part of the eye

Answer: 3

Test-Taking Strategy:
Remember to read the question carefully, noting the subject of the question and the strategic words. In this question the strategic words and the subject are a side effect of the medication. Eliminate options 2 and 4 first because they are comparable or alike and both indicate the presence of hepatitis, an adverse effect of the medication. From the remaining options, eliminate option 1 because of the word *severe.* Remember that the question asks about a side effect, not an adverse effect.

Tip for the Beginning Nursing Student

Erythromycin (E-Mycin) is in a group of medications called macrolide antibiotics. Macrolide antibiotics slow the growth of, or sometimes kill, sensitive bacteria by reducing the production of important proteins needed by the bacteria to survive. Erythromycin is used to treat many different types of infections caused by bacteria. You will learn about this medication in your pharmacology course and in your medical-surgical nursing course when you study the immune system.

Adverse Effect

An adverse effect is more severe than a side effect and is always an undesirable effect. For example, an adverse effect of a sulfonamide is hypersensitivity that may be evidenced by a rash, fever, and shortness of breath. An adverse effect can range from a mild effect to a severe effect, such as anaphylaxis. Adverse effects are always reported to the health care provider. A sample question that asks about an adverse effect is provided.

ADVERSE EFFECT

More severe than a side effect
Always an undesirable effect
Always reported to the health care provider

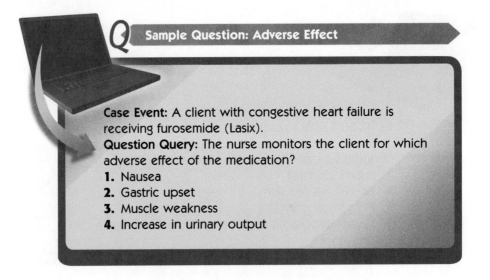

Sample Question: Adverse Effect

Case Event: A client with congestive heart failure is receiving furosemide (Lasix).
Question Query: The nurse monitors the client for which adverse effect of the medication?

1. Nausea
2. Gastric upset
3. Muscle weakness
4. Increase in urinary output

Answer: 3

Test-Taking Strategy:

Read the question carefully, noting the subject of the question and the strategic words. In this question the strategic words and the subject are an adverse effect of the medication. Eliminate options 1 and 2 first because they are comparable or alike and both relate to the gastrointestinal system. From the remaining options, eliminate option 4 because it is an intended effect of the medication. Also, recall that furosemide is a diuretic and can cause electrolyte imbalances and that muscle weakness is an indication of hypokalemia. Remember that the question asks about an adverse effect.

Tip for the Beginning Nursing Student

Furosemide (Lasix) is a potent diuretic (water pill) that works by blocking the absorption of salt and fluid in the kidney tubules, causing a profound increase in urine output (diuresis). The diuretic effect of furosemide can cause body water and electrolyte depletion. It is used to treat excessive fluid accumulation and swelling (edema) of the body caused by heart failure, cirrhosis, chronic kidney failure, and nephrotic syndrome. It is sometimes used in conjunction with other blood pressure pills to treat high blood pressure. You will learn about this medication in your pharmacology course and in your medical-surgical nursing course when you study the cardiovascular system.

Toxic Effect

A toxic effect (toxicity) of a medication occurs when the medication level in the body exceeds the therapeutic level either from overdosing or medication accumulation. Always report toxic effects to the health care provider. Toxic effects are most often identified by monitoring the plasma (serum) therapeutic range of the medication. For example, the therapeutic blood level of digoxin (Lanoxin) is 0.5 to 2 ng/mL; if the blood level is greater than 2 ng/mL, the client experiences toxicity. The client will normally exhibit certain signs and symptoms (depending on the medication) that indicate toxicity, and the nurse needs to monitor for these signs and symptoms. For example, in digoxin toxicity, the client may experience gastrointestinal disturbances, such as anorexia, nausea, and vomiting; or ocular disturbances, such as photophobia, light flashes, or halos around bright objects. Table 10-1 lists medications commonly used in the clinical setting and their therapeutic blood level; a sample question that asks about a toxic effect follows.

TOXIC EFFECT

The medication level in the body exceeds the therapeutic level.

TABLE 10-1 THERAPEUTIC BLOOD MEDICATION LEVELS

Therapeutic Medication	Range
Acetaminophen (Tylenol)	10-20 mcg/mL
Carbamazepine (Tegretol)	5-12 mcg/mL
Digoxin (Lanoxin)	0.5-2 ng/mL
Gentamicin (Garamycin)	5-10 mcg/mL
Lithium (Lithobid)	0.5-1.3 mEq/L
Magnesium sulfate	4-7 mg/dL
Phenytoin (Dilantin)	10-20 mcg/mL
Salicylate	100-250 mcg/mL
Theophylline (Theo-Dur)	10-20 mcg/mL

Sample Question: Toxic Effect

Case Event: The nurse reviews the results of a therapeutic blood level that was drawn from a client taking theophylline (Theo-24) and notes that the level is 21 mcg/mL.

Question Query: The nurse would most appropriately:

1. Report the result to the health care provider.
2. Administer the next scheduled dose of theophylline.
3. Place the results of the blood test in the client's medical record.
4. Ask the laboratory to draw another blood specimen to verify the result.

Answer: 1

Test-Taking Strategy:

Remember to read the question carefully, noting the subject of the question and the strategic words. In this question the strategic words are *most appropriately,* and the subject is a toxic effect of the medication. Recalling that the therapeutic blood level of theophylline is 10 to 20 mcg/mL will assist in determining that the client is experiencing toxicity. Remember that toxic effects are always reported to the health care provider.

Tip for the Beginning Nursing Student

Theophylline (Theo-24) is an oral bronchodilator medication used to treat symptoms of asthma, chronic bronchitis, and emphysema. It opens the airways by relaxing the smooth muscle of the airways and blood vessels in the lungs. It is indicated for the treatment of the symptoms of reversible airflow obstruction associated with chronic asthma and other chronic lung diseases, such as emphysema and chronic bronchitis. You will learn about this medication in your pharmacology course and in your medical-surgical nursing course when you study the respiratory system.

MEDICATION NAMES
Do You Need to Memorize Both the Generic Name and the Trade Name of a Medication?

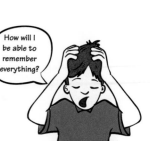

How will I be able to remember everything?

No memorizing is necessary! When a pharmacology question appears on the computer screen, both the generic name and the trade name will appear. This will assist you in answering the question correctly. One medication name, perhaps the generic name, may be unfamiliar to you, but you may recognize the trade name. For example, a question may ask about a medication named furosemide (Lasix). You may not be familiar with the medication name furosemide, but it is very likely that you will be familiar with the medication name Lasix because it is a commonly administered medication.

How Will Medical Terminology Skills Help to Answer a Pharmacology Question?

If a pharmacology question appears on your examination that contains the name of a medication with which you are unfamiliar, try to break the generic or trade name of the medication into parts and use medical terminology to assist in determining the medication action. Following is a pharmacology question that illustrates how this strategy works.

BREAK THE WORD DOWN!

Q **Sample Question: Medical Terminology Skills**

Case Event: Metoprolol (Lopressor) has been prescribed for a client.
Question Query: The nurse performs which most important assessment before administering the medication to the client?
1. Takes the client's temperature
2. Checks the client's lung sounds
3. Takes the client's blood pressure
4. Checks the client for peripheral edema

Answer: 3
Test-Taking Strategy:
Remember to read the question carefully, noting the subject of the question and the strategic words. In this question the strategic words are *most important,* and the subject is an assessment. Focus on the name of the medication; if you are unfamiliar with the medication, try to break the name of the medication into parts and use medical terminology to assist in determining the medication action. For example, Lopressor lowers (lo) the blood pressure (pressor).

Tip for the Beginning Nursing Student

Metoprolol (Lopressor) is a beta-adrenergic blocking agent that is used for treating high blood pressure, heart pain (angina pectoris), abnormal rhythms of the heart, and some neurological conditions. It blocks the action of the sympathetic nervous system by blocking beta receptors on sympathetic nerves. Because the sympathetic nervous system is responsible for increasing the heart rate, by blocking the action of these nerves, metoprolol reduces the heart rate and is useful in treating abnormally rapid heart rhythms. Metoprolol also reduces the force of contraction of heart muscle and thereby lowers blood pressure. By reducing the heart rate and the force of muscle contraction, metoprolol reduces the need for oxygen by heart muscle. Because heart pain (angina pectoris) occurs when oxygen demand of the heart muscle exceeds the supply of oxygen, metoprolol is helpful in treating heart pain (angina pectoris). You will learn about this medication in your pharmacology course and in your medical-surgical nursing course when you study the cardiovascular system.

▲ MEDICATION CLASSIFICATIONS
How Will It Help to Identify a Medication by the Classification to Which It Belongs?

Medications that belong to a particular classification have similar medication actions and usually have commonalities in their side effects and nursing interventions related to administration. It is nearly impossible to learn every feature about every individual medication. Learning medications by a "classification system method" groups several medications with similar properties together and makes the amount of information that needs to be learned condensed and manageable.

With regard to side effects and nursing interventions, do not try to memorize every side effect and every nursing intervention for every medication. It is best if you associate side effects with nursing interventions. Learn to recognize the common side effects associated with each medication classification, and then relate the appropriate nursing interventions to each side effect. For example, if a side effect is hypertension, then the associated nursing intervention would be to monitor blood pressure; if a side effect is hypokalemia, then the associated nursing interventions are to monitor the client for signs of hypokalemia and to monitor the client's potassium blood level. Again, this makes the vast amount of information that you need to remember manageable.

Relate nursing interventions to the side effects of a medication!

How Can You Determine the Medication Classification if You Are Unfamiliar With the Medication?

If you are presented with a pharmacology question that contains the name of a medication with which you are unfamiliar, some strategies to use include the following:

1. Note whether the question identifies the client's diagnosis. For example, if the question states: "Cyclophosphamide (Cytoxan) has been prescribed for a client with metastatic breast cancer," focusing on the client's diagnosis will help you to determine that cyclophosphamide is an antineoplastic medication.
2. Break down the name of the medication (either the generic or trade name) into parts. For example, if the question states: "Terbutaline sulfate (Brethine) has been prescribed for a client," think about "breath" when you look at the medication name Brethine to help you determine that it is a respiratory medication.
3. Note the letters in the medication name, and look for those letters that identify a particular medication classification.

COMMONALITIES IN MEDICATION NAMES

Learning commonalities in medication names that belong to a particular classification will also help in answering a question. If you note a medication name in a test question and are unfamiliar with the medication, if you can at least associate the medication with a classification you will be able to determine the medication's action, side effects, and nursing interventions. A list of commonalities in medication names is provided below and in Appendix C. Sample questions follow.

1. Androgens: Most medication names end with the letters -*terone*, such as testosterone (Androderm, Testoderm).
2. Angiotensin-converting enzyme (ACE) inhibitors: Most medication names end with the letters -*pril*, such as enalapril (Vasotec).
3. Antidiuretic hormones: Most medication names end with the letters -*pressin*, such as desmopressin (DDAVP).
4. Antilipemic medications: Most medication names end with the letters -*statin*, such as atorvastatin (Lipitor).
5. Antiviral medications: Most antiviral medications contain *vir* in their names, such as ritonavir (Norvir).
6. Benzodiazepines: Benzodiazepines include alprazolam (Xanax), chlordiazepoxide (Librium), clorazepate (Tranxene), estazolam (ProSom), and triazolam (Halcion); most other benzodiazepines names end with the letters -*pam*, such as diazepam (Valium).
7. β-Adrenergic blockers: Most medication names end with the letters -*lol*, such as atenolol (Tenormin).
8. Calcium channel blockers: Most medication names end with the letters -*pine*, such as amlodipine (Norvasc); some exceptions include diltiazem (Cardizem, Cardizem SR) and verapamil (Calan, Isoptin).
9. Carbonic anhydrase inhibitors: Most medication names end with the letters -*mide*, such as acetazolamide (Diamox).
10. Estrogens: Most estrogen medications contain *est* in their names, such as conjugated estrogen (Premarin).
11. Glucocorticoids and corticosteroids: Most medication names end with the letters -*sone*, such as prednisone (Deltasone).

12. Histamine H$_2$ receptor antagonists: Most medication names end with the letters *-dine*, such as cimetidine (Tagamet).
13. Nitrates: Most medications contain *nitr* in their names, such as nitroglycerin (Nitrostat).
14. Pancreatic enzyme replacements: Most medications contain *pancre* in their names, such as pancrelipase (Pancrease).
15. Phenothiazines: Most medication names end with the letters *-zine*, such as chlorpromazine (Thorazine).
16. Proton pump inhibitors: Most medication names end with the letters *-zole*, such as lansoprazole (Prevacid).
17. Sulfonamides: Most medications include *sulf* in their names, such as sulfasalazine (Azulfidine).
18. Sulfonylureas: Most medication names end with the letters *-mide*, such as chlorpropamide (Diabinese).
19. Thiazide diuretics: Most medication names end with the letters *-zide*, such as hydrochlorothiazide (HydroDIURIL).
20. Thrombolytic medications: Most medication names end with the letters *-ase*, such as alteplase (Activase).
21. Thyroid hormones: Most medications contain *thy* in their names, such as levothyroxine (Synthroid).
22. Xanthine bronchodilators: Most medication names end with the letters *-line*, such as theophylline.

Q | **Sample Question: Commonalities in Medication Names**

Case Event: A nurse is collecting data from a client who is taking pantoprazole (Protonix).

Question Query: The nurse determines that the medication is effective if the client states relief of which of the following symptoms?

1. Heartburn
2. Constipation
3. A nighttime cough
4. Migraine headaches

Answer: 1

Test-Taking Strategy:
Remember to read the question carefully, noting the subject of the question and the strategic words. In this question the strategic words are *is effective* and *relief of*, and the subject is an intended effect. Remembering that most proton pump inhibitor medication names end with the suffix *-zole* will direct you to option 1.

Tip for the Beginning Nursing Student

Pantoprazole (Protonix) is in a group of medications called proton pump inhibitors that decreases the amount of acid produced in the stomach. It is used to treat erosive esophagitis (damage to the esophagus from stomach acid) and other conditions involving excess stomach acid, such as a condition known as Zollinger-Ellison syndrome. You will learn about this medication in your pharmacology course and in your medical-surgical nursing course when you study gastrointestinal disorders.

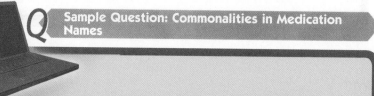

Q Sample Question: Commonalities in Medication Names

Case Event: A nurse is collecting a health history on a client seen at the health care clinic for the first time. When the nurse asks the client about current prescribed medications, the client tells the nurse that he takes indinavir (Crixivan) twice daily.

Question Query: Based on this finding, the nurse suspects the presence of which condition?

1. Diverticulitis
2. Peptic ulcer disease
3. Inflammatory bowel disease
4. Human immunodeficiency virus (HIV)

Answer: 4

Test-Taking Strategy:
Remember to read the question carefully, noting the subject of the question and the strategic words. In this question the strategic words are *suspects the presence,* and the subject is the nurse's finding. Remembering that many antiviral medication names contain the letters *vir* will direct you to option 4. Also note that options 1, 2, and 3 are comparable or alike and relate to a gastrointestinal disorder.

Tip for the Beginning Nursing Student

Indinavir (Crixivan) is a protease inhibitor. Protease inhibitors block the part of HIV called protease. When protease is blocked or inhibited, HIV is unable to infect new cells. Protease inhibitors are almost always used in combination with at least two other anti-HIV medications. You will learn about this medication in your pharmacology course and in your medical-surgical nursing course when you study immune disorders.

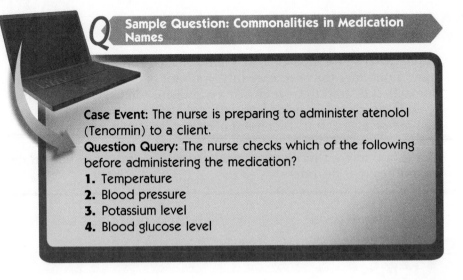

Sample Question: Commonalities in Medication Names

Case Event: The nurse is preparing to administer atenolol (Tenormin) to a client.

Question Query: The nurse checks which of the following before administering the medication?

1. Temperature
2. Blood pressure
3. Potassium level
4. Blood glucose level

Answer: 2

Test-Taking Strategy:

Remember to read the question carefully, noting the subject of the question and the strategic words. In this question the strategic words are *before administering,* and the subject is an assessment. Note the name of the medication, *atenolol.* Recalling that most β-blocker medication names end with the letters *-lol* and that these medications are used to control blood pressure will direct you to option 2.

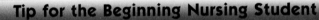

Tip for the Beginning Nursing Student

Atenolol (Tenormin) is a β-adrenergic blocking agent that is used for treating high blood pressure, heart pain (angina pectoris), abnormal rhythms of the heart, and some neurological conditions. It blocks the action of the sympathetic nervous system by blocking beta receptors on sympathetic nerves. Because the sympathetic nervous system is responsible for increasing the heart rate, by blocking the action of these nerves, atenolol reduces the heart rate and is useful in treating abnormally rapid heart rhythms. Atenolol also reduces the force of contraction of heart muscle and thereby lowers blood pressure. You will learn about this medication in your pharmacology course and in your medical-surgical nursing course when you study the cardiovascular system.

REFERENCES

Hodgson, B., & Kizior, R. (2008). *Saunders nursing drug handbook 2008.* Philadelphia: Saunders.

Lehne, R. (2007). *Pharmacology for nursing care* (6th ed.). Philadelphia: Saunders.

Lilley, L., Harrington, S., & Snyder, J. (2007). *Pharmacology and the nursing process* (5th ed.). St. Louis: Mosby.

Linton, A., & Maebius, N. (2007). *Introduction to medical-surgical nursing* (4th ed.). Philadelphia: Saunders.

Monahan, F., Sands, J., Marek, J., Neighbors, M., & Green, C. (2007). *Phipps' medical-surgical nursing: Health and illness perspectives* (8th ed.). St. Louis: Mosby.

National Council of State Boards of Nursing Web site: www.ncsbn.org

Potter, P., & Perry, A. (2009). *Fundamentals of nursing* (7th ed.). St. Louis: Mosby.

Skidmore-Roth, L. (2007). *2007 Mosby's nursing drug reference* (20th ed.). St. Louis: Mosby.

Varcarolis, E., Carlson, V., & Shoemaker, N. (2006). *Foundations of psychiatric mental health nursing* (5th ed.). Philadelphia: Saunders.

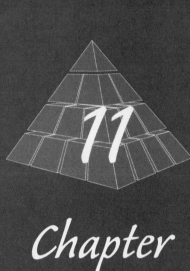

11

Chapter

Additional Pyramid Strategies

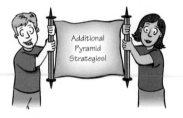

In addition to all the test-taking strategies that you have reviewed so far in this book, you can use other helpful strategies to assist in the process of elimination and answering questions correctly. This chapter reviews these helpful strategies and provides sample questions to illustrate how these strategies are used. Also included in this chapter are useful strategies for answering questions that relate to medication and intravenous (IV) calculations, laboratory values, client positioning, therapeutic diets, and disaster planning. Some additional pyramid strategies include:

1. Eliminating options that contain close-ended words
2. Eliminating options that contain medical rather than nursing interventions
3. Eliminating comparable or alike options
4. Ensuring that all components of an option are correct
5. Selecting the umbrella option
6. Visualizing the information in the case event, question query, and options
7. Looking for concepts in the question that are comparable or alike to a concept in one of the options

▲ ELIMINATING OPTIONS THAT CONTAIN CLOSE-ENDED WORDS: HOW WILL THIS HELP?

In most situations, if an option contains a close-ended word, it is incorrect. As you read each option, if you note a word that is close ended, eliminate that option. Conversely, as you read an option and note an open-ended word, then that may be the correct option. A list of close-ended and open-ended words follows.

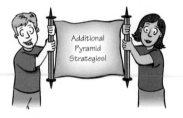

Close-Ended Words

All
Always
Cannot
Every
Must
Never
None
Not
Only
Will not

Open-Ended Words

Generally
May
Possibly
Usually

> Close-ended words may indicate an incorrect option!
> Open-ended words may indicate a correct option!

Following are sample questions that illustrate the strategy of close-ended versus open-ended words.

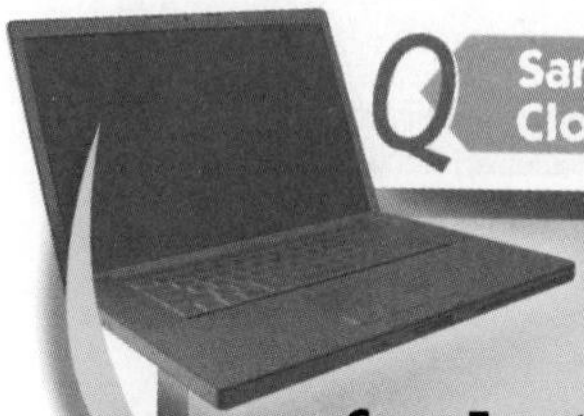

Q Sample Question: Eliminating Options That Contain Close-Ended Words

Case Event: A nurse is providing dietary instructions to a client about a low-fat diet.
Question Query: The nurse tells the client to:
1. Never use butter for cooking.
2. Drink fluids only if they are fat free.
3. Eat only foods that have less than 1% fat content.
4. Read the labels on food items to determine the fat content.

Answer: 4
Test-Taking Strategy:
Read every word in each option carefully. Note the close-ended words *never* in option 1 and *only* in options 2 and 3. These options should be eliminated because they are incorrect. Remember that the use of a close-ended word in an option will most likely make the option incorrect!

Tip for the Beginning Nursing Student

For a regular healthy diet it is usually recommended that of the total calories eaten, no more than 30% should come from fat. A low-fat diet may require even a greater restriction. Low-fat diets may be prescribed for a variety of conditions, including gastrointestinal disorders such as liver disease or gallbladder disease, cardiovascular disorders, or obesity. You will learn about the various types of diets in your fundamentals of nursing course and in your medical-surgical nursing course.

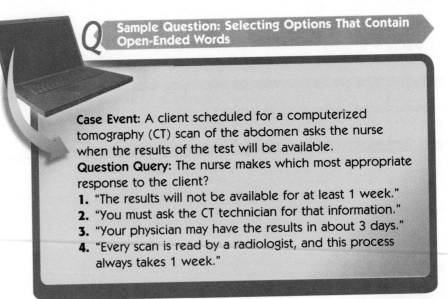

Sample Question: Selecting Options That Contain Open-Ended Words

Case Event: A client scheduled for a computerized tomography (CT) scan of the abdomen asks the nurse when the results of the test will be available.

Question Query: The nurse makes which most appropriate response to the client?

1. "The results will not be available for at least 1 week."
2. "You must ask the CT technician for that information."
3. "Your physician may have the results in about 3 days."
4. "Every scan is read by a radiologist, and this process always takes 1 week."

Answer: 3

Test-Taking Strategy:
Read every word in each option carefully, and note the strategic words *most appropriate.* If you were unable to answer this question using nursing knowledge, note the use of the open-ended word *may* in option 3. Also, note the close-ended words *will not* in option 1, *must* in option 2, and *every* and *always* in option 4. These options should be eliminated, because they are incorrect. Remember that the use of a close-ended word in an option will most likely make the option incorrect and the use of an open-ended word in an option tends to make the option correct.

Tip for the Beginning Nursing Student

A CT scan is an x-ray procedure that combines x-ray images with the aid of a computer to generate cross-sectional views and, if needed, three-dimensional images of the internal organs and structures of the body. A CT scan is used to define normal and abnormal structures in the body and/or assist in procedures by helping to accurately guide the placement of instruments or treatments. You will learn about this diagnostic procedure during your nursing education, most likely in your medical-surgical nursing course.

ELIMINATING OPTIONS THAT CONTAIN MEDICAL RATHER THAN NURSING INTERVENTIONS: HOW WILL THIS HELP?

Doctor   Nurse

An important point to remember is that the NCLEX exam is a nursing examination, not a medical one. Therefore focus on nursing, and select the option that relates to a nursing intervention rather than a medical one. The only situation in which you may need to select a medical intervention is if the question indicates to do so. For example, if the question query states, "Which intervention does the nurse to prescribe?" then you may need to select the option that contains a medical action or prescription. Following is a review with sample questions that illustrate this strategy.

Focus on nursing rather than medical interventions!

Q Sample Question: Eliminating Options That Contain Medical Rather Than Nursing Interventions

Case Event: A nurse is caring for a client with a diagnosis of heart failure who suddenly experiences severe dyspnea and suspects that pulmonary edema has developed.
Question Query: The nurse immediately:
1. Inserts a Foley catheter
2. Places the client in high-Fowler's position
3. Obtains a vial of furosemide (Lasix) and a syringe
4. Obtains a dose of morphine sulfate from the opioid (narcotic) medication drawer

Answer: 2
Test-Taking Strategy:
Note the strategic word *immediately,* and note the subject of the question—a nursing action. Although options 1, 3, and 4 are interventions that would be done in this situation, they all require a medical order from

the physician. Option 2 is a nursing action that does not require a medical order. Remember that your exams are nursing examinations, not medical examinations!

Tip for the Beginning Nursing Student

Heart failure is an inability of the heart to maintain adequate circulation to meet the metabolic needs of the body because of an impaired pumping ability. Heart failure can progress to pulmonary edema, a condition in which fluid accumulates in lung tissue. This is a medical emergency. If this occurs the immediate action of the nurse is to place the client in an upright (high-Fowler's) position. You will learn about heart failure and pulmonary edema when you learn about cardiac disorders. One important thing to remember is that with all clients, airway is the priority.

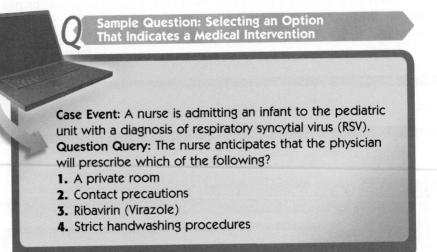

Q Sample Question: Selecting an Option That Indicates a Medical Intervention

Case Event: A nurse is admitting an infant to the pediatric unit with a diagnosis of respiratory syncytial virus (RSV).
Question Query: The nurse anticipates that the physician will prescribe which of the following?
1. A private room
2. Contact precautions
3. Ribavirin (Virazole)
4. Strict handwashing procedures

Answer: 3

Test-Taking Strategy:
Note the subject of the question—the intervention that the physician will prescribe. Although the physician may document options 1, 2, and 4 on the medical order sheet, these are interventions that the nurse can implement for an infant with RSV. That is, a physician's order is not required for these interventions. In contrast, option 3 requires a physician's order. Remember that your exam is a nursing examination, not a medical examination, and the only situation in which you may need to select a medical intervention is if the question indicates to do so!

Tip for the Beginning Nursing Student

RSV is a viral infection that is a common cause of acute bronchiolitis, bronchopneumonia, and the common cold in infants and young children. Symptoms include fever, cough, and severe malaise. Treatment includes rest, humidity, adequate fluid intake, oxygen, and the administration of ribavirin (Virazole). You will learn about this virus when you study respiratory infections in your pediatrics course.

ELIMINATING COMPARABLE OR ALIKE OPTIONS: HOW WILL THIS HELP?

An important point for you to remember is that multiple-choice questions have only one correct option. As you read the options, if you note options that are comparable or alike with regard to their context, eliminate these options. The correct answer to the question will be the option that is different. Following is a sample question that illustrates this strategy of eliminating comparable or alike options.

> Eliminate comparable or alike options!

Sample Question: Eliminating Comparable or Alike Options

Case Event: A nurse is preparing a plan of care for a client who will be receiving a blood transfusion.

Question Query: The nurse writes which intervention in the plan that relates to monitoring for a transfusion reaction?

1. Weigh the client before and after the transfusion.
2. Check the client's lung sounds hourly for crackles.
3. Monitor the client's temperature during the transfusion.
4. Monitor the client's intake and output during the transfusion.

Answer: 3

Test-Taking Strategy:
Note the subject of the question—a transfusion reaction. If you know the signs of a transfusion reaction, you can answer this question easily. If you do not know these signs, read the options carefully. Note that options 1, 2, and 4 are comparable or alike in that they relate to the complication of fluid overload. Because they are all comparable or alike, they are incorrect and need to be eliminated. Remember that the correct answer to the question will be the option that is different!

Tip for the Beginning Nursing Student

A blood transfusion involves the IV administration of a component of blood, such as packed red blood cells, to replace blood or one of its components lost as a result of trauma, surgery, or a disease. One complication that can occur when administering blood is a blood transfusion reaction. Some signs and symptoms of this complication include fever; facial flushing; rapid, thready pulse; cold, clammy skin; itching; dizziness; difficulty breathing; or low back or chest pain. You will learn about blood transfusions, the complications, and the nursing care involved with the administration of blood during your medical-surgical nursing course when you study hematological disorders.

ENSURING THAT ALL PARTS OF AN OPTION ARE CORRECT: HOW WILL THIS HELP?

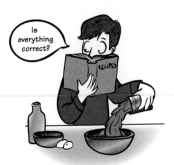

Some questions on exams or on the NCLEX exam may contain options that include two parts, and each part of the option is separated by the word *and*. Read the question carefully, note the strategic words, and focus on the subject. As you read the options, read both parts of the option. If you note that one part of the option is incorrect, then the entire option is incorrect; therefore eliminate that option. In these types of questions, it is important to ensure that both parts of the option are correct. Following is a sample question that illustrates this strategy of ensuring that all parts of an option are correct.

Ensure that all parts of an option are correct!

Sample Question: Ensuring That All Parts of an Option Are Correct

Case Event: A nurse is performing an assessment on a client diagnosed with a cataract of the right eye.
Question Query: The nurse would expect to obtain which data on assessment?
1. A cloudy white pupil and reports of eye pain
2. Reports of a frontal headache and photophobia
3. Reports of a gradual loss of vision and photophobia
4. Reports of blurred vision and excessive tearing of the eye

Answer: 3

Test-Taking Strategy:
The options in this question contain two parts, and each part of the option is separated by the word *and.* Read the question carefully, note the strategic words, and focus on the subject. The strategic words are *expect to obtain*, and the subject of the question is assessment data noted in a client with a cataract. In this question, knowledge regarding the differences between the signs and symptoms of a cataract versus glaucoma will assist in answering the question correctly. Although a cloudy white pupil and photophobia occur in a client with a cataract, eye pain and frontal headaches do not. Therefore options 1 and 2 are not entirely correct and need to be eliminated. Eye pain and frontal headaches occur in the client with glaucoma. From the remaining two options, recalling that excessive tearing occurs in the client with glaucoma, not the client with a cataract, will assist in eliminating option 4. Remember that all parts of the option need to be correct for the option to be correct!

 Tip for the Beginning Nursing Student

Cataract is a condition that affects the lens of the eye. On assessment the nurse would note a cloudy white pupil. Symptoms include a gradual loss of vision, photophobia, painless blurring and distortion of objects, and glare from bright lights. You will learn about cataracts, their treatment, and the nursing care involved during your medical-surgical nursing course when you study eye disorders.

SELECTING THE UMBRELLA OPTION: HOW WILL THIS HELP?

The umbrella option is a general statement that may incorporate the content of the other options within it. When you are answering a question and note that more than one option appears to be correct, look for the umbrella option. The umbrella option will be the correct answer. Following is a sample question that illustrates this strategy.

Look for the umbrella option!

Case Event: In a telephone call from emergency medical services, a nurse in the emergency department is told that several victims who survived a plane crash and are suffering from cold exposure will be transported to the hospital.

Question Query: The initial nursing action of the emergency department nurse is which of the following?

1. Call the nursing supervisor to activate the agency disaster plan.
2. Supply the trauma rooms with bottles of sterile water and normal saline.
3. Call the intensive care unit to request that nurses be sent to the emergency room.
4. Call the laundry department to request as many warm blankets as possible for the emergency room.

Answer: 1

Test-Taking Strategy:

Note the strategic word *initial*, and focus on the subject—the nursing action in the event of a disaster. As you read each option, you will note that all options are correct. In this type of question, look for the umbrella option. Option 1 is the umbrella option. Activating the agency disaster plan will ensure that the interventions in options 2, 3, and 4 will occur. Remember that the umbrella option incorporates the ideas of the other options within it.

Tip for the Beginning Nursing Student

A disaster preparedness plan is a structured and formal plan of action that is implemented when a disaster occurs in the health care agency or external to the agency, such as in the community. The plan provides a coordinated plan of action for all members of the health care team. You will learn about disasters and disaster preparedness plans during your community nursing course.

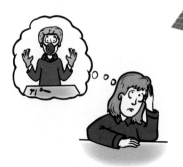

▲ VISUALIZING THE INFORMATION IN THE CASE EVENT, QUESTION QUERY, AND OPTIONS: HOW WILL THIS HELP?

As you read the question, it is helpful to visualize the case event. Forming a mental image of the situation places you as the nurse into the scenario. This may be useful because as you create the mental image, you may recall a similar situation that you experienced in the actual clinical area and recall what the nurse did in the situation. In addition, visualize each option as you read it. This process will assist in determining the correct option. Visualizing and relating the case event to a similar clinical experience can be a valuable strategy as you attempt to eliminate incorrect options. Following is a sample question that illustrates this strategy of visualizing the information.

> Visualize the information!

Sample Question: Visualizing the Information in the Case Event, Question Query, and Options

Case Event: A nurse prepares to perform a sterile dressing change on an abdominal incision.

Question Query: The nurse explains the procedure to the client, washes her hands, and sets up the sterile field. The nurse takes which action next?

1. Dons sterile gloves.
2. Assesses the integrity of the abdominal incision.
3. Dons clean gloves and removes the old dressing.
4. Cleans the wound with povidone-iodine (Betadine) solution as prescribed.

Answer: 3

Test-Taking Strategy:
Note the strategic word *next.* Form a mental image of this procedure, and visualize the steps that you would take in this procedure. You cannot clean the wound or assess the wound unless you remove the old dressing; therefore eliminate options 2 and 4. From the remaining options, recall that sterile gloves are necessary for cleaning and dressing the incision once the old dressing is removed. This will direct you to option 3. Remember that visualizing and relating the case event to a similar clinical experience can be a valuable strategy as you attempt to eliminate incorrect options!

Tip for the Beginning Nursing Student

A sterile procedure, such as a sterile dressing change, is one that involves taking measures so that no microorganisms come in contact with the wound or anything that is used to perform the procedure. There is a special technique that is used to maintain sterility when performing this procedure; you will learn this technique and how to perform sterile dressing changes during your fundamentals of nursing course.

▲ LOOKING FOR CONCEPTS IN THE QUESTION THAT ARE COMPARABLE OR ALIKE TO A CONCEPT IN ONE OF THE OPTIONS: HOW WILL THIS HELP?

Read the question carefully, noting the strategic words and the subject of the question. As you read each option, look for the option that contains comparable or alike concepts or has a relationship to those identified in the question. This strategy may help as you are eliminating the incorrect options. Following is a sample question that illustrates this strategy of looking for comparable or alike concepts.

> Look for a concept in the question that is comparable or alike to a concept in one of the options!

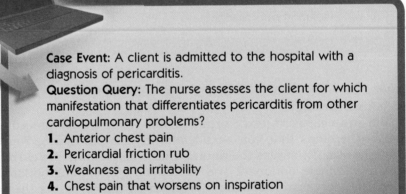

Q Sample Question: Looking for Comparable or Alike Concepts in the Question and in One of the Options

Case Event: A client is admitted to the hospital with a diagnosis of pericarditis.
Question Query: The nurse assesses the client for which manifestation that differentiates pericarditis from other cardiopulmonary problems?
1. Anterior chest pain
2. Pericardial friction rub
3. Weakness and irritability
4. Chest pain that worsens on inspiration

Answer: 2
Test-Taking Strategy:
Note the strategic word *differentiates*, and focus on the subject—a manifestation that differentiates pericarditis from other cardiopulmonary problems. This tells you that the correct option will be one that is unique to this health problem. Note the relationship between the word *pericarditis* in the question and the word *pericardial* in the correct option. Also recall that a pericardial friction rub is heard when there is inflammation of the pericardial sac, during the inflammatory phase of pericarditis. Remember to look for the option that contains a comparable or alike concept or has a relationship to the information in the question!

Tip for the Beginning Nursing Student

Pericarditis is an inflammation of the pericardium (the sac that surrounds the heart) and can be associated with trauma, infection, myocardial infarction, malignant disease, or other disorders. The client exhibits fever, substernal chest pain, difficulty breathing, a dry nonproductive cough, and a rapid pulse rate. On auscultation of the lungs and chest, a pericardial friction rub and a muffled heartbeat over the apex of the heart would be heard. You will learn about auscultation of the lungs and chest during your physical assessment course and about pericarditis during your medical-surgical nursing course when you study cardiac disorders.

WHAT STRATEGIES WILL HELP WHEN ANSWERING MEDICATION AND INTRAVENOUS CALCULATION QUESTIONS?

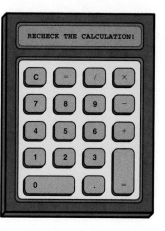

When a medication or IV calculation question is presented, always use the appropriate formula to solve the problem. Shortcuts should not be used in making these calculations. The problem and the answer should be expressed in the correct units of measure. Always be careful with decimal points. It is important to place the decimal points in the correct places, or the answer will be incorrect. When solving a medication calculation problem, always determine whether the answer is within reason and makes sense. Following are two sample questions related to medication and IV calculations. Appendix D provides commonly used units of measures and formulas for calculating medication doses and IV flow rates.

✓ NCLEX® Exam Tip

On the NCLEX exam, medication and IV calculation questions will most likely be in a multiple-choice or a fill-in-the-blank format. You will be provided with an on-screen calculator for these medication and IV problems. Even if you use the calculator to calculate dosages and flow rates, it is important to recheck the calculation before selecting an option or typing the answer. Follow the formula, place the decimal points in the correct places, and check the accuracy of the calculation. Read the question carefully, because many of these questions will ask you to round the answer to the nearest tenth position or to the nearest whole number. Also remember to place a zero before a decimal point and to avoid placing trailing zeros after the numeric value in the answer.

MEDICATION AND INTRAVENOUS CALCULATIONS

Use the on-screen calculator.
Convert the unit of measure if necessary.
Follow the formula.
Place the decimal point in the correct place.
Place a zero before a decimal point, and avoid trailing zeros.
Recheck the accuracy of the calculation.

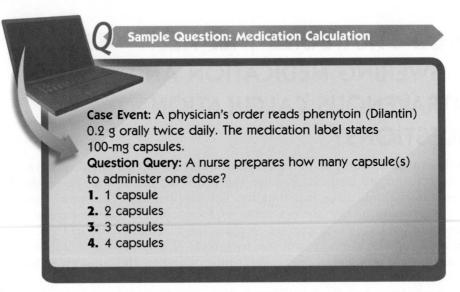

Sample Question: Medication Calculation

Case Event: A physician's order reads phenytoin (Dilantin) 0.2 g orally twice daily. The medication label states 100-mg capsules.
Question Query: A nurse prepares how many capsule(s) to administer one dose?
1. 1 capsule
2. 2 capsules
3. 3 capsules
4. 4 capsules

Answer: 2 capsules

Test-Taking Strategy:
Use the medication calculation formula. In this medication calculation problem, it is necessary to first convert grams to milligrams. In the metric system, to convert larger to smaller multiply by 1000 or move the decimal three places to the right; therefore 0.2 g = 200 mg.

Formula:

$$\frac{D\,(desired)}{A\,(available)} \times Q\,(quantity) = X$$

$$\frac{200\text{ mg}}{100\text{ mg}} \times 1\text{ tablet} = 2\text{ tablets}$$

Use the on-screen calculator to perform the calculation, and then recheck your work, making sure that the answer makes sense before selecting an option or typing the answer!

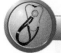

Tip for the Beginning Nursing Student

You will learn about nursing math in your fundamentals of nursing course or in another course specifically designed to teach you about nursing math. You will be using nursing math to perform calculations when you prepare medications in the clinical setting. Be sure to learn the formulas and how to perform the calculations, because the formulas are critical steps in the process of preparing a safe dose of a medication.

Q Sample Question: Intravenous Calculation

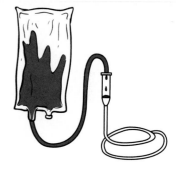

Case Event: A physician orders 1000 mL 0.45% normal saline to infuse over 8 hours. The drop factor is 15 gtt/mL. **Question Query:** The nurse sets the flow rate at how many drops per minute (gtt/min)? (Round the answer to the nearest whole number.)

Answer: 31 gtt/min

Test-Taking Strategy:

This question is in the fill-in-the-blank format. Use the formula for calculating IV flow rates when answering the question, and note that the question asks you to round the answer to the nearest whole number.

Formula:

$$\frac{\text{Total volume to infuse} \times \text{Drop (gt) factor}}{\text{Time in minutes}} = \text{Drops/minute}$$

$$\frac{1000 \times 15}{480 \, (8 \text{ hours} \times 60 \text{ minutes})} = 31.25 \text{ or } 31 \text{ gtt/min}$$

Use the on-screen calculator. Remember to follow the formula, recheck your answer, and make sure that the answer makes sense before typing it!

Tip for the Beginning Nursing Student

You will learn about calculating IV flow rates in your fundamentals of nursing course or in another course specifically designed to teach you about IV therapy. You will be using this formula for calculating an IV flow rate in the clinical setting when you care for a client receiving IV therapy. Be sure to learn this formula and how to determine the accurate flow rate, because it is critical for the safe administration of IV fluids to a client.

▲ WHAT STRATEGIES WILL HELP WHEN ANSWERING QUESTIONS RELATED TO LABORATORY VALUES?

LEARN NORMAL LABORATORY VALUES!

The questions on a nursing exam or the NCLEX exam related to laboratory values will require you to identify whether the laboratory value is normal or abnormal, and then think critically about the effects of the laboratory value in terms of the client. If you know the normal values, you will be able to determine if an abnormality exists when a laboratory value is presented in a question. Pyramid points to review are the normal values for the most common laboratory tests, therapeutic serum medication levels of commonly prescribed medications, and determination of the need to implement specific actions based on the findings. Remember that most blood specimens should not be drawn during hemodialysis or from an extremity that has an IV solution running. Table 10-1 provides the therapeutic serum medication levels of commonly prescribed medications. Appendix E lists the most commonly prescribed laboratory tests and their normal values.

When a question is presented on your exams regarding a specific laboratory value, note the disorder presented in the question and the associated body organ that is affected. This will help you determine the correct option. For example, if the question asks you about the immune status of a client receiving chemotherapy, assessment of laboratory values will focus on the white blood cell count. You will need to analyze the results as possibly being low and determine the specific client need, which in this case would be the risk for infection. In the client receiving chemotherapy who has a low white blood cell count, your plan should center on the immune system, specifically protecting that client from infection. Interventions focus on preventive interventions related to infection, perhaps even protective isolation measures, such as neutropenic precautions. Evaluation may focus on maintaining a normal temperature in the client. Following is a sample question that relates to a laboratory test.

LABORATORY VALUES

Note the disorder presented in the question!
Identify whether the laboratory value is normal or abnormal!
Identify the associated body organ that is affected as a result of the disorder!

Q Sample Question: Laboratory Values

Case Event: A client with a diagnosis of sepsis is receiving antibiotics by the IV route.
Question Query: The nurse assesses for nephrotoxicity by monitoring which laboratory value most closely?
1. Lipase level
2. Platelet count
3. Blood urea nitrogen
4. White blood cell count

Answer: 3

Test-Taking Strategy:

Note the strategic words *most closely.* Focus on the information in the question, and note that the subject is nephrotoxicity. Read each option carefully, and note that option 3 is the only option that relates to kidney function. Option 1 relates to pancreatic function. Option 2 relates to the hematological system. Option 4 relates to the immune system. Remember to note the disorder or subject presented in the question and the associated body organ that is affected as a result!

Tip for the Beginning Nursing Student

Sepsis refers to a systemic infection that can occur as a result of a localized or other type of infection in the body. This serious infection needs to be treated aggressively with antibiotics, and usually blood cultures are done to determine the antibiotic of choice. Nephrotoxicity, which refers to the destruction of kidney cells, is a complication that can occur with the use of antibiotics. To monitor for nephrotoxicity the nurse would check the results of the blood urea nitrogen and creatinine level. You will learn about antibiotics in a pharmacology course or in your medical-surgical nursing course when you study infections and immune disorders.

WHAT STRATEGIES WILL HELP WHEN ANSWERING QUESTIONS RELATED TO CLIENT POSITIONING?

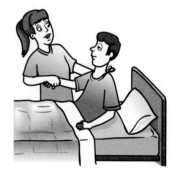

Nursing responsibility includes positioning clients in a safe and appropriate manner to provide safety and comfort. Knowledge regarding the client position required for a certain procedure or condition is expected. It is the nurse's responsibility to reduce the likelihood and prevent the development of complications related to an existing condition, prescribed treatment, or medical or surgical procedure. It is imperative that the nurse review the physician's orders after treatments or procedures and take note of instructions regarding positioning and mobility.

When you are presented with a question that relates to positioning a client, focus on the information in the question, the client's diagnosis, and the anatomical location of the client's diagnosis, and consider the pathophysiology of the disorder and the goals of care. That is, think about what complications you want to prevent. Some guidelines to remember when answering questions related to positioning are listed below and are also noted in Appendix F.

CLIENT POSITIONING

Always review the physician's orders!
Focus on the client's diagnosis!
Identify the anatomical location of the client's disorder!
Consider the pathophysiology of the disorder and the goals of care!
Think about what complications you want to prevent!

Guidelines Related to Positioning

Elevation of an affected body part reduces edema.

Clients who have had neck or head surgery are placed in semi-Fowler's or Fowler's position.

After a liver biopsy the client is placed in a right lateral (side-lying) position to provide pressure to the site and prevent bleeding.

Clients receiving irrigations or feedings through a nasogastric, gastrostomy, or jejunostomy tube are placed in semi-Fowler's or Fowler's position to prevent aspiration.

The left Sims' position is used to administer a rectal enema or irrigation to allow the solution to flow by gravity in the natural direction of the colon.

Clients with a respiratory disorder or cardiovascular disorder are placed in semi-Fowler's or Fowler's position.

Clients with peripheral arterial disease may be advised to elevate their feet and legs at rest, because swelling can prevent arterial blood flow, but they should not raise their legs above the level of the heart because extreme elevation slows arterial blood flow; some clients may be advised to maintain a slightly dependent position to promote perfusion.

Clients with peripheral venous disease are usually advised to elevate their feet and legs above heart level.

Clients with a head injury are placed in semi-Fowler's or Fowler's position.

If a client develops autonomic dysreflexia, the head of the bed is elevated.

In clients with hemorrhagic strokes the head of the bed is usually elevated to 30 degrees to reduce intracranial pressure and to facilitate venous drainage.

For clients with ischemic strokes the head of the bed is usually kept flat.

After craniotomy the client should NOT be positioned on the operated site, especially if the bone flap has been removed, because the brain has no bony covering on the affected site; semi-Fowler's to Fowler's position is maintained with the head in a midline, neutral position to facilitate venous drainage from the head, and extreme hip and neck flexion is avoided.

With increased intracranial pressure, the client is placed in semi-Fowler's to Fowler's position; the head is maintained in a midline, neutral position to facilitate venous drainage from the head, and extreme hip and neck flexion is avoided.

In a spinal cord injury the client is immobilized on a spinal backboard, with the head in a neutral position, to prevent incomplete injury from becoming complete; head flexion, rotation, or extension is avoided; and the client is logrolled.

In the client who underwent a total hip replacement, positioning will depend on the surgical techniques used, the method of implantation, the prosthesis, and the physician's preference; extreme internal and external rotation and adduction are avoided, and side-lying on the operative side is not allowed (unless specifically prescribed by the physician).

The following question relates to positioning a client.

Sample Question: Client Positioning

Case Event: A nurse assists a physician in performing a liver biopsy.
Question Query: After the biopsy the nurse plans to place the client in which of the following positions?
1. Supine
2. Prone
3. A left side-lying position with a small pillow or folded towel under the puncture site
4. A right side-lying position with a small pillow or folded towel under the puncture site

Answer: 4

Test-Taking Strategy:
Focus on the information in the question and the anatomical location of the procedure, and think about what complication you want to prevent. In this situation you want to prevent bleeding. Remember that the liver is on the right side of the body and that the application of pressure on the right side will minimize the escape of blood or bile through the puncture site, because this position compresses the liver against the chest wall at the biopsy site. Remember to focus on the information in the question, the client's diagnosis, and the anatomical location of the client's diagnosis, and consider the pathophysiology of the disorder and the goals of care!

Tip for the Beginning Nursing Student

A liver biopsy is a diagnostic procedure in which local anesthesia is administered followed by the introduction of a special needle into the liver to obtain a specimen for pathological examination. Bleeding is a concern following the procedure, and this is the reason why the client will be placed on the right side. This position provides pressure at the biopsy site by compressing the liver against the chest wall. You will learn about a liver biopsy in your medical-surgical nursing course when you study gastrointestinal disorders.

WHAT STRATEGIES WILL HELP WHEN ANSWERING QUESTIONS RELATED TO THERAPEUTIC DIETS?

On nursing examinations, you may be asked questions about diet therapy and certain food items that are allowed with certain diets. You may also be asked about a particular diet that may be prescribed for a client

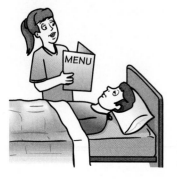

with a certain disorder. Therefore nutritional therapy and knowing the nutritional components of various food items are essential. Some strategies that you can use to help you answer these questions if you are unsure of the answer are listed below and are followed by a practice question that relates to a therapeutic diet. In addition, Appendix G lists therapeutic diets, their indications for use, and associated nursing considerations.

Strategies for Answering Questions Related to Therapeutic Diets

1. Focus on the data in the question.
2. Note the subject of the question: Is the question asking about a specific diet or a specific food item?
3. Note the diagnosis of the client, and think about the organ system that is affected.
4. Think about the pathophysiology associated with the client's disorder.
5. Look at the options that are provided, and try to relate the client's disorder to the correct option.

Q Sample Question: Therapeutic Diet

Case Event: The nurse is providing dietary instructions to an older client who is immobile and experiencing frequent episodes of constipation. The client complains that the constipation is uncomfortable.

Question Query: The nurse should tell the client that which food item would be most helpful to include in the diet?

1. Pasta
2. Cabbage
3. White bread
4. Whole-grain bread

Answer: 4

Test-Taking Strategy:
Focus on the data in the question, and note the client's diagnosis. Think about the body organ affected in this disorder and the associated pathophysiology. A client with constipation needs to include high-fiber foods in the diet. The only food item that is high in fiber is whole grains. Also note that options 1 and 3 are comparable or alike in that they are low-fiber foods. Option 2 is a gas-forming food and needs to be avoided, because it will increase any discomfort that the client may be experiencing. Remember to focus on the data in the question, note the client's diagnosis, and think about the body organ affected and the associated pathophysiology.

Tip for the Beginning Nursing Student

Constipation is a condition in which the client is having difficulty passing stool or is experiencing the incomplete or infrequent passage of hard stool. If immobility is the cause, one intervention is to include adequate amounts of fiber and fluids in the diet. You will learn about constipation in your fundamentals of nursing course when you study elimination patterns and in your medical-surgical nursing course when you study gastrointestinal disorders.

WHAT STRATEGIES WILL HELP WHEN ANSWERING QUESTIONS RELATED TO DISASTERS?

A disaster is any human-made or natural event that causes destruction and devastation and requires assistance from others. For a health care agency a disaster can be external or internal. External disasters include those that occur outside the health care agency, and internal disasters include those that occur inside the health care agency. If a disaster occurs, the agency disaster preparedness plan (emergency response plan) is immediately activated by the health care agency and the nurse responds by following the directions identified in the plan. In the community setting, if the nurse is the first responder to a disaster, the nurse cares for the victims by attending to those with life-threatening problems first; once rescue workers arrive at the scene, immediate plans for triage should begin.

TYPES OF DISASTERS

HUMAN-MADE DISASTERS

Dam failures resulting in flooding
Hazardous substance accidents, such as pollution, chemical spills, or toxic gas leaks
Accidents that result in the release of radiological materials
Resource shortages, such as food, water, and electricity
Structural collapse, fire, or explosions
Terrorist attacks, such as bombings, riots, and bioterrorism
Transportation accidents

NATURAL DISASTERS

Blizzards
Communicable disease epidemics
Cyclones
Droughts
Earthquakes
Floods
Forest fires
Hailstorms
Hurricanes
Landslides
Mudslides
Tornadoes
Tsunamis (tidal waves)
Volcanic eruptions

The NCLEX exam may contain questions about disasters and will focus on nursing interventions. A question may identify the nurse as the first responder to a disaster site and will ask you to identify the victim that the nurse would attend to first. If the question identifies a site outside the hospital environment, select the option that identifies a victim that the nurse could realistically save. Think about survivability and ask yourself, "Who can I save?" Also use prioritizing skills. Ask yourself, "Which victims sustained injuries that are not critical or life threatening and could wait to be cared for?"

An NCLEX question may also identify the nurse as the leader of a nursing unit and ask which clients in the unit could be discharged to free up beds for victims of a disaster brought to the emergency department who need to be admitted to the hospital. In this situation, read each client's description carefully and determine if the client can safely return home and if there are home care and community resources that could care for the client and meet the client's needs. These types of questions require the use of prioritizing skills.

> When triaging victims of a disaster at a disaster site, think survivability!
> Determine which victims sustained life-threatening injuries and need immediate treatment to sustain life!

Q **Sample Question: Human-Made Disaster**

Case Event: The nurse is the first responder to the site of a disaster in which several people were injured in a train accident.

Question Query: Which victim of the accident would the nurse attend to first?

1. A victim with a fractured arm
2. A victim with multiple bruises on the legs
3. A victim with a severe head injury who is not breathing
4. A victim with an upper leg injury who is bleeding profusely

Answer: 4

Test-Taking Strategy:
Focus on the data in the question, and note that the disaster site is outside the hospital environment. Therefore determine which victim has a life-threatening injury and requires immediate treatment to sustain life. Think survivability. The victims described in options 1 and 2 sustained injuries that are not critical or life threatening and could wait for care. Outside the hospital environment, resources are limited. Therefore it is

unlikely that the nurse could help the victim with a severe head injury who is not breathing. The nurse could apply pressure to the leg of the victim who is bleeding profusely and could save this victim's life.

Tip for the Beginning Nursing Student

Disaster management is an important role of the nurse. An important point to remember is that the nurse needs to use prioritizing skills to determine how best to proceed in a disaster situation. Many types of disasters can occur, but the principles of care remain the same. The immediate priority of the nurse is to attend to the victim who has immediate and life-threatening needs and who could be saved. You will learn about disaster management and the nurse's roles and responsibilities in your community nursing course.

REFERENCES

Chernecky, C., & Berger, B. (2008). *Laboratory tests and diagnostic procedures* (5th ed.). Philadelphia: Saunders.

Ignatavicius, D., & Workman, M. (2006). *Medical-surgical nursing: Critical thinking for collaborative care* (5th ed.). Philadelphia: Saunders.

Kee, J., & Marshall, S. (2009). *Clinical calculations: With applications to general and specialty areas* (6th ed.). Philadelphia: Saunders.

Linton, A., & Maebius, N. (2007). *Introduction to medical-surgical nursing* (4th ed.). Philadelphia: Saunders.

National Council of State Boards of Nursing (eds.). (2007). *2007 NCLEX-RN® Detailed Test Plan.* Chicago: Author.

National Council of State Boards of Nursing (eds.). (2008). *2008 Detailed Test Plan for the NCLEX-PN® Examination.* Chicago: Author.

Potter, P., & Perry, A. (2009). *Fundamentals of nursing* (7th ed.). St. Louis: Mosby.

Schlenker, E., & Long, S. (2007). *Williams' essentials of nutrition & diet therapy* (9th ed.). St. Louis: Mosby.

Silvestri, L. (2010). *Saunders comprehensive review for the NCLEX-PN® examination* (4th ed.). St. Louis: Saunders.

Silvestri, L. (2008). *Saunders comprehensive review for the NCLEX-RN® examination* (4th ed.). St. Louis: Saunders.

Wong, D., Perry, S., Hockenberry, M., Lowdermilk, D., & Wilson, D. (2006). *Maternal-child nursing care* (3rd ed.). St. Louis: Mosby.

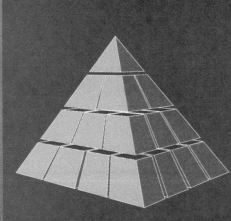

Part III

Practice Test

Fundamental Skills Questions

Chapter 12

1. A nurse develops a plan of care for a newly hospitalized client who reports difficulty sleeping. The nurse plans to implement which best intervention?
   1 Offer the client a sleeping pill at night.
   2 Provide the client with a snack at bedtime.
   3 Ask the client what the client does to prepare for sleep.
   4 Leave the television on in the client's room at a very low volume.

Level of Cognitive Ability: Application
Client Needs: Physiological Integrity
Integrated Process: Nursing Process/ Assessment/Data Collection
Content Area: Fundamental Skills

Answer: 3
Rationale: The best intervention is to ask the client what the client does to prepare for sleep. The nurse needs to assess habits that are beneficial to the client compared with those that disturb sleep. Options 1, 2, and 4 provide interventions without assessing what measures would be helpful to the client.

Test-Taking Strategy: Note the strategic word *best*, and use the steps of the nursing process. The only option that addresses assessment/data collection is option 3. Review care of the client who has difficulty sleeping if you had difficulty with this question.

Tip for the Beginning Nursing Student: You will learn about sleep patterns and measures to promote sleep in your fundamentals of nursing course. An important point to remember is that you always want to determine what measures the client takes at home to sleep and incorporate these measures in the plan of care during hospitalization.

References
Christensen, B., & Kockrow, E. (2006). *Foundations of nursing* (5th ed., pp. 417-418). St. Louis: Mosby.
Potter, P., & Perry, A. (2009). *Fundamentals of nursing* (7th ed., pp. 1039-1040). St. Louis: Mosby.

2. A nurse notes documentation in a client's medical record that the client is experiencing anuria. Based on this notation, the nurse determines that the client:

Answer: 1
Rationale: Anuria is the term used to describe an inability to produce urine. Oliguria is a diminished capacity to form urine and is most likely the result of a decrease in renal perfusion. Options 3 and 4 do not relate to urinary tract dysfunction.

1 Is unable to produce urine
2 Has a diminished capacity to form urine
3 Has difficulty having a bowel movement
4 Has episodes of alternating constipation and diarrhea

Level of Cognitive Ability:
    Comprehension
Client Needs: Physiological Integrity
Integrated Process: Nursing Process/Assessment/Data Collection
Content Area: Fundamental Skills

Test-Taking Strategy: Note the word *anuria,* and use medical terminology skills to answer the question. Recalling that the prefix *an-* refers to absence and the suffix *-uria* refers to urine will direct you to option 1. Review the description of anuria and the various test-taking strategies if you had difficulty with this question.

Tip for the Beginning Nursing Student: You will learn about the terminology used to describe conditions related to the renal system in your fundamentals of nursing course and your medical-surgical nursing course when you study renal disorders. It is important to remember that the client should maintain a urinary output of at least 30 mL/hour and the nurse should monitor for this occurrence. A decline in urine output could indicate kidney dysfunction or failure, hypovolemia, or an obstruction in the renal system. This occurrence needs to be reported.

References
deWit, S. (2009). *Medical-surgical nursing: Concepts & practice* (p. 825). St. Louis: Saunders.
Ignatavicius, D., & Workman, M. (2010). *Medical-surgical nursing: Patient-centered collaborative care* (6th ed., p. 1535). Philadelphia: Saunders.

---

3. A nurse is caring for a client who has a fever and is diaphoretic. The nurse monitors the client's intake and output and expects that:
    1 The client's urine will be dilute.
    2 The client's output will be decreased.
    3 The client's urine production will be increased.
    4 The majority of the client's fluid will be excreted through the skin.

Level of Cognitive Ability:
    Comprehension
Client Needs: Physiological Integrity
Integrated Process: Nursing Process/Assessment/Data Collection
Content Area: Fundamental Skills

Answer: 2
Rationale: Febrile conditions affect urine production. The client who is diaphoretic loses fluids through insensible water loss, which decreases urine production. However, the increased body temperature associated with fever increases accumulation of body wastes. Although urine volume may be reduced, it is highly concentrated. Options 1, 3, and 4 are incorrect.

Test-Taking Strategy: Noting that the client has a fever and is diaphoretic will direct you to option 2 because this client will also be losing some (not the majority) fluid through the skin. Review the conditions that affect fluid balance and the various test-taking strategies if you had difficulty with this question.

Tip for the Beginning Nursing Student: You will learn about fluid balance and monitoring intake and output in your fundamentals of nursing course. An important point to remember is that fluid can be lost through the skin, the lungs during breathing, the kidneys, and the gastrointestinal tract. Normally most fluid is lost through the kidneys, but if the client has a fever and is diaphoretic (sweating), more than the normal amount is lost through the skin and less than the normal amount is lost through the kidneys.

Reference
Potter, P., & Perry, A. (2009). *Fundamentals of nursing* (7th ed., p. 505). St. Louis: Mosby.

4. A nurse provides instructions to a female client regarding the procedure for collecting a midstream urine sample. The nurse tells the client to do which of the following?
   1 Douche before collecting the specimen.
   2 Cleanse the perineum from front to back.
   3 Collect the urine in the cup as soon as the urine flow begins.
   4 Collect the specimen before bedtime, and bring it to the laboratory the next morning.

Level of Cognitive Ability: Application
Client Needs: Safe and Effective Care Environment
Integrated Process: Teaching and Learning
Content Area: Fundamental Skills

Answer: 2

Rationale: As part of correct procedure, the client should cleanse the perineum from front to back with the antiseptic swabs that are packaged with the specimen kit. The client should begin the flow of urine, collecting the sample after starting the flow of urine. The specimen should be sent to the laboratory as soon as possible and not allowed to stand. Improper specimen handling can yield inaccurate test results. It is not normal procedure to douche before collecting the specimen.

Test-Taking Strategy: Noting the name of the type of sample—*midstream*—will assist in eliminating option 3. Recalling that the specimen should be sent or brought to the laboratory immediately after collection will assist in eliminating option 4. From the remaining options, use basic principles related to hygiene to assist in directing you to option 2. Review the procedure for collecting a midstream urine sample and the various test-taking strategies if you had difficulty with this question.

Tip for the Beginning Nursing Student: You will learn about basic hygiene principles, asepsis, and collecting urine specimens in your fundamentals of nursing course. An important client teaching point to remember is that the female client is taught to always wipe or cleanse the perineum from front to back to prevent the spread of microorganisms from the rectal area to the labial area, which could result in a urinary tract infection.

References
Christensen, B., & Kockrow, E. (2006). *Foundations of nursing* (5th ed., pp. 502-503). St. Louis: Mosby.
Ignatavicius, D., & Workman, M. (2010). *Medical-surgical nursing: Patient-centered collaborative care* (6th ed., p. 1540). Philadelphia: Saunders.

5. A nurse provides dietary instructions to a client diagnosed with iron deficiency anemia. The nurse tells the client to increase the intake of which of the following foods?
   1 Plums
   2 Red apples
   3 Egg whites
   4 Kidney beans

Level of Cognitive Ability: Application
Client Needs: Physiological Integrity
Integrated Process: Teaching and Learning
Content Area: Fundamental Skills

Answer: 4

Rationale: The client with iron deficiency anemia should increase intake of foods that are naturally high in iron, including kidney beans, soybeans, chickpeas, lima beans, cooked Swiss chard, red meat, liver and other organ meats, blackstrap molasses, lentils, egg yolk, spinach, kale, turnip tops, beet greens, carrots, raisins, and apricots. The food items in options 1, 2, and 3 are not high in iron.

Test-Taking Strategy: Focus on the subject—a food high in iron. Eliminate options 1 and 2 first because they are comparable or alike and are fruit items. From the remaining options recall either that beans are high in iron or that egg yolk (not egg white) is high in iron. This will direct you to option 4. Review foods high in iron and the various test-taking strategies if you had difficulty with this question.

Tip for the Beginning Nursing Student: Iron deficiency anemia is a condition in which the client lacks sufficient red blood cells. One cause is an insufficient intake of dietary iron. You will learn about anemia in your fundamentals of nursing course and in your medical-surgical nursing course when you study hematological disorders. You will also learn about the foods high in iron when you study nutrition. These food items are important to know because you will be teaching your client about a high-iron diet.

References
deWit, S. (2009). *Medical-surgical nursing: Concepts & practice* (p. 385). St. Louis: Saunders.

Ignatavicius, D., & Workman, M. (2010). *Medical-surgical nursing: Patient-centered collaborative care* (6th ed., p. 899). Philadelphia: Saunders.

Schlenker, E. & Long, S. (2007). *Williams' essentials of nutrition & diet therapy* (9th ed., pp. 166, 169). St. Louis: Mosby.

---

6. A client asks a nurse about the use of a complementary or alternative measure that will assist in promoting sleep. The nurse suggests which of the following?
1 Herbal therapy
2 Acupuncture sessions
3 Muscle relaxation techniques
4 Traditional Chinese medicine sessions

Level of Cognitive Ability: Application
Client Needs: Physiological Integrity
Integrated Process: Nursing Process/ Implementation
Content Area: Fundamental Skills

Answer: 3
Rationale: A simple relaxation technique, such as muscle relaxation, can help reduce any existing anxiety and promote sleep. Acupuncture is an invasive procedure that stimulates certain points on the body by the insertion of special needles to modify the perception of pain, normalize physiological functions, or treat or prevent disease. Traditional Chinese medicine focuses on restoring and maintaining a balanced flow of vital energy; interventions include acupressure, acupuncture, herbal therapies, diet, meditation, and tai chi and qi gong (exercise that focuses on breathing, visualization, and movement). Herbal therapy involves the use of herbs (plant or a plant part). Some herbs have been determined to be safe, but other herbs, even in small amounts, can be toxic and the nurse would not recommend their use to a client. The client who is taking prescription medications should consult the health care provider regarding the use of herbs because serious herb-medication interactions can occur.

Test-Taking Strategy: Note the relationship between the words *promoting sleep* and option 3. Also note that options 1, 2, and 4 are comparable or alike in that they include invasive measures. Review complementary and alternative therapies that will assist in promoting sleep and the various test-taking strategies if you had difficulty with this question.

Tip for the Beginning Nursing Student: Complementary and alternative therapies include nontraditional and non-Western medical forms of treatment and may be prescribed to supplement existing medical therapies. They must be prescribed by the health care provider. You will learn about complementary and alternative therapies in your fundamentals of nursing course and your pharmacology course. An important point to remember is that the nurse would not recommend the use of these treatments, especially invasive ones, without first consulting the health care provider. Some of these therapies can harm the client.

References
Christensen, B., & Kockrow, E. (2006). *Foundations of nursing* (5th ed., pp. 432-433). St. Louis: Mosby.
Potter, P., & Perry, A. (2009) *Fundamentals of nursing* (7th ed., pp. 775-776). St. Louis: Mosby.

---

7. A nurse instructs a client taking a potassium-sparing diuretic about foods high in potassium. The nurse determines that the client needs further instruction if the client states that which food is high in potassium?
  1 Kiwi
  2 Celery
  3 Oranges
  4 Dried fruit

Level of Cognitive Ability:
  Comprehension
Client Needs: Physiological Integrity
Integrated Process: Teaching and Learning
Content Area: Fundamental Skills

Answer: 2
Rationale: Meats, some dairy products, dried fruits, bananas, cantaloupe, kiwi, and oranges are high in potassium. Vegetables that are high in potassium include avocados, broccoli, dried beans or peas, lima beans, mushrooms, potatoes, seaweed, soybeans, and spinach. Celery is a vegetable that is low in potassium.

Test-Taking Strategy: Note the strategic words *needs further instruction.* These words indicate a negative event query and indicate that you need to select the option that is an incorrect client response. Eliminate options 1, 3, and 4 because they are comparable or alike and are fruit items. Review the foods that are high and low in potassium content and the various test-taking strategies if you had difficulty with this question.

Tip for the Beginning Nursing Student: A diuretic is a medication that promotes the formation and excretion of urine and leads to an increase in urine output. These medications are used for clients with excess body fluid, such as those with hypertension or heart failure. Many diuretics cause the loss of potassium in the urine. A potassium-sparing diuretic does not, and the client tends to retain potassium rather than lose it. The client is taught about diet and the foods that are high and low in potassium. Both a low potassium level and a high potassium level can cause serious problems for the client; therefore potassium imbalances are important to learn. You will learn about potassium imbalances and nutrition in your fundamentals of nursing course, and you will learn about diuretics in your pharmacology course.

References
deWit, S. (2009). *Medical-surgical nursing: Concepts & practice* (p. 48). St. Louis: Saunders.
Ignatavicius, D., & Workman, M. (2010). *Medical-surgical nursing: Patient-centered collaborative care* (6th ed., p. 187). Philadelphia: Saunders.
Schlenker, E., & Long, S. (2007). *Williams' essentials of nutrition & diet therapy* (9th ed., p. 159). St. Louis: Mosby.

---

8. A clear liquid diet has been prescribed for a client. The nurse offers which item to the client?
  1 Apple juice
  2 Orange juice
  3 Tomato juice
  4 Ice cream without nuts

Answer: 1
Rationale: A clear liquid diet consists of foods that are relatively transparent. The food items in options 2, 3, and 4 would be included in a full liquid diet.

Test-Taking Strategy: Eliminate options 2, 3, and 4 because they are comparable or alike and are items allowed

Level of Cognitive Ability: Application
Client Needs: Physiological Integrity
Integrated Process: Nursing Process/
   Implementation
Content Area: Fundamental Skills

on a full liquid diet. Remember that a clear liquid diet consists of foods that are relatively transparent. Option 1 is the only food item that is transparent. Review food items allowed on a clear liquid diet and full liquid diet and the various test-taking strategies if you had difficulty with this question.

Tip for the Beginning Nursing Student: A clear liquid diet may be prescribed to provide fluids to treat or prevent dehydration, to provide complete bowel rest, to feed a malnourished person or a person who has not had any oral intake for some time, in preparation for surgery or tests, or as a postsurgical diet. A clear liquid diet consists of foods that are relatively transparent. You will learn about this type of diet and other diets in your fundamentals of nursing course.

References

Christensen, B., & Kockrow, E. (2006). *Foundations of nursing* (5th ed., pp. 635-636). St. Louis: Mosby.

Grodner, M., Long, S., & Walkinshaw, B. (2007). *Foundations and clinical applications of nutrition: A nursing approach* (4th ed., pp. 322-323). St. Louis: Mosby.

---

9. Oxygen by nasal cannula at 4 L/ minute is prescribed for a hospitalized client. The nurse avoids which action in the care of the client?
   1 Humidifies the oxygen
   2 Applies water-soluble lubricant to the nares
   3 Instructs the client to breath through the nose only
   4 Instructs the client and family about the purpose of the oxygen

Level of Cognitive Ability: Application
Client Needs: Physiological Integrity
Integrated Process: Nursing Process/
   Implementation
Content Area: Fundamental Skills

Answer: 3
Rationale: The nasal cannula provides for lower concentrations of oxygen and can even be used with mouth breathers because movement of air through the oropharynx pulls oxygen from the nasopharynx. It is not necessary to instruct a client to breathe only through the nose. Options 1, 2, and 4 are correct interventions.

Test-Taking Strategy: Note the strategic word *avoids*. This is a negative event query and indicates that you need to look for the incorrect nursing action. Noting that option 3 contains the close-ended word *only* will direct you to this option. Review care of the client receiving oxygen and the various test-taking strategies if you had difficulty with this question.

Tip for the Beginning Nursing Student: Oxygen therapy is a treatment measure that needs to be prescribed by the physician and is used when a client is not able to take in sufficient oxygen on his or her own to adequately provide nutrients to the cells of the body. You will learn about oxygen therapy in your fundamentals of nursing course and in your medical-surgical nursing course when you study respiratory disorders.

References

Christensen, B., & Kockrow, E. (2010). *Foundations of nursing* (5th ed., pp. 560-561). St. Louis: Mosby.

Ignatavicius, D., & Workman, M. (2006). *Medical-surgical nursing: Critical thinking for collaborative care* (6th ed., p. 574). Philadelphia: Saunders.

10. A nurse is caring for a client who is dying. The nurse develops the plan of care understanding that which intervention would be inappropriate in the care of the client?
    1 Offer to contact the clergy to support the client's spiritual needs.
    2 Make referrals to other disciplines based on the client's stated needs.
    3 Plan to balance the client's need for assistance with that for independence.
    4 Provide extremely thorough answers to each question asked by the client or family.

Level of Cognitive Ability:
Comprehension
Client Needs: Psychosocial Integrity
Integrated Process: Caring
Content Area: Fundamental Skills

Answer: 4

Rationale: In planning care for the dying client, the nurse provides information and answers questions to the extent most helpful to the client and family. The nurse makes referrals to other disciplines and clergy based on an identified need and tries to balance the client's need for assistance with the need to maintain some measure of independence. Also it is very helpful to spend time with the client.

Test-Taking Strategy: Note the strategic word *inappropriate.* This indicates a negative event query and that you need to select the option that is an incorrect intervention. Eliminate options 1 and 2 first because they are comparable or alike. From the remaining options, note the exaggerated detail of response implied in option 4, which makes it inappropriate. Review the psychosocial needs of the dying client and the various test-taking strategies if you had difficulty with this question.

Tip for the Beginning Nursing Student: The client who is dying has many physical and psychosocial needs, and you will learn about these needs and how to care for the dying client in your fundamentals of nursing course. Another point to remember is that the client's family may also need some supportive care. Simply letting the family know that you are there to assist them if they should need anything can be quite supportive. Use therapeutic communication techniques to focus on the client's and family's feelings. You will learn about these techniques in your fundamentals of nursing course.

References
deWit, S. (2009). *Medical-surgical nursing: Concepts & practice* (pp. 186-187). St. Louis: Saunders.

Ignatavicius, D., & Workman, M. (2006). *Medical-surgical nursing: Patient-centered collaborative care* (6th ed., pp. 115-116). Philadelphia: Saunders.

11. A nurse is calculating the client's fluid intake during a 12-hour period. The client consumed 4 oz of juice, 8 oz of coffee, and 6 oz of milk at breakfast. At lunchtime the client consumed 8 oz of iced tea and 6 oz of water. At dinnertime the client consumed 8 oz of coffee and 6 oz of lemonade. The client also consumed 4 oz of water at 10:00 AM, at 2:00 PM, and again at 6:00 PM when he received his oral medications. At 8:00 AM and 2:00 PM the client received an intravenous

Answer: 1840

Rationale: There are 30 mL in 1 oz. The client consumed 4 oz of juice, 8 oz of coffee, and 6 oz of milk at breakfast. This totals 18 oz and equals 540 mL. At lunchtime the client consumed 8 oz of iced tea and 6 oz of water. This totals 14 oz and equals 420 mL. At dinnertime the client consumed 8 oz of coffee and 6 oz of lemonade. This totals 14 oz and equals 420 mL. The client also consumed 4 oz of water at 10:00 AM, at 2:00 PM, and again at 6:00 PM when he received his oral medications. This totals 12 oz and equals 360 mL. At 8:00 AM and 2:00 PM the client received an intravenous antibiotic diluted in 50 mL of normal saline. This totals 100 mL. Therefore 540 mL, 420 mL, 420 mL, 360 mL, and 100 mL equal 1840 mL.

antibiotic diluted in 50 mL of normal saline. The nurse determines that the client's total intake in milliliters is:

Answer: _____mL

Level of Cognitive Ability: Application
Client Needs: Physiological Integrity
Integrated Process: Nursing Process/ Assessment/Data Collection
Content Area: Fundamental Skills

Test-Taking Strategy: Note that the question requires you to convert ounces to milliliters. Remember that there are 30 mL in 1 oz. Read the question carefully, note the amount of oral intake in ounces, and then convert the total to milliliters. Use a calculator to assist in answering the question. Also remember to add the amount of intravenous intake. Review the procedure for calculating fluid intake and the various test-taking strategies if you had difficulty with this question.

Tip for the Beginning Nursing Student: Calculating intake and output will be a nursing measure that you will be implementing for many of your clients. It involves knowing how many milliliters are contained in various eating and drinking utensils and knowing that there are 30 mL in 1 oz. If you can remember this conversion and learn about the amount of milliliters in various eating and drinking utensils, then simple addition will be all that is necessary to determine intake and output. You will learn about calculating intake and output in your fundamentals of nursing course.

References

deWit, S. (2009). *Medical-surgical nursing: Concepts & practice* (p. 867). St. Louis: Saunders.

Perry, A., & Potter, P. (2010). *Clinical nursing skills & techniques* (7th ed., p. 514-515). St. Louis: Mosby.

---

12. A nurse is teaching a client about a low-fat diet. The nurse tells the client to avoid which food item?
    1 Watermelon
    2 Tomato soup
    3 Low-fat yogurt
    4 Cream of mushroom soup

Level of Cognitive Ability: Application
Client Needs: Physiological Integrity
Integrated Process: Teaching and Learning
Content Area: Fundamental Skills

Answer: 4

Rationale: One cup of cream of mushroom soup contains 14 g of fat, whereas tomato soup contains 2 g. Low-fat yogurt contains 2 g of fat. Fresh fruits and vegetables are low in fat.

Test-Taking Strategy: Note the strategic word *avoid.* Eliminate option 1 first because it is a fruit and option 3 because of the words *low-fat.* From the remaining options, noting the word *cream* in option 4 will direct you to this option. Review the foods high in fat and the various test-taking strategies if you had difficulty with this question.

Tip for the Beginning Nursing Student: You will learn about nutrition and the various types of diets in your fundamentals of nursing course. Remember that most fruits and vegetables are low in fat. Also some protein foods such as chicken and turkey are low in fat, whereas red meats tend to contain higher fat contents.

References

Christensen, B., & Kockrow, E. (2006). *Foundations of nursing* (5th ed., p. 648). St. Louis: Mosby.

Grodner, M., Long, S., & Walkinshaw, B. (2007). *Foundations and clinical applications of nutrition: A nursing approach* (4th ed., pp. 96-97). St. Louis: Mosby.

13. An antibiotic is diluted in 100 mL normal saline (NS) and is to be administered piggyback over 30 minutes. The drop factor is 10 drops(gtt)/mL. A nurse sets the flow rate at how many drops per minute? (Round to the nearest whole number.)

Answer: _____ gtt/minute

Level of Cognitive Ability: Application
Client Needs: Physiological Integrity
Integrated Process: Nursing Process/ Implementation
Content Area: Fundamental Skills

Answer: 33

Rationale: Use the intravenous (IV) flow rate formula:

$$\frac{\text{Total volume} \times \text{drop factor}}{\text{Time in minutes}} = \text{Drops/minute}$$

$$\frac{100 \text{ mL} \times 10 \text{ gtt}}{30 \text{ minutes}} = \frac{1000}{30} = 33.3, \text{ or } 33 \text{ gtt/minute}$$

Test-Taking Strategy: Use the formula for calculating IV flow rates. Use a calculator, follow the formula, recheck your answer, and make sure that the answer makes sense before documenting the answer. Remember to round the answer to the nearest whole number. Review the IV calculation formula and test-taking strategies for answering IV calculation questions if you had difficulty with this question.

Tip for the Beginning Nursing Student: You will learn about calculating IV flow rates in your fundamentals of nursing course or in another course specifically designed to teach you about IV therapy. You will be using this formula for calculating an IV flow rate in the clinical setting when you care for a client receiving IV therapy. Be sure to learn this formula and how to determine the accurate flow rate because it is critical for the safe administration of IV fluids to a client.

Reference
Potter, P., & Perry, A. (2009). *Fundamentals of nursing* (7th ed., pp. 1007-1008). St. Louis: Mosby.

---

14. A nurse is preparing to assist in performing a venipuncture to initiate continuous intravenous (IV) therapy with 0.9% normal saline solution. The nurse gathers the needed supplies and plans to assist with which of the following before performing the venipuncture?

1 Applying a tourniquet below the chosen venipuncture site
2 Placing an armboard at the joint located above the venipuncture site
3 Placing cool compresses over the vein to be used for the venipuncture
4 Inspecting the 0.9% normal saline solution for particles or contamination

Level of Cognitive Ability: Application
Client Needs: Physiological Integrity

Answer: 4

Rationale: All IV solutions should be free of particles or precipitates. A tourniquet is applied above the chosen venipuncture site, not below. Cool compresses cause vasoconstriction, making the vein less visible. Armboards are applied only if necessary and after the IV line is started.

Test-Taking Strategy: Visualizing the procedure for preparing to initiate an IV infusion will help eliminate options 1 and 2. From the remaining options, use principles related to heat and cold to eliminate option 3. Review the procedure for performing a venipuncture and the various test-taking strategies if you had difficulty with this question.

Tip for the Beginning Nursing Student: A venipuncture is the insertion of a special needle or cannula into a client's vein to provide access for administering fluids and medications. You will learn about the procedure for performing a venipuncture during your nursing education. One extremely important point to remember when you are preparing to infuse or administer any solution by the IV route is that you need to inspect the solution for particles or

Integrated Process: Nursing Process/
Implementation
Content Area: Fundamental Skills

precipitates. If these are noted then you would not use the solution for administration and would contact the pharmacy and return the solution to the department.

References
Linton, A. (2007). *Introduction to medical-surgical nursing* (4th ed., p. 281). Philadelphia: Saunders.
Potter, P., & Perry, A. (2009). *Fundamentals of nursing* (7th ed., p. 1445). St. Louis: Mosby.

---

15. A physician has prescribed vitamin K (AquaMEPHYTON) 1.5 mg intramuscularly. The nurse reads the label on the medication vial and administers how many milliliters to the client?

```
NDC 0006-7780
1 mL INJECTION
AquaMEPHYTON®
(PHYTONADIONE)
10 mg per mL
Dist. by:
MERCK & CO.,INC.
West Point, PA 19486, USA
7442309
Lot      Exp.
```

Fig. 12-1 From Kee, J., & Marshall, S. (2009). *Clinical calculations: With applications to general and specialty areas* (6th ed.). Philadelphia: Saunders.

Answer: _____mL

Level of Cognitive Ability: Application
Client Needs: Physiological Integrity
Integrated Process: Nursing Process/
Implementation
Content Area: Fundamental Skills

Answer: 0.15
Rationale: Use the following formula for calculating medication doses.

$$\frac{\text{Desired}}{\text{Available}} \times mL = mL \text{ per dose}$$

$$\frac{1.5 \text{ mg}}{10 \text{ mg}} \times 1 \text{ mL} = 0.15 \text{ mL}$$

Test-Taking Strategy: Follow the formula for the calculation of the correct dose. It is not necessary to perform a conversion with this problem. Label the formula including the answer. Remember to use a calculator, follow the formula, recheck your answer, and make sure that the answer makes sense before documenting the answer. Review the test-taking strategies for answering medication calculation questions and the various test-taking strategies if you had difficulty with this question.

Tip for the Beginning Nursing Student: You will learn about nursing math in your fundamentals of nursing course or in another course specifically designed to teach you about nursing math. You will use nursing math to perform calculations when you prepare medications in the clinical setting. Be sure to learn the formulas and how to perform the calculations because the formulas are critical steps in preparing a safe dose of a medication.

References
Kee, J., & Marshall, S. (2009). *Clinical calculations: With applications to general and specialty areas* (6th ed., pp. 86, 375). Philadelphia: Saunders.
Potter, P., & Perry, A. (2009). *Fundamentals of nursing* (7th ed., pp. 696-699). St. Louis: Mosby.

---

16. A nurse receives a telephone call from the hospital admission office and is told that a client with human immunodeficiency virus (HIV) will be admitted to the nursing unit. In planning infection control measures for the client, the nurse prepares to institute:

1 Droplet precautions

Answer: 3
Rationale: HIV is a retrovirus that causes acquired immunodeficiency syndrome (AIDS). The HIV virus is transmitted through anal or oral sexual contact with infected semen or vaginal secretions, through contact with infected blood or blood products, by transmission of the virus from mother to fetus during childbirth, through breast feeding, or from other infected body fluids. Standard precautions, which include blood and body fluid precautions, will prevent contact with infectious matter and protect a health care

2 Contact precautions
3 Standard precautions
4 Airborne precautions

Level of Cognitive Ability: Application
Client Needs: Safe and Effective Care Environment
Integrated Process: Nursing Process/ Planning
Content Area: Fundamental Skills

provider from contracting the virus when providing care. Droplet, contact, and airborne precautions are more specific types of precautions and are known as transmission-based precautions. Droplet precautions require the use of a mask and are used when organisms can be spread by respiratory droplets but are unable to remain in the air farther than 3 feet (e.g., influenza). Contact precautions are used when caring for clients who have an infection that can be spread by direct or indirect contact (e.g., draining wounds). Airborne precautions require the use of a special particulate filter mask. These precautions are used to prevent infection when infectious organisms remain in the air for prolonged periods of time and can be transported in the air for distances greater than 3 feet (e.g., tuberculosis). No data in the question indicate that these types of precautions alone are necessary.

Test-Taking Strategy: Read each option carefully. Note that option 3 is the umbrella option. Review the methods of transmission of HIV, isolation techniques, and the various test-taking strategies if you had difficulty with this question.

Tip for the Beginning Nursing Student: Standard precautions are actions developed by the Centers for Disease Control and Prevention (CDC) that include hand hygiene and the use of other barrier precautions designed to reduce the transmission of infectious organisms. These actions are used for the care of every client regardless of whether an infection is present. Standard precautions are specific to the task and include the use of gloves, water-impermeable gowns, masks, and eye protection. You will learn about these types of precautions in your fundamentals of nursing course.

References
deWit, S. (2009). *Medical-surgical nursing: Concepts & practice* (p. 120). St. Louis: Saunders.
Harkreader, H., Hogan, M.A., & Thobaben, M. (2007). *Fundamentals of nursing: Caring and clinical judgment* (3rd ed., pp. 514-515). Philadelphia: Saunders.

---

17. A client with heart disease says to the nurse, "I guess I'll never be able to eat ice cream again." The nurse appropriately responds by stating:
1 "Why do you say that?"
2 "There are lots of other foods you can eat."
3 "You do not think you will be able to eat ice cream at all?"
4 "Ice cream has too much fat content, so why would you even want to eat it?"

Answer: 3
Rationale: The nurse most appropriately responds by rephrasing the client's statement. Option 3 is a therapeutic response and rephrases the client's statement. Options 1, 2, and 4 are examples of nontherapeutic communication techniques. Option 1 requests an explanation from the client. Options 2 and 4 give advice. In addition, option 4 lectures the client.

Test-Taking Strategy: Use therapeutic communication techniques. Option 3 is the only therapeutic response and rephrases the client's statement. Review therapeutic communication techniques and the test-taking strategies for answering communication questions if you had difficulty with this question.

Level of Cognitive Ability: Application
Client Needs: Psychosocial Integrity
Integrated Process: Communication
and Documentation
Content Area: Fundamental Skills

Tip for the Beginning Nursing Student: Therapeutic communication techniques promote and encourage the client to communicate and share his or her feelings with the nurse. Nontherapeutic communication techniques block the communication process and are not methods that the nurse would use when caring for a client. You will learn about therapeutic and nontherapeutic communication techniques in your fundamentals of nursing course.

References
Christensen, B., & Kockrow, E. (2006). *Adult health nursing* (5th ed., pp. 363-364). St. Louis: Mosby.
deWit, S. (2009). *Medical-surgical nursing: Concepts & practice* (p. 9). St. Louis: Saunders.
Lewis, S., Heitkemper, M., Dirksen, S., & Bucher, L. (2007). *Medical-surgical nursing: Assessment and management of clinical problems* (7th ed., p. 791). St. Louis: Mosby.

---

18. A client scheduled for an operative procedure states to the nurse, "I am not sure if I should have this surgery." Which of the following responses by the nurse is appropriate?
1 "It is your decision."
2 "Do not worry. Everything will be fine."
3 "Why do you not want to have this surgery?"
4 "Tell me what concerns you have about the surgery."

Level of Cognitive Ability: Application
Client Needs: Psychosocial Integrity
Integrated Process: Communication
and Documentation
Content Area: Fundamental Skills

Answer: 4
Rationale: The nurse needs to gather more data and assist the client in exploring his or her feelings about the surgery. Options 1, 2, and 3 are nontherapeutic. Option 1 is a blunt response and does not address the client's concern. Option 2 provides false reassurance. Option 3 can make the client feel defensive.

Test-Taking Strategy: Use therapeutic communication techniques. Option 4 is the only option that addresses the client's concern. Review therapeutic communication techniques and the test-taking strategies for answering communication questions if you had difficulty with this question.

Tip for the Beginning Nursing Student: Regardless of the type of surgery that the client is having, the nurse needs to address any concerns that the client may have. Always focus on the client's feelings and concerns. The nurse would use therapeutic communication techniques to promote and encourage the client to communicate and share his or her feelings with the nurse. Nontherapeutic communication techniques block the communication process and are not methods that the nurse would use when caring for a client. You will learn about therapeutic and nontherapeutic communication techniques in your fundamentals of nursing course.

References
Christensen, B., & Kockrow, E. (2006). *Adult health nursing* (5th ed., pp. 348-349). St. Louis: Mosby.
deWit, S. (2009). *Medical-surgical nursing: Concepts & practice* (p. 9). St. Louis: Saunders.
Ignatavicius, D., & Workman, M. (2010). *Medical-surgical nursing: Patient-centered collaborative care* (6th ed., pp. 259-260). Philadelphia: Saunders.

19. A 15-year-old female seeks treatment for a sexually transmitted infection at a local clinic. With regard to informed consent, the nurse does which of the following?
1 Asks the client to sign the informed consent form
2 Tells the client that a court order for treatment is needed
3 Tells the client that parental consent for treatment is needed
4 Calls the client's mother to obtain telephone consent for treatment

Level of Cognitive Ability: Application
Client Needs: Safe and Effective Care Environment
Integrated Process: Nursing Process/ Implementation
Content Area: Fundamental Skills

Answer: 1

Rationale: Parents normally must give informed consent for treatment of a minor. Some exceptions to this include the need for emergency treatment; when the consent of the minor is sufficient, such as for treatment of a sexually transmitted infection; or when a court order or other legal authorization has been made. Therefore options 2, 3, and 4 are incorrect.

Test-Taking Strategy: Note the strategic words *15-year-old female* and *sexually transmitted infection.* Eliminate options 2, 3, and 4 because they are comparable or alike and indicate the need for informed consent from someone other than the client. Review the laws regarding consent for treatment of minors and the various test-taking strategies if you had difficulty with this question.

Tip for the Beginning Nursing Student: Informed consent involves obtaining permission from the client to perform a treatment or procedure. The many types of informed consent include those needed to administer anesthesia, perform surgery, or administer blood; it is the physician's responsibility to explain the treatment or procedure to the client. The issues surrounding informed consent in the health care environment are extremely important ones, and you need to be sure that you understand these issues. You will learn about obtaining informed consent in your fundamentals of nursing course.

References

Christensen, B., & Kockrow, E. (2006). *Foundations of nursing* (5th ed., p. 25). St. Louis: Mosby.
Potter, P., & Perry, A. (2009). *Fundamentals of nursing* (7th ed., p. 333). St. Louis: Mosby.

20. A client will be receiving long-term, continuous parenteral nutrition (PN) at home. The nurse formulates which priority nursing diagnosis for the client?
1 *Hopelessness*
2 *Social isolation*
3 *Ineffective coping*
4 *Risk for situational low self-esteem*

Level of Cognitive Ability: Analysis
Client Needs: Psychosocial Integrity
Integrated Process: Nursing Process/ Planning
Content Area: Fundamental Skills

Answer: 2

Rationale: The client will be receiving long-term, continuous PN at home. Therefore the client will be socially isolated from stimuli outside the home. No data in the question support options 1, 3, or 4.

Test-Taking Strategy: Focus on the data provided in the question, and note the strategic words *long-term, continuous,* and *at home.* Eliminate options 1, 3, and 4 because no data in the question support these options. Review care of the client receiving PN and the various test-taking strategies if you had difficulty with this question.

Tip for the Beginning Nursing Student: Parenteral nutrition is a solution containing a high concentration of nutrients and glucose and is administered intravenously (usually through the subclavian vein) to a client who has a disorder in which he or she is unable to obtain adequate nutrition orally. The nursing diagnosis *Social isolation* indicates that the client's ability to socialize with others will be limited as a result of the client's condition. You will learn about nursing diagnoses in your fundamentals of nursing course and about parenteral nutrition when you study nutrition and gastrointestinal disorders.

References

Lewis, S., Heitkemper, M., Dirksen, S., & Bucher, L. (2007). *Medical-surgical nursing: Assessment and management of clinical problems* (7th ed., p. 968). St. Louis: Mosby.

Linton, A. (2007). *Introduction to medical-surgical nursing* (4th ed., p. 744). Philadelphia: Saunders.

---

21. A nurse is having a conversation with a client and responds to the client's statement by saying, "You say that your mother left you when you were 6 years old." The nurse is using which therapeutic communication technique?

1 Focusing
2 Restating
3 Summarizing
4 Sharing observations

Level of Cognitive Ability: Application
Client Needs: Psychosocial Integrity
Integrated Process: Communication and Documentation
Content Area: Fundamental Skills

Answer: 2

Rationale: In restating the nurse repeats the main thought that the client expressed. This therapeutic communication technique indicates that the nurse is listening to the client. In this technique the nurse validates, reinforces, or calls attention to something important that the client said. Therefore options 1, 3, and 4 are incorrect.

Test-Taking Strategy: Focus on the nursing statement. Noting the strategic words *"You say that. ..."* in the nursing statement will assist in identifying the technique that the nurse is using. Review therapeutic communication techniques and the test-taking strategies for answering communication questions if you had difficulty with this question.

Tip for the Beginning Nursing Student: Therapeutic communication techniques promote and encourage the client to communicate and share his or her feelings with the nurse. Nontherapeutic communication techniques block the communication process and are not methods that the nurse would use when caring for a client. You will learn about therapeutic and nontherapeutic communication techniques in your fundamentals of nursing course.

References

Fortinash, K., & Holoday-Worret, P. (2008). *Psychiatric mental health nursing* (4th ed., pp. 69-73). St. Louis: Mosby.

Varcarolis, E., Carlson, V., & Shoemaker, N. (2006). *Foundations of psychiatric mental health nursing* (5th ed., pp. 185-190). Philadelphia: Saunders.

---

22. A physician's order reads morphine sulfate gr ⅛ intramuscularly stat. The medication ampule reads morphine sulfate 10 mg per mL. A nurse prepares how many milliliters to administer the correct dose?
Answer: _____ mL

Level of Cognitive Ability: Application
Client Needs: Physiological Integrity
Integrated Process: Nursing Process/Implementation
Content Area: Fundamental Skills

Answer: 0.75

Rationale: It is necessary to convert gr ⅛ to milligrams. After converting grains to milligrams, use the formula to calculate the correct dose.

Conversion using ratio and proportion:

$$60 \text{ mg:gr } 1 :: x \text{ mg:gr } \tfrac{1}{8}$$

$$1x = 1/8 \times 60/1$$

$$x = 60/8 = 7.5 \text{ mg}$$

Formula:

$$\frac{\text{Desired}}{\text{Available}} \times mL = mL \text{ per dose}$$

$$\frac{7.5 \text{ mg}}{10 \text{ mg}} \times 1 \text{ mL} = 0.75 \text{ mL}$$

Test-Taking Strategy: In this medication calculation problem, it is necessary to first convert grains to milligrams. Next use a calculator and follow the formula for the calculation of the correct dose. Recheck your work, making sure that the answer makes sense. Review the medication calculation formula and the test-taking strategies for answering medication calculation questions if you had difficulty with this question.

Tip for the Beginning Nursing Student: You will learn about nursing math in your fundamentals of nursing course or in another course specifically designed to teach you about nursing math. You will be using nursing math to perform calculations when you prepare medications in the clinical setting. Be sure to learn the formulas and how to perform the calculations because the formulas are critical steps in the process of preparing a safe dose of a medication.

Reference
Potter, P., & Perry, A. (2009). *Fundamentals of nursing* (7th ed., pp. 697-700). St. Louis: Mosby.

---

23. A nurse instructs a client on a tyramine-restricted diet about foods that need to be avoided. The nurse tells the client to avoid which of the following items in the diet?
1 Apples
2 Chicken
3 Tomatoes
4 Homemade bread

Level of Cognitive Ability: Application
Client Needs: Physiological Integrity
Integrated Process: Teaching and Learning
Content Area: Fundamental Skills

Answer: 4
Rationale: Some foods that are naturally high in tyramine include aged cheeses, yogurt, canned meats, beef or chicken liver, sausage, dried fish, beer and some wines, sherry, and chocolate. The client should also avoid yeast and any products made with yeast, such as homemade bread. Most fruits and vegetables are acceptable. The fruits and vegetables that should be avoided are bananas, figs, broad leaf beans and pea pods, eggplant, and mixed Chinese vegetables.

Test-Taking Strategy: Note the strategic word *avoid* in the query of the question. Eliminate options 1 and 3 first because they are fruit items. From the remaining options it is necessary to know that yeast and yeast products need to be avoided. Review foods that need to be avoided in a tyramine-restricted diet and the various test-taking strategies if you had difficulty with this question.

Tip for the Beginning Nursing Student: A healthy and balanced diet is important for all individuals. In the clinical setting a major responsibility will be to ensure that your clients are receiving adequate nutrition to heal and to maintain health. Many times specific diets are prescribed for clients, and you will be responsible for teaching the client about the diet, what can be eaten, and what food items should be restricted. Tyramine is an amino acid that stimulates the release of the catecholamines epinephrine and norepinephrine. Tyramine may be restricted in certain disorders, but it is very important that individuals taking monoamine oxidase inhibitors avoid the ingestion of foods and beverages containing tyramine. Monoamine oxidase inhibitors are antidepressants that you will learn about in your pharmacology course and in your mental health nursing course. You will learn about other various therapeutic diets in your fundamentals of nursing course or in a nutrition course.

Reference
Schlenker, E., & Long, S. (2007). *Williams' essentials of nutrition & diet therapy* (9th ed., p. 729). St. Louis: Mosby.

24. A client's medication is available for injection in an ampule. Which of the following would the nurse do when drawing up this medication?
1 Shake the ampule gently to mix the contents.
2 Snap the top of the ampule backward toward the nurse.
3 Wipe the neck of the ampule with gauze after snapping it open.
4 Place an alcohol wipe around the neck of the ampule before snapping it open.

Level of Cognitive Ability: Application
Client Needs: Safe and Effective Care Environment
Integrated Process: Nursing Process/ Implementation
Content Area: Fundamental Skills

Answer: 4
Rationale: Basic procedure for drawing up medication from an ampule involves tapping the top chamber until the medication lies in the lower area, placing an alcohol wipe around the neck of the ampule, snapping the top toward the nurse so that it opens away from the nurse, and withdrawing the medication without injecting air into the ampule. Snapping the ampule so that it opens away from the nurse prevents injury from possible shattered glass fragments. The neck is not wiped with the gauze because first, it is unnecessary and could contaminate the contents of the ampule and second, it could injure the nurse's fingers from sharp glass edges.

Test-Taking Strategy: Visualize this procedure and each of the options. Eliminate option 1 because of the word *shake.* Next eliminate option 2 because it is unsafe and could harm the nurse. From the remaining options use principles of both asepsis and safety to direct you to option 4. Review medication preparation from an ampule and the various test-taking strategies if you had difficulty with this question.

Tip for the Beginning Nursing Student: An ampule is a small container usually made of glass that contains a single dose of a medication. This is one type of container that contains medication that you will be using in the clinical setting. You will be administering injections and will be drawing medication from an ampule and other types of containers to prepare the injection. You will be learning about special procedures for drawing medication from containers and for preparing and administering injections to a client in your fundamentals of nursing course.

References

Christensen, B., & Kockrow, E. (2006). *Foundations of nursing* (5th ed., p. 724). St. Louis: Mosby.

Potter, P., & Perry, A. (2009). *Fundamentals of nursing* (7th ed., p. 739). St. Louis: Mosby.

25. The client has a platelet count of 60,000 cells/mm^3. The nurse would implement which measure in the care of this client?

1 Using a straight razor for shaving the client

2 Providing vigorous skin care avoiding the use of lotions

3 Measuring the temperature using a tympanic thermometer

4 Encouraging the client to use a firm-bristle toothbrush for mouth care

Level of Cognitive Ability: Application
Client Needs: Safe and Effective Care Environment
Integrated Process: Nursing Process/ Implementation
Content Area: Fundamental Skills

Answer: 3

Rationale: The client with a low platelet count is at risk for bleeding. Therefore the nurse institutes measures that will minimize the risk of injury or bleeding. The nurse would measure the temperature using a tympanic thermometer. Rectal thermometers are avoided because of the risk of bleeding, and oral thermometers are avoided if there is oral soreness or bleeding. The nurse would avoid vigorous washing or rubbing of the skin to avoid causing ecchymosis and would use lotions to prevent dryness and cracking of the skin. In addition, the nurse would avoid the use of straight razors or firm-bristle toothbrushes, which could also cause bleeding.

Test-Taking Strategy: Focus on the subject—a platelet count of 60,000 cells/mm^3. Recalling the normal platelet count and determining that a platelet count of 60,000 cells/mm^3 is low, placing the client at risk for bleeding, will assist in eliminating options 1, 2, and 4. Also noting the words *straight razor, vigorous,* and *firm* in these options, respectively, will assist in eliminating them. If you had difficulty with this question, review the bleeding precautions associated with clients at risk for bleeding and the various test-taking strategies.

Tip for the Beginning Nursing Student: Platelets are a component of the blood and are formed in the bone marrow. They are essential for the coagulation of blood and in the maintenance of hemostasis. Therefore, if the platelet count is low, the coagulation of blood will not occur as it should and the client is at risk for bleeding. The normal platelet count is 150,000 to 400,000 cells/mm^3. If the count is low then the nurse institutes measures to protect the client from injury and resultant bleeding. You will be learning about normal and abnormal laboratory values in your fundamentals of nursing course. You will also learn about the platelet count when you study hematological disorders in your medical-surgical nursing course.

References

Christensen, B., & Kockrow, E. (2006). *Foundations of nursing* (5th ed., p. 243). St. Louis: Mosby.

deWit, S. (2009). *Medical-surgical nursing: Concepts & practice* (pp. 181-182). St. Louis: Saunders.

Potter, P., & Perry, A. (2009). *Fundamentals of nursing* (7th ed., pp. 513-514). St. Louis: Mosby.

13 Chapter

Adult Health Questions

26. A nurse is monitoring a client who had a pleural biopsy. The nurse determines that the client is experiencing a complication if the client exhibits:

1 Diaphoresis
2 Warm, dry skin
3 Mild pain at the biopsy site
4 Capillary refill of 2 seconds

Level of Cognitive Ability: Analysis
Client Needs: Physiological Integrity
Integrated Process: Nursing Process/
    Evaluation
Content Area: Adult Health

Answer: 1
Rationale: The nurse observes the client for dyspnea (difficulty breathing), excessive pain, pallor, or diaphoresis (profuse sweating) following pleural biopsy. These could indicate the presence of complications, such as pneumothorax, hemothorax, or intercostal nerve injury. Mild pain is expected, because the procedure itself is painful. Abnormal signs and symptoms should be reported to the physician. Options 2 and 4 are normal findings.

Test-Taking Strategy: Focus on the subject—a complication. Eliminate options 2 and 4 because they are normal findings. From the remaining options noting the word *mild* in option 3 will assist in eliminating this option. Review the complications associated with a pleural biopsy and the various test-taking strategies if you had difficulty with this question.

Tip for the Beginning Nursing Student: A pleural biopsy is an invasive procedure that involves the insertion of a needle into the pleural cavity or pleural space to obtain tissue or fluid for pathological examination. This procedure is diagnostic and may be done if suspicious lesions are present. The nurse monitors for signs of respiratory distress or bleeding following a biopsy. You will learn about care of the client following pleural biopsy and the important client assessments in your medical-surgical nursing course when you study respiratory disorders.

References
deWit, S. (2009). *Medical-surgical nursing: Concepts & practice* (pp. 288-289). St. Louis: Saunders.
Ignatavicius, D., & Workman, M. (2010). *Medical-surgical nursing: Patient-centered collaborative care* (6th ed., p. 569). Philadelphia: Saunders.

27. A nurse caring for a client following a bowel resection notes that the client is restless. The nurse takes the client's vital signs and notes that the client's pulse rate has increased and that the blood pressure has dropped significantly since the previous readings. The nurse suspects that the client is going into shock and immediately:
1 Checks the client's oxygen saturation level
2 Rechecks the vital signs to verify the findings
3 Slows the rate of the intravenous (IV) fluid infusing
4 Raises the client's legs above the level of the heart

Level of Cognitive Ability: Application
Client Needs: Physiological Integrity
Integrated Process: Nursing Process/ Implementation
Content Area: Adult Health

Answer: 4

Rationale: In addition to hypotension, manifestations of shock include tachycardia; restlessness and apprehension; and cold, moist, pale, or cyanotic skin. If a client develops signs of shock the nurse would immediately raise the client's legs above the level of the heart to improve venous return and immediately notify the surgeon. The nurse would also plan to administer oxygen or increase its rate of delivery, increase the rate of IV fluids (unless contraindicated), administer medications as prescribed, and continue to monitor the client and the client's response to interventions.

Test-Taking Strategy: Note the strategic word *immediately.* Use the ABCs—airway, breathing, and circulation—to answer the question. This will direct you to option 4. Raising the client's legs above the level of the heart will assist in providing blood flow to body tissues. Review the interventions for shock and the test-taking strategies for answering prioritizing questions if you had difficulty with this question.

Tip for the Beginning Nursing Student: Shock is an abnormal condition of inadequate blood flow to the body's tissues resulting in an inadequate delivery of oxygen and nutrients to the tissues. There are different types of shock, but the most common is hypovolemic shock. It is caused by any condition that results in hypovolemia, such as hemorrhage. Fluid volume must be restored immediately to oxygenate perfusion-deprived tissues. This condition can be life threatening if not immediately treated. You will learn about shock as a postoperative complication in your fundamentals of nursing course and in your medical-surgical nursing course.

References
Christensen, B., & Kockrow, E. (2006). *Adult health nursing* (5th ed., p. 54). St. Louis: Mosby.
Ignatavicius, D., & Workman, M. (2010). *Medical-surgical nursing: Patient-centered collaborative care* (6th ed., pp. 833, 836). Philadelphia: Saunders.

28. A nurse is performing an assessment on a client with a diagnosis of a brain tumor that is located in the brainstem and notes that the client is assuming the posture in Figure 13-1. The nurse contacts the physician and reports that the client is exhibiting:
1 Opisthotonos
2 Flaccid quadriplegia
3 Decorticate posturing
4 Decerebrate posturing

Answer: 4

Rationale: In decerebrate posturing the upper extremities are stiffly extended and adducted with internal rotation and pronation of the palms. The lower extremities are stiffly extended with plantar flexion. The teeth are clenched, and the back is hyperextended. Decerebrate posturing indicates a lesion in the brainstem at the midbrain or upper pons. In decorticate posturing the upper extremities (arms, wrists, and fingers) are flexed with adduction of the arms. The lower extremities are extended with internal rotation and plantar flexion. Decorticate posturing indicates a hemispheric lesion of the cerebral cortex. Flaccid quadriplegia is complete loss of muscle tone and paralysis of all four

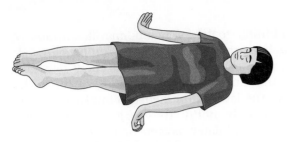

Fig. 13-1 From Ignatavicius, D., & Workman, M. (2006). *Medical-surgical nursing: Critical thinking for collaborative care* (5th ed., p. 1630). Philadelphia: Saunders.

Level of Cognitive Ability: Analysis
Client Needs: Physiological Integrity
Integrated Process: Nursing Process/ Assessment/Data Collection
Content Area: Adult Health

extremities, indicating a completely nonfunctional brainstem. Opisthotonos is a prolonged arching of the back with the head and heels bent backward. It indicates meningeal irritation.

Test-Taking Strategy: Note the position of the client and that the extremities are stiffly extended. Also, noting the client's diagnosis and recalling that this posture indicates a lesion in the brainstem at the midbrain or upper pons will assist in answering the question. Review abnormal postures and the various test-taking strategies if you had difficulty with this question.

Tip for the Beginning Nursing Student: A brain tumor refers to a lesion in the brain. The clinical manifestations that the client exhibits depend on the location of the tumor. If a client has a tumor in the brain, one concern is increased intracranial pressure occurring because of the tumor. Another concern is deterioration in the client's condition as a result of the tumor pressing on structures in the brain. The nurse needs to monitor the neurological status of the client closely. If the nurse notes posturing, this indicates deterioration in the client's condition and needs to be reported immediately. You will learn about brain tumors, the signs of increased intracranial pressure, and posturing in your medical-surgical nursing course when you study neurological disorders.

References
Christensen, B., & Kockrow, E. (2006). *Adult health nursing* (5th ed., p. 703). St. Louis: Mosby.
Lewis, S., Heitkemper, M., Dirksen, S., & Bucher, L. (2007). *Medical-surgical nursing: Assessment and management of clinical problems* (7th ed., p. 1472). St. Louis: Mosby.
Linton, A., & Maebius, N. (2007). *Introduction to medical-surgical nursing* (4th ed., pp. 441-442). Philadelphia: Saunders.

29. A client newly diagnosed with type 1 diabetes mellitus is taking NPH insulin at 7:00 AM daily. The nurse monitors the client closely for which signs and symptoms in the late afternoon?
 1 Increased appetite and abdominal pain
 2 Hunger, shakiness, and cool, clammy skin
 3 Thirst, red dry skin, and fruity breath odor
 4 Increased urination and rapid deep breathing

Level of Cognitive Ability: Analysis
Client Needs: Physiological Integrity
Integrated Process: Nursing Process/ Implementation
Content Area: Adult Health

Answer: 2
Rationale: The client taking NPH insulin would experience peak effects of the medication from approximately 6 to 12 hours after administration. At this time the client is at risk of hypoglycemia if food intake is insufficient. The nurse would teach the client to watch for signs and symptoms of hypoglycemia during this time frame, which include hunger, shakiness, cold sweating, headache, anxiety, increased pulse, blurred vision, confusion, and difficulty concentrating. The other options list various manifestations of hyperglycemia.

Test-Taking Strategy: Note that the client is taking NPH insulin at 7:00 AM. Also note the strategic words *signs and symptoms in the late afternoon.* Recall that hypoglycemic reactions can occur at peak insulin times. Also recall that NPH is an intermediate-acting insulin and peaks during the afternoon. Therefore you are looking for the option that identifies signs and symptoms of a hypoglycemic reaction. Eliminate options 1, 3, and 4 because they are comparable or alike and identify signs and symptoms of hyperglycemia. Remember the *3 Ps* of hyperglycemia—polyuria, polydipsia, and polyphagia. Review the signs and symptoms of hypoglycemia and the various test-taking strategies if you had difficulty with this question.

Tip for the Beginning Nursing Student: Both injectable and oral insulins are used to treat the client with diabetes mellitus, and these medications can cause hypoglycemia. Two important complications of diabetes mellitus are hypoglycemia and hyperglycemia. It is important to know the signs and symptoms of each and the interventions needed if either occurs and to teach this information to the client. You will learn about these complications and the other complications of diabetes mellitus when you study endocrine disorders in your medical-surgical nursing course.

References
deWit, S. (2009). *Medical-surgical nursing: Concepts & practice* (p. 932). St. Louis: Saunders.

Lewis, S., Heitkemper, M., Dirksen, S., & Bucher, L. (2007). *Medical-surgical nursing: Assessment and management of clinical problems* (7th ed., pp. 1281-1282). St. Louis: Mosby.

Linton, A., & Maebius, N. (2007). *Introduction to medical-surgical nursing* (4th ed., p. 1013). Philadelphia: Saunders.

---

30. The nurse is developing a teaching plan for the client with viral hepatitis. The nurse lists which item in the plan?
1 Consume three large meals daily.
2 The diet should be low in calories.
3 Activity should be limited to prevent fatigue.
4 Alcohol intake should be limited to 2 oz per day.

Level of Cognitive Ability: Application
Client Needs: Physiological Integrity
Integrated Process: Teaching and Learning
Content Area: Adult Health

Answer: 3
Rationale: The client with viral hepatitis should limit activity to avoid fatigue during the recuperation period. The diet should be optimal in calories, protein, and carbohydrates. The client should take in several small meals per day rather than three large meals. Alcohol is restricted not limited.

Test-Taking Strategy: Eliminate option 4 first using general principles related to client teaching. Next focus on the client's diagnosis, and recall that the liver needs rest during the healing process. This will direct you to option 3. Review care of the client with hepatitis and the various test-taking strategies if you had difficulty with this question.

Tip for the Beginning Nursing Student: Viral hepatitis is a viral inflammatory disease of the liver caused by one of the hepatitis viruses. It can be transmitted orally, sexually, through contaminated water or food, or through exposure to infected blood; the mode of transmission varies depending on the type of hepatitis virus. You will learn about viral hepatitis when you study gastrointestinal disorders in your medical-surgical nursing course.

References
Ignatavicius, D., & Workman, M. (2010). *Medical-surgical nursing: Patient-centered collaborative care* (6th ed., p. 1360). Philadelphia: Saunders.

Linton, A., & Maebius, N. (2007). *Introduction to medical-surgical nursing* (4th ed., p. 806). Philadelphia: Saunders.

31. A nurse is reading the results of the client's Mantoux test and palpates a 4-mm area of induration at the test site. The nurse documents that the result:
1 Confirms tuberculosis
2 Is positive for tuberculosis
3 Is negative for tuberculosis
4 Provides a conclusive determination of tuberculosis

Level of Cognitive Ability: Application
Client Needs: Safe and Effective Care Environment
Integrated Process: Communication and Documentation
Content Area: Adult Health

Answer: 3

Rationale: More than 5 mm of induration is considered a positive result for clients with known or suspected human immunodeficiency infection, intravenous drug users, people in close contact with a known case of tuberculosis, or clients with a chest radiograph suggestive of previous tuberculosis. More than 10 mm of induration indicates exposure to and infection with tuberculosis. However, the infection may not be an active one, and the result could indicate the presence of inactive (dormant) disease.

Test-Taking Strategy: Eliminate options 1, 2, and 4 because they are comparable or alike and indicate that tuberculosis is present. Review the Mantoux test and the various test-taking strategies if you had difficulty with this question.

Tip for the Beginning Nursing Student: Tuberculosis is an infection caused by an acid-fast bacillus known as *Mycobacterium tuberculosis.* It is usually transmitted by the inhalation or ingestion of infected droplets and usually affects the lungs. The Mantoux test is a skin test that consists of an intradermal injection of a purified protein derivative of the tubercle bacillus. This test is used to assist in establishing a diagnosis of tuberculosis. You will learn about this test and tuberculosis when you study respiratory disorders in your medical-surgical nursing course.

References

deWit, S. (2009). *Medical-surgical nursing: Concepts & practice* (p. 325). St. Louis: Saunders.
Ignatavicius, D., & Workman, M. (2010). *Medical-surgical nursing: Patient-centered collaborative care* (6th ed., p. 669). Philadelphia: Saunders.

32. An emergency room nurse initiates cardiopulmonary resuscitation (CPR) on a victim who was in a motor vehicle crash. The nurse uses the method shown in Figure 13-2 to open the airway in which of the following situations?
1 If the client is unconscious
2 If neck trauma is suspected
3 In all situations requiring CPR
4 If the client has a history of headaches

Answer: 2

Rationale: The jaw thrust without head tilt maneuver is used when head and/or neck trauma is suspected. This maneuver opens the airway while maintaining proper head and neck alignment, thus reducing the risk of further damage to the neck. In situations requiring CPR, the client will be unconscious. Options 3 and 4 are both incorrect. In addition, it is unlikely that the nurse will be able to obtain data from the client.

Test-Taking Strategy: Focus on the data in the question. Eliminate option 3 because of the close-ended word *all.* Noting that the client requires CPR will assist in eliminating options 1 and 4. Review CPR guidelines and the various test-taking strategies if you had difficulty with this question.

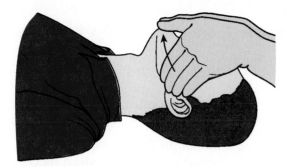

Fig. 13-2 From Harkreader, H., Hogan, M.A., & Thobaben, M. (2007). *Fundamentals of nursing: Caring and clinical judgment* (3rd ed.). Philadelphia: Saunders. Based on American Heart Association. (2005). The American Heart Association 2005 guidelines for cardiopulmonary resuscitation and emergency cardiovascular care. *Circulation, 112* (24, Suppl.). Available at http://www.americanheart.org.

Level of Cognitive Ability: Application
Client Needs: Physiological Integrity
Integrated Process: Nursing Process/
  Implementation
Content Area: Adult Health

Tip for the Beginning Nursing Student: Review the guidelines for performing CPR to ensure that you are ready to perform the procedure if an emergency situation arises. Remember that if the client is a victim of injury such as from a motor vehicle crash or a fall from a ladder, and you suspect a neck injury, the jaw thrust maneuver is used to open the airway. As a health care provider, you will be required to remain current with your CPR certification. You will also review the CPR guidelines in your medical-surgical nursing course when you study cardiac disorders.

References

Linton, A., & Maebius, N. (2007). *Introduction to medical-surgical nursing* (4th ed., p. 226). Philadelphia: Saunders.
Monahan, F., Sands, J., Marek, J., Neighbors, M., & Green, C. (2007). *Phipps' medical-surgical nursing: Health and illness perspectives* (8th ed., p. 800). St. Louis: Mosby.
Perry, A., & Potter, P. (2010). *Clinical nursing skills & techniques* (7th ed., p. 731). St. Louis: Mosby.

---

33. The client has been diagnosed with polycystic kidney disease. The nurse assesses the client for which manifestation that is most common for this disorder?
1 Headache
2 Hypotension
3 Flank pain and hematuria
4 Complaints of low pelvic pain

Level of Cognitive Ability: Application
Client Needs: Physiological Integrity
Integrated Process: Nursing Process/
  Assessment/Data Collection
Content Area: Adult Health

Answer: 3

Rationale: The most common findings with polycystic kidney disease are hematuria and flank or lumbar pain that is either colicky in nature or dull and aching. Other common findings include proteinuria, calculi, uremia, and palpable kidney masses. Hypertension is another common finding and may be associated with cardiomegaly and heart failure. The client may complain of a headache, but this is not a specific assessment finding in polycystic kidney disease.

Test-Taking Strategy: Note the strategic words *most common.* Note the relationship between the word *kidney* in the name of the disorder and the word *flank* in the correct option. Review the manifestations of polycystic kidney disease and the various test-taking strategies if you had difficulty with this question.

Tip for the Beginning Nursing Student: Polycystic kidney disease is an abnormal condition in which the kidneys are enlarged and contain many cysts. The three forms of the disease are childhood polycystic disease, congenital polycystic disease, and adult polycystic disease. Kidney failure can result that can progress to uremia and death. Treatment is symptomatic or may include dialysis or renal transplant. You will learn about this disease in your pediatrics nursing course or your medical-surgical nursing course when you study renal disorders.

References
Christensen, B., & Kockrow, E. (2006). *Adult health nursing* (5th ed., p. 492). St. Louis: Mosby.
Lewis, S., Heitkemper, M., Dirksen, S., & Bucher, L. (2007). *Medical-surgical nursing: Assessment and management of clinical problems* (7th ed., p. 1176). St. Louis: Mosby.

---

34. A client is tested for human immunodeficiency virus (HIV) with an enzyme-linked immunosorbent assay (ELISA) test, and the test result is positive. The client is very upset and asks the nurse if this means that he definitely has HIV. The nurse appropriately tells the client that:

1 He definitely has HIV.
2 Another test will be done to determine if he has HIV.
3 False-positive results are reported all of the time and that he should not be worried.
4 A positive ELISA means that the infection was diagnosed early in the initial infection period.

Level of Cognitive Ability: Application
Client Needs: Physiological Integrity
Integrated Process: Nursing Process/ Implementation
Content Area: Adult Health

Answer: 2
Rationale: The normal value for an ELISA test is negative. If the ELISA is positive, a second test, the Western blot, is performed to confirm a positive HIV status. The other options are incorrect. In addition, the nurse would not tell a client that "he should not be worried." If testing is performed too early in the initial infection period, a false-negative result may occur.

Test-Taking Strategy: Use therapeutic communication techniques to eliminate options 1 and 3. Next, careful reading of option 4 will assist in eliminating this option. Remember that if testing is performed too early in the initial infection period, a false-negative result may occur. Review interpretations of results of an ELISA test and the various test-taking strategies if you had difficulty with this question.

Tip for the Beginning Nursing Student: HIV is a retrovirus that causes acquired immunodeficiency syndrome (AIDS). The HIV virus is transmitted through anal or oral sexual contact with infected semen or vaginal secretions, through contact with infected blood or blood products, by transmission of the virus from mother to fetus during childbirth, through breast-feeding, or through other infected body fluids. Various blood tests done to confirm the diagnosis include the ELISA and the Western blot. You will learn about these blood tests and HIV when you study immune disorders in your medical-surgical nursing course.

References
Ignatavicius, D., & Workman, M. (2010). *Medical-surgical nursing: Patient-centered collaborative care* (6th ed., pp. 373-374). Philadelphia: Saunders.
Linton, A. (2007). *Introduction to medical-surgical nursing* (4th ed., p. 620). Philadelphia: Saunders.

---

35. The nurse monitors for which acid-base disorder that can likely occur in a client with an ileostomy?

1 Metabolic acidosis
2 Metabolic alkalosis
3 Respiratory acidosis
4 Respiratory alkalosis

Level of Cognitive Ability: Analysis
Client Needs: Physiological Integrity
Integrated Process: Nursing Process/ Assessment/Data Collection
Content Area: Adult Health

Answer: 1
Rationale: Intestinal secretions are high in bicarbonate because of the effects of pancreatic secretions. These fluids may be lost from the body before they can be reabsorbed with conditions such as diarrhea or creation of an ileostomy. The decreased bicarbonate level creates the actual base deficit of metabolic acidosis. The client with an ileostomy is not at risk for developing the acid-base disorders identified in options 2, 3, and 4.

Test-Taking Strategy: Note that the client has an ileostomy. Because the client does not have a respiratory condition, eliminate options 3 and 4. Next recall that intestinal fluids are alkaline; therefore alkaline secretions are lost in a client with an ileostomy, resulting in an acidotic condition. If you had difficulty with this question, review the causes of metabolic acidosis and the various test-taking strategies.

Tip for the Beginning Nursing Student: An ileostomy is a surgical formation of an opening of the ileum onto the surface of the abdomen, through which fecal matter is emptied. This surgical procedure is performed for conditions such as advanced or recurrent ulcerative colitis, Crohn's disease, or cancer of the large bowel. You will learn about an ileostomy when you study gastrointestinal disorders in your medical-surgical nursing course.

References

Linton, A., & Maebius, N. (2007). *Introduction to medical-surgical nursing* (4th ed., p. 399). Philadelphia: Saunders.

Monahan, F., Sands, J., Marek, J., Neighbors, M., & Green, C. (2007). *Phipps' medical-surgical nursing: Health and illness perspectives* (8th ed., pp. 395, 1256). St. Louis: Mosby.

---

36. A nurse provides instructions to a client who is being discharged 24 hours after undergoing a percutaneous renal biopsy. Which statement by the client indicates a need to reinforce the instructions?
1 "A fever is normal following this procedure."
2 "I should not work out at the gym for about 2 weeks."
3 "I will call the physician if my urine becomes bloody."
4 "I need to avoid any strenuous lifting for about 2 weeks."

Level of Cognitive Ability: Analysis
Client Needs: Physiological Integrity
Integrated Process: Teaching and Learning
Content Area: Adult Health

Answer: 1
Rationale: Following percutaneous renal biopsy the client is instructed to report immediately fever, increasing pain levels (back, flank, or shoulder), bleeding from the puncture site, weakness, dizziness, grossly bloody urine, or dysuria. Activity should be restricted if blood is seen in the urine. The client is also instructed to avoid strenuous lifting, physical exertion, or trauma to the biopsy site for up to 2 weeks after discharge.

Test-Taking Strategy: Note the strategic words *need to reinforce the instructions.* These words indicate a negative event query and the need to select the option that identifies an incorrect client statement. Eliminate options 2 and 4 first because they are comparable or alike. From the remaining options, recall the complications of this procedure. This will direct you to option 1. Review client instructions following a percutaneous renal biopsy and the various test-taking strategies if you had difficulty with this question.

Tip for the Beginning Nursing Student: A percutaneous renal biopsy is performed by the insertion of a needle through the skin into the kidney to obtain a piece of tissue for pathological analysis. Infection and bleeding are concerns following this procedure, and the nurse monitors the client closely for these complications. You will learn about a percutaneous renal biopsy when you study renal disorders in your medical-surgical nursing course.

References

Ignatavicius, D., & Workman, M. (2010). *Medical-surgical nursing: Patient-centered collaborative care* (6th ed., pp. 1547-1548). Philadelphia: Saunders.

Linton, A. (2007). *Introduction to medical-surgical nursing* (4th ed., p. 845). Philadelphia: Saunders.

37. A client being treated for respiratory failure has the following arterial blood gas (ABG) results: pH 7.30, $Paco_2$ 58 mm Hg, Pao_2 75 mm Hg, HCO_3^- 27 mEq/L. The nurse interprets that the client has which of the following acid-base disturbances?
 1 Metabolic acidosis
 2 Metabolic alkalosis
 3 Respiratory acidosis
 4 Respiratory alkalosis

Level of Cognitive Ability: Analysis
Client Needs: Physiological Integrity
Integrated Process: Nursing Process/ Assessment/Data Collection
Content Area: Adult Health

Answer: 3
Rationale: Acidosis is defined as a pH of less than 7.35, whereas alkalosis is defined as a pH of greater than 7.45. In a respiratory condition an opposite effect will be seen between the pH and the $Paco_2$. In respiratory acidosis the pH is decreased and the $Paco_2$ is elevated. The normal HCO_3^- is 22 to 27 mm Hg. Metabolic acidosis is present when the HCO_3^- is less than 22 mEq/L, whereas metabolic alkalosis is present when the HCO_3^- is greater than 27 mEq/L. This client's ABG results are consistent with respiratory acidosis.

Test-Taking Strategy: Focus on the client's diagnosis, and recall that this client will have difficulty exchanging oxygen and carbon dioxide. This will assist in eliminating options 1 and 2. From the remaining options, remember that the pH is decreased with acidosis. This will direct you to option 3. Review the steps related to reading blood gas values and the various test-taking strategies if you had difficulty with this question.

Tip for the Beginning Nursing Student: Respiratory failure is the inability of the cardiovascular and pulmonary system to maintain an adequate exchange of oxygen and carbon dioxide in the lungs. Respiratory failure can be caused by various conditions that affect oxygenation or ventilation, such as emphysema, infection, pneumonia, or lung cancer. You will learn about respiratory failure and ABG values when you study respiratory disorders in your medical-surgical nursing course.

References
deWit, S. (2009). *Medical-surgical nursing: Concepts & practice* (p. 54). St. Louis: Saunders.
Ignatavicius, D., & Workman, M. (2010). *Medical-surgical nursing: Patient-centered collaborative care* (6th ed., pp. 206, 208). Philadelphia: Saunders.

38. A client with a family history of cervical cancer has made an appointment to have a Papanicolaou smear done. The nurse who schedules the appointment tells the client that:
 1 Sexual intercourse needs to be avoided for 24 hours before the test.
 2 If the client is menstruating, douching will be required right before the test.
 3 A vaginal hygiene spray should be used for 2 consecutive days before the scheduled test.
 4 The test is very uncomfortable, but a local anesthetic will be injected into the vaginal area.

Answer: 1
Rationale: A Papanicolaou smear cannot be performed during menstruation. The test is usually painless but may be slightly uncomfortable with placement of the speculum or while a cervical scraping is obtained. A local anesthetic is not injected into the vaginal area. The client is instructed to avoid sexual intercourse, douching, or using vaginal hygiene sprays or deodorants for 24 hours before the test.

Test-Taking Strategy: Eliminate option 4 first because of the words *very uncomfortable.* From the remaining options, think about the test and its purpose to direct you to option 1. Review client preparation for a Papanicolaou test and the various test-taking strategies if you had difficulty with this question.

Level of Cognitive Ability: Application
Client Needs: Health Promotion and
   Maintenance
Integrated Process: Teaching and
   Learning
Content Area: Adult Health

Tip for the Beginning Nursing Student: A Papanicolaou smear is a simple test in which cells are scraped from the cervix to obtain a specimen for examination. This test is usually done annually and permits early diagnosis of cervical cancer. You will learn about this screening test when you study oncological disorders in your medical-surgical nursing course.

References

deWit, S. (2009). *Medical-surgical nursing: Concepts & practice* (p. 950). St. Louis: Saunders.
Ignatavicius, D., & Workman, M. (2010). *Medical-surgical nursing: Patient-centered collaborative care* (6th ed., p. 1652). Philadelphia: Saunders.

---

39. A client with a diagnosis of multiple myeloma is admitted to the hospital. When collecting data from the client, the nurse asks which question that specifically relates to a clinical manifestation of this disorder?
   1 "Do you have diarrhea?"
   2 "Are you having any bone pain?"
   3 "Have you noticed an increase in appetite?"
   4 "Do you have feelings of anxiety and nervousness, along with difficulty sleeping?"

Level of Cognitive Ability: Analysis
Client Needs: Physiological Integrity
Integrated Process: Nursing Process/
   Assessment/Data Collection
Content Area: Adult Health

Answer: 2
Rationale: Multiple myeloma is characterized by an abnormal proliferation of plasma B cells. These cells infiltrate the bone marrow and produce abnormal and excessive amounts of immunoglobulin. The most common presenting complaint is bone pain. Hypercalcemia occurs as a result of release of calcium from the deteriorating bone tissue, and subsequently the client presents with confusion, somnolence, constipation, nausea, and thirst.

Test-Taking Strategy: Focus on the client's diagnosis, and use medical terminology to answer the question. Also, recalling the pathophysiology of multiple myeloma and the effects it produces on the body will direct you to option 2. Review the manifestations associated with multiple myeloma and the various test-taking strategies if you had difficulty with this question.

Tip for the Beginning Nursing Student: Multiple myeloma is a malignant tumor of the bone marrow. The tumor disrupts normal bone marrow function, destroys osseous tissue, and causes pain, fractures, hypercalcemia, and skeletal deformities. You will learn about multiple myeloma when you study oncologic disorders in your medical-surgical nursing course.

References

Christensen, B., & Kockrow, E. (2006). *Adult health nursing* (5th ed., p. 316). St. Louis: Mosby.
Monahan, F., Sands, J., Marek, J., Neighbors, M., & Green, C. (2007). *Phipps' medical-surgical nursing: Health and illness perspectives* (8th ed., p. 457). St. Louis: Mosby.

---

40. A nurse has provided instructions to a client scheduled for an exercise electrocardiogram (stress test) at 9:00 AM on the following day. The nurse determines that the client needs additional instructions if the client states:
   1 "I should not go to the gym to lift weights today."

Answer: 4
Rationale: For the procedure the client should wear rubber-soled, supportive shoes, such as sneakers, and light, loose, comfortable clothing. A shirt that buttons in front is helpful for electrocardiogram (ECG) lead placement. The client should not do strenuous physical activity for at least 12 hours before testing.

2 "I should wear sneakers when I come for the test."

3 "I will wear light, loose, comfortable clothing for the procedure."

4 "I can eat breakfast before the procedure as long as I eat by 8:00 AM."

Level of Cognitive Ability: Analysis
Client Needs: Physiological Integrity
Integrated Process: Teaching and Learning
Content Area: Adult Health

Test-Taking Strategy: Note the strategic words *needs additional instructions.* These words indicate a negative event query and the need to select the option that is an incorrect client statement. Recall what this test entails. Select the option that could interfere with testing and test results, namely, digestion. Review client teaching related to a stress test and the strategies for answering negative event questions if you had difficulty with this question.

Tip for the Beginning Nursing Student: An exercise electrocardiogram (stress test) measures the function of the cardiopulmonary system as the body is subjected to carefully controlled amounts of physiological stress. In this test a cardiac monitoring device is attached to the client and the cardiopulmonary system is monitored while the client performs some type of exercise, such as walking on a treadmill. The results of this test provide valuable information for the physician to determine cardiopulmonary problems or the effectiveness of medications or other treatments. You will learn about this type of stress test when you study cardiovascular disorders in your medical-surgical nursing course.

References

deWit, S. (2009). *Medical-surgical nursing: Concepts & practice* (p. 412). St. Louis: Saunders.

Ignatavicius, D., & Workman, M. (2010). *Medical-surgical nursing: Patient-centered collaborative care* (6th ed., p. 724). Philadelphia: Saunders.

---

41. A client has undergone pericardiocentesis to treat cardiac tamponade. The nurse monitors the client for which sign to determine whether the tamponade is recurring?

1 Facial flushing
2 Decreasing pulse
3 Paradoxical pulse
4 Rising blood pressure

Level of Cognitive Ability: Analysis
Client Needs: Physiological Integrity
Integrated Process: Nursing Process/ Evaluation
Content Area: Adult Health

Answer: 3

Rationale: Cardiac tamponade is a life-threatening situation caused by the accumulation of fluid in the pericardium. The fluid accumulates rapidly and in sufficient quantity to compress the heart and restrict blood flow in and out of the ventricles. Hypotension, tachycardia, jugular vein distension, cyanosis of the lips and nails, dyspnea, muffled heart sounds, diaphoresis, and paradoxical pulse (a decrease in systolic arterial pressure exceeding 10 mm Hg during inspiration) are indications of this emergency situation. The emergency intervention of choice is pericardiocentesis, a procedure in which fluid is aspirated from the pericardial sac. Options 1, 2, and 4 are not indications of cardiac tamponade.

Test-Taking Strategy: Note the strategic word *recurring.* This tells you that the correct option is a symptom of the original problem, which is cardiac tamponade. Recalling the pathophysiology associated with cardiac tamponade will direct you to option 3. Review these signs and the various test-taking strategies if you had difficulty with this question.

Tip for the Beginning Nursing Student: When cardiac tamponade occurs, the heart becomes compressed by the accumulation of fluid in the pericardium. In order to sustain life, this fluid needs to be removed. Pericardiocentesis involves a surgical puncture into the pericardial space between the serous membranes for aspiration of the fluid from the pericardial sac. You will learn about cardiac tamponade and pericardiocentesis when you study cardiovascular disorders in your medical-surgical nursing course.

References

Chernecky, C., & Berger, B. (2008). *Laboratory tests and diagnostic procedures* (5th ed., p. 863). Philadelphia: Saunders.

Christensen, B., & Kockrow, E. (2006). *Adult health nursing* (5th ed., p. 371). St. Louis: Mosby.

Ignatavicius, D., & Workman, M. (2010). *Medical-surgical nursing: Patient-centered collaborative care* (6th ed., p. 786). Philadelphia: Saunders.

---

42. A client has undergone cardiac catheterization using the right femoral artery for access. The nurse determines that the client is experiencing a complication of the procedure if which of the following is(are) noted?
1 Urine output 40 mL/hour
2 Blood pressure 118/76 mm Hg
3 Pallor and coolness of the right leg
4 Respirations 18 breaths per minute

Level of Cognitive Ability: Analysis
Client Needs: Physiological Integrity
Integrated Process: Nursing Process/ Evaluation
Content Area: Adult Health

Answer: 3

Rationale: Potential complications after cardiac catheterization include allergic reaction to the dye, cardiac dysrhythmias, and a number of vascular complications, such as hemorrhage, thrombosis, or embolism. The nurse detects these complications by monitoring for signs and symptoms of allergic reaction, decreased urine output, hematoma or hemorrhage at the insertion site, or signs of decreased circulation to the affected leg. Options 1, 2, and 4 are normal findings.

Test-Taking Strategy: Note the strategic words *experiencing a complication.* This tells you that the correct option is an abnormal piece of assessment data. Eliminate options 1, 2, and 4 because they are normal findings. Pallor and coolness indicate thrombosis or hematoma and should be further assessed and reported. Review the signs of complications following a cardiac catheterization if you had difficulty with this question.

Tip for the Beginning Nursing Student: A cardiac catheterization is a diagnostic procedure in which a catheter is introduced through an incision into a large blood vessel and threaded through the circulatory system of the heart. This procedure is primarily done to assess the status of the coronary arteries in the heart and to determine if any blockage is present and if so, the extent of the blockage. Postprocedure monitoring for complications is a primary nursing responsibility. You will learn about cardiac catheterization and important nursing interventions when you study cardiovascular disorders in your medical-surgical nursing course.

References

Chernecky, C., & Berger, B. (2008). *Laboratory tests and diagnostic procedures* (5th ed., pp. 295-297). Philadelphia: Saunders.

Ignatavicius, D., & Workman, M. (2010). *Medical-surgical nursing: Patient-centered collaborative care* (6th ed., p. 724). Philadelphia: Saunders.

43. The nurse in the emergency room is performing an assessment on a client who sustained a right finger laceration from a fish hook while fishing. The nurse asks the client which priority question?

1 "When was your last physical examination?"
2 "Have you had a chest x-ray in the last year?"
3 "When did you receive your last tetanus immunization?"
4 "Have you ever sustained this type of injury in the past?"

Level of Cognitive Ability: Application
Client Needs: Physiological Integrity
Integrated Process: Nursing Process/ Assessment/Data Collection
Content Area: Adult Health

Answer: 3

Rationale: A client who sustains a laceration is at risk of developing complications such as osteomyelitis, gas gangrene, and tetanus. During the assessment the nurse asks the client about the date of the last tetanus immunization to ensure that the client has tetanus prophylaxis. Although options 1 and 4 may be components of the assessment, these questions are not the priority. Option 2 is unrelated to the data in the question.

Test-Taking Strategy: Focusing on the data in the question will assist in eliminating option 2. From the remaining options noting the word *laceration* will direct you to option 3. Review emergency care for the client who sustains a laceration and the various test-taking strategies if you had difficulty with this question.

Tip for the Beginning Nursing Student: Tetanus toxoid is an active immunizing agent prepared from detoxified tetanus toxin that produces an antigenic response in the body. It provides immunity to tetanus, an acute, potentially fatal infection of the central nervous system caused by an anaerobic bacillus, *Clostridium tetani.* The bacillus may enter the body through a wound, such as a laceration. If a client sustains an injury that involves a laceration or other type of wound, a booster shot of tetanus toxoid is given if the client was previously immunized. People known to have been adequately immunized within 5 years of the injury (or a time period determined by the physician) do not usually require immunization. You will learn about treatment of injuries when you study integumentary disorders in your medical-surgical nursing course.

References

Black, J., & Hawks, J. (2009). *Medical-surgical nursing: Clinical management for positive outcomes* (8th ed., pp. 2209-2210). St. Louis: Saunders.
Christensen, B., & Kockrow, E. (2006). *Foundations of nursing* (5th ed., p. 768). St. Louis: Mosby.

44. A client has been admitted to the hospital with a fractured pelvis sustained in a motor vehicle accident. The nurse monitors for complications and assesses the client closely for which of the following in the early posttrauma period?

1 Pain
2 Fever
3 Hematuria
4 Bradycardia

Level of Cognitive Ability: Analysis
Client Needs: Physiological Integrity

Answer: 3

Rationale: One complication of a pelvic fracture is damage to the kidneys and lower urinary tract. Therefore the nurse would monitor for signs of this complication, which would include bloody urine. This client is also at risk for hypovolemic shock. Bone fragments can damage blood vessels, leading to hemorrhage into the abdominal cavity and the thigh area. Signs of hypovolemic shock include tachycardia and hypotension. Although infection is also a complication (indicated by a fever), it is not generally noted in the early posttrauma period.

Test-Taking Strategy: Note the strategic words *early posttrauma period.* This will assist in eliminating option 2. Next focus on the anatomical location of the injury to

Integrated Process: Nursing Process/
Assessment/Data Collection
Content Area: Adult Health

direct you to option 3 from the remaining options. Review the complications following this type of injury and the various test-taking strategies if you had difficulty with this question.

Tip for the Beginning Nursing Student: Pelvic fractures usually occur as a result of motor vehicle accidents, falls, and crush injuries. Hemorrhage is a primary concern because the force from the impact can rupture blood vessels surrounding the pelvic ring. You will learn about pelvic fractures, the complications, and the nursing interventions in the care of the client when you study musculoskeletal disorders in your medical-surgical nursing course.

References

Christensen, B., & Kockrow, E. (2006). *Adult health nursing* (5th ed., p. 163). St. Louis: Mosby.

Lewis, S., Heitkemper, M., Dirksen, S., & Bucher, L. (2007). *Medical-surgical nursing: Assessment and management of clinical problems* (7th ed., p. 1652). St. Louis: Mosby.

---

45. A client has just had a plaster cast removed from the right arm. The nurse assesses the skin to ensure intactness and then does which of the following?
1 Soaks the arm in warm water for 1 hour
2 Washes the skin gently and applies skin lotion
3 Scrubs the skin vigorously with soap and water
4 Instructs the client that continuous skin soaking will be necessary for the next 24 hours to remove debris

Level of Cognitive Ability: Application
Client Needs: Health Promotion and Maintenance
Integrated Process: Nursing Process/ Implementation
Content Area: Adult Health

Answer: 2

Rationale: The skin under a casted area may be discolored and crusted with dead skin layers. Once the skin is inspected for intactness, the nurse would gently wash the skin and apply a generous coating of lotion, gently massaging it into the skin. The client is instructed that it may take several days for the entire residue and debris to be removed from the skin. Lengthy or continuous soaks may cause excessive skin softening that could result in skin breakdown.

Test-Taking Strategy: Eliminate option 3 first because of the word *vigorously.* Next eliminate options 1 and 4 because they are comparable or alike and would lead to excessive skin softening that could result in skin breakdown. Also noting the word *gently* in option 2 will direct you to this option. Review client instructions regarding skin care following removal of a cast and the various test-taking strategies if you had difficulty with this question.

Tip for the Beginning Nursing Student: A plaster cast is a solid and stiff dressing formed with plaster of paris around a limb or other body part to immobilize it. You will learn about casts and the nursing interventions in the care of the client when you study musculoskeletal disorders in your medical-surgical nursing course.

References

Ignatavicius, D., & Workman, M. (2010). *Medical-surgical nursing: Patient-centered collaborative care* (6th ed., p. 1194). Philadelphia: Saunders.

Linton, A., & Maebius, N. (2007). *Introduction to medical-surgical nursing* (4th ed., p. 922). Philadelphia: Saunders.

46. A home care nurse is assessing a client who began using peritoneal dialysis 1 week ago. The nurse would suspect the onset of peritonitis if which of the following is noted on assessment?
1 Anorexia
2 Cloudy dialysate output
3 Mild abdominal discomfort
4 Oral temperature of 99.0° F

Level of Cognitive Ability: Analysis
Client Needs: Physiological Integrity
Integrated Process: Nursing Process/ Assessment/Data Collection
Content Area: Adult Health

Answer: 2
Rationale: Typical symptoms of peritonitis include fever, nausea, malaise, rebound abdominal tenderness, and cloudy dialysate output. The very slight temperature elevation in option 4 is not the clearest indicator of infection. The complaint of anorexia is too vague to indicate peritonitis. Some mild abdominal discomfort may occur initially with peritoneal dialysis. Peritonitis would cause cloudy dialysate output.

Test-Taking Strategy: Focus on the subject—peritonitis. Use medical terminology to recall that the suffix *-itis* indicates inflammation or infection. Eliminate option 1 first because it is a vague symptom. Next eliminate option 3 because of the word *mild*. From the remaining options, note that the temperature is only slightly elevated and recall that infection would cause white blood cells to be present in the dialysate output, which would yield cloudiness. Review the signs of peritonitis in the client receiving peritoneal dialysis and the various test-taking strategies if you had difficulty with this question.

Tip for the Beginning Nursing Student: Peritoneal dialysis is a procedure used for clients with kidney failure to remove toxins and other wastes that are normally removed by the kidneys from the body. It is a procedure that uses the peritoneum (membrane that lines the abdominal cavity) as the membrane to filter out these toxins and wastes. Fluid (dialysate) flows into the abdominal cavity, filters out these toxins and wastes, and flows out. One complication of peritoneal dialysis is peritonitis, an inflammation and infection of the peritoneum. One indication of peritonitis is cloudy output because output should be clear in consistency. You will learn about peritoneal dialysis and its complications in your medical-surgical nursing course when you study renal (kidney) disorders.

References
Ignatavicius, D., & Workman, M. (2010). *Medical-surgical nursing: Patient-centered collaborative care* (6th ed., p. 1629). Philadelphia: Saunders.
Linton, A., & Maebius, N. (2007). *Introduction to medical-surgical nursing* (4th ed., p. 875). Philadelphia: Saunders.

47. Following right eye cataract surgery, a client is taught to avoid strain on the operative eye. Which statement by the client indicates a need for further teaching?
1 "I should not rub my eye."
2 "I can lie on my right side to sleep at night."
3 "I need to take stool softeners to prevent straining."
4 "I should avoid bending over lower than my waist level."

Answer: 2
Rationale: Following cataract surgery, the client needs to be instructed to lie on the nonoperated side to prevent swelling and pressure in the operated area. Options 1, 3, and 4 are correct measures to take following cataract surgery to reduce strain on the operated eye.

Test-Taking Strategy: Note the strategic words *need for further teaching.* These words indicate a negative event query and the need to select the option that is an incorrect client statement. Recalling that it is necessary to prevent pressure and strain on the operated site will assist in directing you to option 2. If you had difficulty with this

Level of Cognitive Ability: Analysis
Client Needs: Physiological Integrity
Integrated Process: Teaching and
    Learning
Content Area: Adult Health

question, review the client teaching points related to post-operative cataract surgery and the various test-taking strategies.

Tip for the Beginning Nursing Student: A cataract is an abnormal progressive clouding of the lens of the eye that leads to visual loss if untreated. Surgical removal of the lens is done only after vision is compromised. Lens implants may be inserted to restore vision. Following surgery, teaching focuses on proper use and administration of eye medications, protecting the eye, activity restrictions, and preventing infection. You will learn about cataract surgery in your medical-surgical nursing course when you study eye disorders.

References

deWit, S. (2009). *Medical-surgical nursing: Concepts & practice* (p. 643). St. Louis: Saunders.

Lewis, S., Heitkemper, M., Dirksen, S., & Bucher, L. (2007). *Medical-surgical nursing: Assessment and management of clinical problems* (7th ed., p. 428). St. Louis: Mosby.

---

48. The wife of a man who sustained an eye injury calls the emergency room and speaks to a nurse. The wife reports that her husband was hit in the eye area by a piece of board while building a shed in the backyard. The nurse advises the wife to immediately:

1 Call an ambulance.
2 Apply ice to the affected eye.
3 Irrigate the eye with cool water.
4 Bring the husband to the emergency room.

Level of Cognitive Ability: Application
Client Needs: Physiological Integrity
Integrated Process: Nursing Process/
    Implementation
Content Area: Adult Health

Answer: 2

Rationale: Treatment for a contusion ideally begins at the time of injury and includes applying ice to the site. The husband should also receive a thorough eye examination to rule out the presence of other injuries, but this is not the immediate action. Irrigating the eye with cool water may be implemented for injuries that involve a splash of an irritant into the eye. It is not necessary to call an ambulance.

Test-Taking Strategy: Eliminate options 1 and 4 first because they are comparable or alike. From the remaining options, focusing on the type of injury sustained will direct you to option 2. Review initial treatment following an eye contusion and the various test-taking strategies if you had difficulty with this question.

Tip for the Beginning Nursing Student: An eye contusion is an injury caused by a blow to the eye area. A contusion does not disrupt the integrity of the skin but causes swelling, pain, and bruising. Ice is immediately applied to limit swelling, pain, and bruising. You will learn about eye injuries in your medical-surgical nursing course when you study eye disorders.

References

Christensen, B., & Kockrow, E. (2006). *Adult health nursing* (5th ed., p. 178). St. Louis: Mosby.

Ignatavicius, D., & Workman, M. (2010). *Medical-surgical nursing: Patient-centered collaborative care* (6th ed., p. 1103). Philadelphia: Saunders.

49. A nurse employed in an eye clinic checks a client's intraocular pressure and notes that the pressure is 16 mm Hg in the right eye and 18 mm Hg in the left eye. The nurse tells the client that the pressure is:
1 Normal in both eyes
2 Elevated in the left eye
3 Elevated in the right eye
4 Low in both eyes, requiring treatment to increase it

Level of Cognitive Ability: Application
Client Needs: Health Promotion and Maintenance
Integrated Process: Nursing Process/Implementation
Content Area: Adult Health

Answer: 1
Rationale: Normal intraocular pressure ranges from 10 to 21 mm Hg. Therefore the client's intraocular pressure is normal, and options 2, 3, and 4 are incorrect.

Test-Taking Strategy: Focus on the data presented in the question. Recalling that normal intraocular pressure ranges from 10 to 21 mm Hg will direct you to option 1. Review this normal finding and the various test-taking strategies if you had difficulty with this question.

Tip for the Beginning Nursing Student: Intraocular pressure is the pressure within the eye and is regulated by the flow of aqueous humor through the trabecular meshwork. An increase in intraocular pressure is associated with a condition known as glaucoma. If glaucoma is untreated, complete and permanent blindness can occur. You will learn about glaucoma and the implications associated with an elevated intraocular pressure in your medical-surgical nursing course when you study eye disorders.

References
deWit, S. (2009). *Medical-surgical nursing: Concepts & practice* (p. 619). St. Louis: Saunders.
Ignatavicius, D., & Workman, M. (2010). *Medical-surgical nursing: Patient-centered collaborative care* (6th ed., p. 1080). Philadelphia: Saunders.

---

50. A stapedectomy is performed on a client with otosclerosis. The nurse prepares the client for discharge and provides the client with which home care instruction?
1 Expect acute vertigo to occur.
2 Lie on the operated ear with the head of the bed flat.
3 You can sneeze or blow your nose as you usually do.
4 Delay plans for air travel for at least 1 month.

Level of Cognitive Ability: Application
Client Needs: Physiological Integrity
Integrated Process: Teaching and Learning
Content Area: Adult Health

Answer: 4
Rationale: Following stapedectomy the client is instructed to lie on the nonoperated ear with the head of the bed elevated. The client should also avoid excessive exercise, straining, and activities that might lead to head trauma. If the client needs to blow the nose, it should be done gently, one nostril at a time, and the client should sneeze with the mouth open. The acute onset of vertigo needs to be reported to the physician. No air travel is allowed for 1 month.

Test-Taking Strategy: Focus on the surgical procedure and its location to direct you to option 4. Also, eliminate option 2 because of the words *lie on the operated ear with the head of the bed flat*, option 1 because of the words *acute vertigo*, and option 3 because of the words *as you usually do*. Review postoperative care following stapedectomy and the various test-taking strategies if you had difficulty with this question.

Tip for the Beginning Nursing Student: Otosclerosis is a condition in which ossification occurs in the ossicles of the middle ear (especially the stapes), leading to hearing loss. Stapedectomy is the removal of the fixed stapes. Insertion of a graft and prosthesis is done to restore hearing. You will learn about otosclerosis and stapedectomy in your medical-surgical nursing course when you study ear disorders.

References

deWit, S. (2009). *Medical-surgical nursing: Concepts & practice* (p. 661). St. Louis: Saunders.

Monahan, F., Sands, J., Marek, J., Neighbors, M., & Green, C. (2007). *Phipps' medical-surgical nursing: Health and illness perspectives* (8th ed., p. 1853). St. Louis: Mosby.

---

51. A nurse is teaching the client taking medications by inhalation about the advantages of a spacer device. The nurse tells the client that the spacer:

1 Disperses medication more deeply and uniformly

2 Reduces the frequency of medication use to only once per day

3 Requires coordinating timing between pressing the inhaler and inhaling

4 Totally eliminates the chance of developing a yeast infection in the mouth

Level of Cognitive Ability: Application
Client Needs: Physiological Integrity
Integrated Process: Teaching and Learning
Content Area: Adult Health

Answer: 1

Rationale: There are key advantages to the use of a spacer device for medications administered by inhalation. One is that it reduces (not totally eliminates) the incidence of yeast infections because large medication droplets are not deposited on oral tissues. The medication is also dispersed more deeply and uniformly than without a spacer. There is less need to coordinate the effort of inhalation with pressing on the canister of the inhaler. Finally, the use of a spacer may decrease either the number or the volume of the puffs taken.

Test-Taking Strategy: Eliminate option 2 because of the close-ended word *only*. Also option 2 is limited by description. Next eliminate option 4 because of the close-ended words *totally eliminates*. From the remaining options visualize this device to assist in eliminating option 3. Review the advantages of the use of the spacer with inhaled medications and the various test-taking strategies if you had difficulty with this question.

Tip for the Beginning Nursing Student: Some medications, particularly respiratory medications, are administered by the inhalation route. To accomplish administration by this route, special inhalation devices are used. A spacer device is a small piece of equipment that can be attached to the inhalation device to make the administration of the medication easier for the client. Teaching the client how to use these devices is an important nursing intervention. You will learn about these devices and how to use them in a pharmacology course or in your medical-surgical nursing course when you study respiratory disorders.

References

Christensen, B., & Kockrow, E. (2006). *Adult health nursing* (5th ed., p. 459). St. Louis: Mosby.

Monahan, F., Sands, J., Marek, J., Neighbors, M., & Green, C. (2007). *Phipps' medical-surgical nursing: Health and illness perspectives* (8th ed., pp. 625-626). St. Louis: Mosby.

---

52. A client diagnosed with acquired immunodeficiency syndrome (AIDS) is hospitalized. The nurse develops a plan of care and determines that which intervention is the priority?

1 Providing emotional support to the client

Answer: 2

Rationale: The client with AIDS has inadequate immune bodies and is at risk for infection. The priority nursing intervention would be to protect the client from infection. The nurse would also provide emotional support to the client, but this is not the priority from the options provided. Discussing the ways that the client contracted the AIDS virus and the ways others can contract AIDS are not appropriate priority interventions.

2 Instituting measures to prevent infection in the client

3 Identifying the ways that AIDS can be contracted by others

4 Discussing the ways that the client contracted the AIDS virus

Level of Cognitive Ability: Application
Client Needs: Physiological Integrity
Integrated Process: Nursing Process/ Planning
Content Area: Adult Health

Test-Taking Strategy: Note the strategic word *priority*. Eliminate options 3 and 4 first because they are comparable or alike. Also use Maslow's Hierarchy of Needs theory to remember that physiological needs are the priority. This will direct you to option 2. Review the priority needs of a client with AIDS and the test-taking strategies for answering prioritizing questions if you had difficulty with this question.

Tip for the Beginning Nursing Student: AIDS is a syndrome that is caused by the human immunodeficiency virus (HIV), a retrovirus that attacks and kills CD4+ lymphocytes (T helper cells). This results in a weakening of the immune system's ability to prevent infection. You will learn about AIDS in your medical-surgical nursing course when you study immune disorders.

References
deWit, S. (2009). *Medical-surgical nursing: Concepts & practice* (p. 253). St. Louis: Saunders.
Monahan, F., Sands, J., Marek, J., Neighbors, M., & Green, C. (2007). *Phipps' medical-surgical nursing: Health and illness perspectives* (8th ed., pp. 490-491). St. Louis: Mosby.

---

53. A client who is recovering from a brain attack (stroke) has residual dysphagia. To assist in assessing the client's swallowing ability the nurse would ask the client to do which of the following?

1 Swallow some water.

2 Produce an audible cough.

3 Suck on a piece of hard candy.

4 Swallow a teaspoon of applesauce.

Level of Cognitive Ability: Application
Client Needs: Safe and Effective Care Environment
Integrated Process: Nursing Process/ Implementation
Content Area: Adult Health

Answer: 2
Rationale: To assess the client's readiness and ability to swallow, the nurse would assess the client's level of consciousness (client needs to be alert), check for a gag reflex (gag reflex must be present), have the client produce an audible cough (client must be able to produce an audible cough), and ask the client to produce a voluntary swallow (client must be able to do this). The nurse would not give the client a liquid or food item and would not ask the client to suck on a piece of hard candy or any other item because of the risk of aspiration.

Test-Taking Strategy: Eliminate options 1, 3, and 4 first because they are comparable or alike and would place the client at risk for aspiration. Also, use the ABCs—airway, breathing, and circulation—to direct you to option 2. Review care of the client with residual dysphagia and the various test-taking strategies if you had difficulty with this question.

Tip for the Beginning Nursing Student: A brain attack (stroke) is an abnormal condition of the brain that is caused by an occlusion from a thrombus, embolus, vasospasm, or hemorrhage. Dysphagia refers to difficulty with swallowing and can occur as a result of the stroke. It places the client at risk for aspiration. You will learn about a brain attack (stroke) and dysphagia in your medical-surgical nursing course when you study neurological disorders.

References

Lewis, S., Heitkemper, M., Dirksen, S., & Bucher, L. (2007). *Medical-surgical nursing: Assessment and management of clinical problems* (7th ed., p. 1460). St. Louis: Mosby.

Linton, A. (2007). *Introduction to medical-surgical nursing* (4th ed., p. 482). Philadelphia: Saunders.

Potter, P., & Perry, A. (2009). *Fundamentals of nursing* (7th ed., pp. 1101, 1104). St. Louis: Mosby.

---

54. A client with chronic renal failure returns to the nursing unit after receiving his second hemodialysis treatment; the nurse is monitoring the client closely for signs of disequilibrium syndrome. What is a sign of this syndrome?
1 Irritability
2 Tachycardia
3 Hypothermia
4 Mental confusion

Level of Cognitive Ability: Analysis
Client Needs: Physiological Integrity
Integrated Process: Nursing Process/ Assessment/Data Collection
Content Area: Adult Health

Answer: 4

Rationale: Disequilibrium syndrome most often occurs in clients who are new to hemodialysis. It is characterized by headache, mental confusion, decreasing level of consciousness, nausea, vomiting, twitching, and possible seizure activity. It results from rapid removal of solutes from the body during hemodialysis and a higher residual concentration gradient in the brain because of the blood-brain barrier. Water goes into cerebral cells because of the osmotic gradient, causing brain swelling and onset of symptoms. It is prevented by dialyzing for shorter times or at reduced blood flow rates. The signs in options 1, 2, and 3 are not associated with disequilibrium syndrome.

Test-Taking Strategy: Focusing on the name of the syndrome will direct you to option 4. This is the only option that addresses a neurological sign. Review the signs of disequilibrium syndrome and the various test-taking strategies if you had difficulty with this question.

Tip for the Beginning Nursing Student: Renal failure is a condition in which the kidneys are unable to excrete wastes, concentrate urine, and conserve electrolytes. A component of treatment is hemodialysis. Hemodialysis requires the use of a dialyzer that is connected to a shunt, fistula, or other device that allows access to the client's bloodstream. The client's blood is transported from the body through the dialyzer, which removes wastes and excess fluids from the blood. The cleaned blood is then returned to the client's body. Disequilibrium syndrome is one complication that car occur as a result of hemodialysis. You will learn about renal failure and disequilibrium syndrome in your medical-surgical nursing course when you study renal disorders.

References

deWit, S. (2009). *Medical-surgical nursing: Concepts & practice* (p. 858). St. Louis: Saunders.

Ignatavicius, D., & Workman, M. (2010). *Medical-surgical nursing: Patient-centered collaborative care* (6th ed., p. 1626). Philadelphia: Saunders.

---

55. A nurse is providing home care instructions to a client with Parkinson's disease about measures to control a right-sided hand tremor. The nurse tells the client to:
1 Sleep on the unaffected side.

Answer: 4

Rationale: The client with a tremor is instructed to use both hands to accomplish a task. The client is also instructed to hold change in a pocket or to squeeze a rubber ball with the affected hand. The client should sleep on the side that has the tremor to control it.

2 Use the left hand only to perform tasks.

3 Use the right hand only to perform tasks.

4 Squeeze a rubber ball with the right hand.

Level of Cognitive Ability: Application
Client Needs: Health Promotion and Maintenance
Integrated Process: Teaching and Learning
Content Area: Adult Health

Test-Taking Strategy: Eliminate options 2 and 3 first because of the close-ended word *only*. From the remaining options visualize each and think about each effect in terms of controlling the tremor. This will direct you to option 4. Review client teaching points for Parkinson's disease and the various test-taking strategies if you had difficulty with this question.

Tip for the Beginning Nursing Student: Parkinson's disease is a progressive neurological disorder that is caused by a depletion of the neurotransmitter dopamine in the brain tissue. It is characterized by resting tremor, pill rolling of the fingers, shuffling gait, mask-like facies, forward flexion of the trunk, muscle rigidity and weakness, and loss of postural reflexes. You will learn about Parkinson's disease in your medical-surgical nursing course when you study neurological disorders.

References

Linton, A. (2007). *Introduction to medical-surgical nursing* (4th ed., p. 448). Philadelphia: Saunders.

Monahan, F., Sands, J., Marek, J., Neighbors, M., & Green, C. (2007). *Phipps' medical-surgical nursing: Health and illness perspectives* (8th ed., p. 1449). St. Louis: Mosby.

---

56. A nurse answers the call bell of a client who has an internal cervical radiation implant. The client states that she thinks that the implant fell out. The nurse checks the client and sees the implant lying in the bed. The nurse immediately uses a long-handled forceps to pick up the implant and places the implant into the lead container in the client's room. Which action would the nurse take next?

1 Ask another nurse to assist in reinserting the implant.

2 Contact the radiation therapist and radiation safety officer.

3 Call for a transport personnel to deliver the lead container to the radiation department.

4 Call a security officer, and ask the officer to send someone to guard the client's room until the situation is resolved.

Level of Cognitive Ability: Application
Client Needs: Safe and Effective Care Environment
Integrated Process: Nursing Process/Implementation
Content Area: Adult Health

Answer: 2

Rationale: A lead container and a pair of long-handled forceps should be kept in the client's room at all times during internal radiation therapy. If the implant becomes dislodged, the nurse should pick up the implant with long-handled forceps and place it in the lead container. The radiation therapist and radiation safety officer are notified immediately of the situation so that they can retrieve and secure the radiation source. The physician is also called after taking action to maintain the safety of the client and others. The nurse does not reinsert a radiation implant device. Options 3 and 4 are incorrect and can expose individuals to the radiation.

Test-Taking Strategy: Note the strategic word *next*. Option 1 can be eliminated first because inserting a radiation device is not a nursing activity. Recalling that the nurse needs to protect himself or herself and others from exposure to the radiation will help eliminate options 3 and 4. Also, these options are comparable or alike. Review the measures related to a dislodged implant and the various test-taking strategies if you had difficulty with this question.

Tip for the Beginning Nursing Student: A cervical radiation implant is a device that is placed in the area of the cervix and emits radiation to the body area. It is a treatment measure for cervical cancer. Because exposure to radiation can be harmful, special precautions are taken to prevent exposure to other individuals. You will learn about cancer and its treatment and about radiation implants in your medical-surgical nursing course when you study oncologic disorders.

References
deWit, S. (2009). *Medical-surgical nursing: Concepts & practice* (p. 175). St. Louis: Saunders.
Ignatavicius, D., & Workman, M. (2010). *Medical-surgical nursing: Patient-centered collaborative care* (6th ed., p. 420). Philadelphia: Saunders.

57. A nurse is caring for a hospitalized client with a diagnosis of acute pancreatitis. The nurse assists the client to which position that will decrease the abdominal pain?

1 Prone
2 Supine with the legs straight
3 Side-lying with the head of the bed flat
4 Upright in a sitting position with the trunk flexed

Level of Cognitive Ability: Application
Client Needs: Physiological Integrity
Integrated Process: Nursing Process/ Implementation
Content Area: Adult Health

Answer: 4

Rationale: Correct positioning will assist in providing comfort to the client with acute pancreatitis. These positions include a side-lying position with the knees curled up to the chest and a pillow pressed against the abdomen or upright in a sitting position with the trunk flexed. Options 1, 2, and 3 are incorrect.

Test-Taking Strategy: Focus on the client's diagnosis, and evaluate each option in terms of the amount of stretching or flexing of the abdominal wall that the action will cause. Also note that options 1, 2, and 3 are comparable or alike in that they are flat positions. Review the positions that will reduce pain in the client with acute pancreatitis and the various test-taking strategies if you had difficulty with this question.

Tip for the Beginning Nursing Student: Pancreatitis is an inflammatory condition of the pancreas and can be acute or chronic. It is characterized by severe epigastric or upper left quadrant abdominal pain radiating to the back, fever, anorexia, nausea, and vomiting. You will learn about pancreatitis in your medical-surgical nursing course when you study gastrointestinal disorders.

References
deWit, S. (2009). *Medical-surgical nursing: Concepts & practice* (p. 759). St. Louis: Saunders.
Ignatavicius, D., & Workman, M. (2010). *Medical-surgical nursing: Patient-centered collaborative care* (6th ed., p. 1374). Philadelphia: Saunders.

58. The nurse provides home care instructions to a client diagnosed with viral hepatitis. The nurse determines that the client understands the instructions if the client makes which statement?

1 "I need to limit my intake of alcohol."
2 "I need to remain in bed for the next 6 weeks."
3 "I can take acetaminophen (Tylenol) for any discomfort."
4 "I need to eat small frequent meals that are low in fat and protein."

Answer: 4

Rationale: Fatigue is a normal response to hepatic cellular damage. During the acute stage, rest is an essential intervention to reduce the liver's metabolic demands and increase its blood supply, but bedrest for 6 weeks is unnecessary. The client should avoid taking all medications, including acetaminophen (which is hepatotoxic), unless prescribed by the physician. The client needs to avoid all alcohol consumption. The client should consume small frequent meals that are low in fat and protein to reduce the workload of the liver.

Test-Taking Strategy: Eliminate option 1 first, recalling that the client needs to avoid (not limit) alcohol intake. Next eliminate option 2 because of the words *next 6 weeks*. From the remaining options recalling that acetaminophen is hepatotoxic will assist in eliminating option 3. Review

Level of Cognitive Ability: Application
Client Needs: Physiological Integrity
Integrated Process: Nursing Process/
   Evaluation
Content Area: Adult Health

instructions for the client with viral hepatitis and the various test-taking strategies if you had difficulty with this question.

Tip for the Beginning Nursing Student: Viral hepatitis is an inflammatory disease of the liver caused by one of the hepatitis viruses. It is characterized by jaundice, anorexia, abdominal and gastric discomfort, hepatomegaly, clay-colored stools, and tea-colored urine. The liver is usually able to regenerate its tissue, and rest is a key component of therapy. You will learn about viral hepatitis when you study gastrointestinal disorders in your medical-surgical nursing course.

References
deWit, S. (2009). *Medical-surgical nursing: Concepts & practice* (p. 746). St. Louis: Saunders.
Ignatavicius, D., & Workman, M. (2010). *Medical-surgical nursing: Patient-centered collaborative care* (6th ed., p. 1360). Philadelphia: Saunders.

---

59. A hospitalized client with chronic renal failure has returned to the nursing unit after a hemodialysis treatment. The nurse checks pre-dialysis and postdialysis documentation of which parameters to determine the effectiveness of the procedure?
  1 Weight and blood urea nitrogen (BUN)
  2 Potassium level and creatinine levels
  3 Blood pressure and weight
  4 BUN and creatinine levels

Level of Cognitive Ability: Analysis
Client Needs: Physiological Integrity
Integrated Process: Nursing Process/
   Evaluation
Content Area: Adult Health

Answer: 3
Rationale: Following hemodialysis the client's vital signs are monitored to determine whether the client is remaining hemodynamically stable and for comparison to predialysis measurements. The client's blood pressure and weight are expected to be reduced as a result of fluid removal. Laboratory studies are done as per protocol but are not necessarily done after the hemodialysis treatment has ended.

Test-Taking Strategy: Focus on the subject—determining the effectiveness of hemodialysis—and note that this is an evaluation-type question. Also remember that when options contain two parts both parts need to be correct in order for the option to be the correct one. Knowing that weight is an important variable allows you to eliminate options 2 and 4. From the remaining options, recalling that vital signs reflect hemodynamic stability will direct you to option 3. Review the parameters that will determine the effectiveness of hemodialysis and the various test-taking strategies if you had difficulty with this question.

Tip for the Beginning Nursing Student: Renal failure is a condition in which the kidneys are unable to excrete wastes, concentrate urine, and conserve electrolytes. A component of treatment is hemodialysis. Hemodialysis requires the use of a dialyzer that is connected to a shunt, fistula, or other device that allows access to the client's bloodstream. The client's blood is transported from the body through the dialyzer, which removes wastes and excess fluids from the blood. The cleaned blood is then returned to the client's body. You will learn about renal failure and hemodialysis in your medical-surgical nursing course when you study renal disorders.

References

Ignatavicius, D., & Workman, M. (2006). *Medical-surgical nursing: Patient-centered collaborative care* (6th ed., p. 1625). Philadelphia: Saunders.

Linton, A. (2007). *Introduction to medical-surgical nursing* (4th ed., p. 870). Philadelphia: Saunders.

60. A nurse is developing a plan of care for a client who is experiencing homonymous hemianopsia following a brain attack (stroke). The nurse documents interventions that will promote a safe environment knowing that in this disorder the client:

1 Has a visual loss in the same half of the visual field of each eye

2 Has lost the ability to recognize familiar objects through the senses

3 Has paralysis of the sympathetic nerves of the eye causing sinking of the eyeball

4 Is unable to carry out a skilled act, such as dressing, in the absence of paralysis

Level of Cognitive Ability: Application
Client Needs: Safe and Effective Care Environment
Integrated Process: Nursing Process/ Planning
Content Area: Adult Health

Answer: 1

Rationale: Homonymous hemianopsia is a visual loss in the same half of the visual field of each eye so the client has only half of normal vision. Option 2 describes agnosia. Option 3 describes Horner's syndrome. Option 4 describes apraxia.

Test-Taking Strategy: Focus on the subject—homonymous hemianopsia. Use medical terminology, noting that *hemi-* means half and *-op-* refers to the eye. This will direct you to option 1. Review care for the client with homonymous hemianopsia and the various test-taking strategies if you had difficulty with this question.

Tip for the Beginning Nursing Student: A brain attack (stroke) is an abnormal condition of the brain that is caused by an occlusion from a thrombus, embolus, vasospasm, or hemorrhage. Homonymous hemianopsia is a visual loss in the same half of the visual field of each eye, so the client has only half of normal vision. This disorder can occur as a result of the stroke and places the client at risk for injury. You will learn about a brain attack (stroke) and homonymous hemianopsia in your medical-surgical nursing course when you study neurological disorders.

References

Christensen, B., & Kockrow, E. (2006). *Adult health nursing* (5th ed., p. 730). St. Louis: Mosby.

Monahan, F., Sands, J., Marek, J., Neighbors, M., & Green, C. (2007). *Phipps' medical-surgical nursing: Health and illness perspectives* (8th ed., pp. 1428, 1436). St. Louis: Mosby.

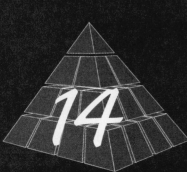

14 Chapter

Mental Health Questions

61. A nurse helps a client with a diagnosis of obsessive-compulsive disorder prepare for bed. One hour later, the client calls the nurse and says he is feeling anxious and asks the nurse to sit and talk for a while. The nurse takes which appropriate initial action?
1 Sits and talks with the client
2 Asks a nursing assistant to sit with the client
3 Asks the client if he would like an antianxiety medication
4 Tells the client that it is time for sleep and that they will talk tomorrow

Level of Cognitive Ability: Application
Client Needs: Psychosocial Integrity
Integrated Process: Caring
Content Area: Mental Health

Answer: 1

Rationale: The appropriate initial nursing action is to sit and talk if the client is expressing anxiety. Antianxiety medication may be necessary, but this is not the initial nursing action. A nursing assistant may not be able to alleviate the client's anxiety. Option 4 is an inappropriate action and places the client's feelings on hold.

Test-Taking Strategy: Note the strategic word *initial*, and use therapeutic communication techniques. Recalling that it is best to address the client's feelings assists in directing you to option 1. Review care of the client with obsessive-compulsive disorder and the various test-taking strategies if you had difficulty with this question.

Tip for the Beginning Nursing Student: Obsessive-compulsive disorder is an anxiety disorder that is characterized by obsessions (ideas, emotions, or impulses that repetitively and insistently force themselves into consciousness) or compulsions (recurrent irresistible impulses to perform some act) that interfere with the individual's normal routine. Therapeutic communication techniques, which promote and encourage the client to communicate and share his or her feelings with the nurse, should be used when caring for a client. You will learn about therapeutic and nontherapeutic communication techniques in your fundamentals of nursing course and about obsessive-compulsive disorder in your mental health nursing course.

References
Keltner, N. Schwecke, L. & Bostro, C. (2007). *Psychiatric nursing* (5th ed., p. 421). St. Louis: Mosby.
Varcarolis, E., Carlson, V., & Shoemaker, N. (2006). *Foundations of psychiatric mental health nursing* (5th ed., p. 290). Philadelphia: Saunders.

62. A nurse is performing an admission interview on a client being admitted to the mental health unit and discovers that the client experienced a severe emotional trauma 1 month ago and is now experiencing paralysis of the right arm. The priority nursing action is to:

1 Refer the client to group therapy.
2 Encourage the client to talk about his feelings.
3 Encourage the client to move and use the arm.
4 Assess the client for organic causes of the paralysis.

Level of Cognitive Ability: Application
Client Needs: Physiological Integrity
Integrated Process: Nursing Process/ Implementation
Content Area: Mental Health

Answer: 4

Rationale: The priority action is to assess for any physiological cause of the paralysis. Although a component of the plan of care is to encourage the client to discuss feelings, this is not the priority action. It is not appropriate to encourage the client to use the arm without ruling out a physiological cause of the paralysis. Although the client may be referred to group therapy, this also is not the initial action.

Test-Taking Strategy: Note the strategic word *priority*. Use Maslow's Hierarchy of Needs theory to remember that physiological needs are the first priority. Option 4 is the only one that addresses a physiological need. Review care of the mental health client who experiences physiological disorders and the test-taking strategies for answering prioritizing questions if you had difficulty with this question.

Tip for the Beginning Nursing Student: A conversion disorder is a somatoform disorder characterized by a loss or alteration of physical functioning without evidence of organic impairment. A conversion disorder can result after a traumatic experience. You will learn about conversion disorders in your mental health nursing course.

References

Linton, A. (2007). *Introduction to medical-surgical nursing* (4th ed., p. 85). Philadelphia: Saunders.
Varcarolis, E., Carlson, V., & Shoemaker, N. (2006). *Foundations of psychiatric mental health nursing* (5th ed., p. 5). Philadelphia: Saunders.

63. A nurse is developing a plan of care for a client admitted to the mental health unit with a diagnosis of obsessive-compulsive disorder who is experiencing severe anxiety. The nurse's priority in the plan of care for this client is to:

1 Monitor for repetitive behavior.
2 Demand active participation in care.
3 Educate the client about self-care demands.
4 Establish a trusting and therapeutic nurse–client relationship.

Level of Cognitive Ability: Application
Client Needs: Psychosocial Integrity
Integrated Process: Caring
Content Area: Mental Health

Answer: 4

Rationale: The priority nursing action is to establish a trusting and therapeutic relationship with the client. The nurse should never demand anything from the client. The remaining options are appropriate components of the plan of care but are not the priority. A trusting nurse–client relationship needs to be established first.

Test-Taking Strategy: Focus on the strategic word *priority*, and note that the client is being admitted to the mental health unit. Recalling that a nurse–client relationship needs to be developed first assists in directing you to option 4. Review care to the client with obsessive-compulsive disorder and the test-taking strategies for answering prioritizing questions if you had difficulty with this question.

Tip for the Beginning Nursing Student: Obsessive-compulsive disorder is an anxiety disorder that is characterized by obsessions (ideas, emotions, or impulses that repetitively and insistently force themselves into consciousness) or compulsions (recurrent irresistible impulses to perform some act) that interfere with the individual's normal routine. The first step to providing therapeutic care for the client is to establish a trusting and therapeutic relationship. If trust is established, the client is more likely to communicate with the nurse. You will learn about the techniques for establishing a trusting and therapeutic relationship with a client in your fundamentals of nursing course and about obsessive-compulsive disorder in your mental health nursing course.

References

Keltner, N. Schwecke, L., & Bostro, C. (2007). *Psychiatric nursing* (5th ed., p. 421). St. Louis: Mosby.

Varcarolis, E., Carlson, V., & Shoemaker, N. (2006). *Foundations of psychiatric mental health nursing* (5th ed., p. 290). Philadelphia: Saunders.

---

64. A nurse is preparing to care for a client admitted to the mental health unit with a diagnosis of dementia and notes a nursing diagnosis of *Self-care deficit* in the plan of care. The nurse plans for which outcome in caring for the client?

1 The client will feed self with cueing within 24 hours.

2 The client will be oriented to place by the time of discharge.

3 The client will be free of hallucinations by the time of discharge.

4 The client will correctly identify objects in his or her room by the time of discharge.

Level of Cognitive Ability: Application
Client Needs: Physiological Integrity
Integrated Process: Nursing Process/ Planning
Content Area: Mental Health

Answer: 1

Rationale: Option 1 identifies an outcome directly related to the client's ability to care for self. Options 2, 3, and 4 are not related to *Self-care deficit*.

Test-Taking Strategy: Note the relationship between the nursing diagnosis *Self-care deficit* and option 1. Also use Maslow's Hierarchy of Needs theory. Option 1 is the only one that addresses a physiological need. Review care of the client with dementia and the various test-taking strategies if you had difficulty with this question.

Tip for the Beginning Nursing Student: Dementia is a term that describes an organic mental disorder characterized by cognitive impairments that are generally of gradual onset and are irreversible. *Self-care deficit* refers to the inability of an individual to care for self. A *Self-care deficit* can occur as a result of dementia, which you will learn about in your mental health nursing course.

References

Keltner, N. Schwecke, L., & Bostro, C. (2007). *Psychiatric nursing* (5th ed., pp. 460-461). St. Louis: Mosby.

Varcarolis, E., Carlson, V., & Shoemaker, N. (2006). *Foundations of psychiatric mental health nursing* (5th ed., p. 443). Philadelphia: Saunders.

---

65. A client experiencing delusions of being poisoned is admitted to the hospital after not eating or drinking for several days. The client shows no evidence of dehydration and malnutrition at this time. The nurse prepares a plan of care for the client and includes which client need as the priority?

1 Self-esteem needs

2 Physiological needs

3 Safety and security needs

4 Love and belonging needs

Answer: 3

Rationale: The maintenance of safety is an important consideration when working with clients who have delusions. No data in the question indicate that options 1, 2, and 4 require immediate attention.

Test-Taking Strategy: Note the strategic words *priority* and *shows no evidence of dehydration and malnutrition*. Use Maslow's Hierarchy of Needs theory. Safety takes precedence if a physiological need does not exist. This will direct you to option 3. Review care of the client experiencing delusions and the test-taking strategies for answering prioritizing questions if you had difficulty with this question.

Level of Cognitive Ability: Application
Client Needs: Safe and Effective Care Environment
Integrated Process: Nursing Process/ Planning
Content Area: Mental Health

Tip for the Beginning Nursing Student: A delusion is a false belief that is firmly maintained by a client even though the belief is not shared by others. The nurse should not attempt to obtain a logical explanation about the delusion from the client. Only the client understands the logic behind the delusion, yet he or she is not able to express it until the delusion has reached conscious awareness. You will learn about delusions and how to deal with a client experiencing them in your mental health nursing course.

References
Keltner, N., Schwecke, L., & Bostro, C. (2007). *Psychiatric nursing* (5th ed., p. 105). St. Louis: Mosby.
Varcarolis, E., Carlson, V., & Shoemaker, N. (2006). *Foundations of psychiatric mental health nursing* (5th ed., p. 400). Philadelphia: Saunders.

---

66. An older woman is admitted to the acute psychiatric unit with a diagnosis of moderate depression. The client is unclean, her hair is uncombed, and she is inappropriately dressed. She is accompanied by her adult daughter who is very upset about her mother's lack of interest in her appearance. The nurse appropriately alleviates the daughter's concern by telling her that:
1 Hygiene is not important to those who are depressed.
2 Client self-esteem needs take priority over appearances.
3 Group peer pressure on the unit will soon have her mother attending to her hygiene needs.
4 The nurse will assist her mother in meeting hygiene needs until she is able to resume self-care.

Level of Cognitive Ability: Application
Client Needs: Psychosocial Integrity
Integrated Process: Caring
Content Area: Mental Health

Answer: 4
Rationale: Both the client and her family should know that the nurse will assist the client until she can resume self-care activities. The client is experiencing psychomotor retardation and decreased energy at this time and requires assistance. Options 1, 2, and 3 will not alleviate the daughter's concern.

Test-Taking Strategy: Focus on the subject—alleviating the daughter's concern—and use Maslow's Hierarchy of Needs theory. Only option 4 addresses the client's physiological needs. Review care of the client with depression and the various test-taking strategies if you had difficulty with this question.

Tip for the Beginning Nursing Student: Depression is a state of sadness or grief and can range from mild and moderate states to severe states. The potential for suicidal behavior should always be assessed in a client experiencing depression. You will learn about depression, its many causes, and the nursing care involved in your mental health nursing course.

References
Fortinash, K., & Holoday-Worret, P. (2008). *Psychiatric mental health nursing* (4th ed., p. 355). St. Louis: Mosby.
Varcarolis, E., Carlson, V., & Shoemaker, N. (2006). *Foundations of psychiatric mental health nursing* (5th ed., p. 336). Philadelphia: Saunders.

---

67. A nurse is preparing to care for a woman victimized by physical abuse. The nurse would plan to first:
1 Support the woman, and facilitate access to a safe environment.

Answer: 1
Rationale: The nurse must provide emotional support to the client and provide measures to ensure a safe environment. Option 2 fosters the notion that the client is at fault. In options 3 and 4 the nurse may be making unreasonable demands, which could cause further distress for the client.

2 Talk to the woman about the fact that she might have provoked the abuse.

3 Reinforce that dealing with the psychological aspects is of the highest priority.

4 Establish firm time lines for the woman to make necessary changes in her life situation.

Level of Cognitive Ability: Application
Client Needs: Safe and Effective Care Environment
Integrated Process: Caring
Content Area: Mental Health

Test-Taking Strategy: Note the strategic word *first.* Use Maslow's Hierarchy of Needs theory to direct you to option 1. Remember that if a physiological need does not exist in one of the options, then a safety need is the priority. Also option 1 provides support to the client. Review care of the client victimized by physical abuse and the test-taking strategies for answering prioritizing questions if you had difficulty with this question.

Tip for the Beginning Nursing Student: Physical abuse is a form of violence. In most states the nurse is required to report abuse to legal authorities if abuse is suspected or occurs in a child or elderly client. If abuse occurs, the priority is to treat any physical injuries sustained. Next it is important to provide support and a safe environment for the victim. You will learn about violence and abuse in your mental health nursing course.

References

Fortinash, K., & Holoday-Worret, P. (2008). *Psychiatric mental health nursing* (4th ed., p. 488). St. Louis: Mosby.

Varcarolis, E., Carlson, V., & Shoemaker, N. (2006). *Foundations of psychiatric mental health nursing* (5th ed., p. 512). Philadelphia: Saunders.

---

68. A client is scheduled for electroconvulsive therapy (ECT). The client says to the nurse, "I am so afraid that it will hurt and will make me worse off than I am." The nurse makes which best statement to the client?

1 "Can you tell me what you understand about the procedure?"

2 "Your fears are a sign that you really should have this procedure."

3 "Try not to worry. This is a well-known and easy procedure for the doctor."

4 "Those are very normal fears, but please be assured that everything will be okay."

Level of Cognitive Ability: Application
Client Needs: Psychosocial Integrity
Integrated Process: Caring
Content Area: Mental Health

Answer: 1

Rationale: Option 1 is a therapeutic communication technique that explores the client's feelings, determines the level of client understanding about the procedure, and displays caring. Option 2 demeans the client and does not encourage further sharing by the client. Option 3 diminishes the client's feelings by directing attention away from the client and to the doctor's importance. Option 4 does not address the client's fears and puts the client's feelings on hold.

Test-Taking Strategy: Use therapeutic communication techniques, and remember to focus on the client's feelings and concerns. Option 1 is the only option that addresses the client's feelings, encourages client verbalization, and displays caring. Review therapeutic communication techniques and the test-taking strategies for answering communication questions if you had difficulty with this question.

Tip for the Beginning Nursing Student: ECT is a treatment in which a tonic-clonic (grand mal) seizure is artificially induced in an anesthetized client by passing an electrical current through electrodes applied to the client's head. A primary indication for using ECT is major depression. Therapeutic communication techniques promote and encourage the client to communicate and share his or her feelings with the nurse. Nontherapeutic communication techniques block the communication process and are not methods that the nurse would use when caring for a client. You will learn about therapeutic and nontherapeutic communication techniques in your fundamentals of nursing course and about ECT in your mental health nursing course.

References

Fortinash, K., & Holoday-Worret, P. (2008). *Psychiatric mental health nursing* (4th ed., pp. 69-73, 535). St. Louis: Mosby.

Varcarolis, E., Carlson, V., & Shoemaker, N. (2006). *Foundations of psychiatric mental health nursing* (5th ed., pp. 185-190, 351-352). Philadelphia: Saunders.

---

69. A woman is treated in the emergency department for a broken clavicle and a black eye. The woman reports that she sustained the injury from falling off a stepstool while trying to change window curtains. If the nurse suspected physical abuse by the client's husband, which statement would best encourage the client to share this information with the nurse?

1 "That black eye looks awfully painful. Did your husband hit you?"

2 "Your black eye sure does not seem as though it could have happened by accident."

3 "If your husband is abusing you, you can take him to court or get a restraining order."

4 "At times I see women who have been hurt by their husband. Have you been hurt by anyone?"

Level of Cognitive Ability: Application
Client Needs: Psychosocial Integrity
Integrated Process: Caring
Content Area: Mental Health

Answer: 4

Rationale: The best approach to asking a woman about violence is to approach the client in a caring and nonthreatening manner. Options 1 and 2 are confrontational, and option 3 assumes that the client desires a restraining order. Option 2 is also incorrect because it is a judgmental statement that is likely to put the client on the defensive. Only option 4 allows the client the right to reject or accept further intervention by the nurse and is a caring response.

Test-Taking Strategy: Use therapeutic communication techniques. Option 4 is the only therapeutic statement, is supportive and displays caring, and provides the client the opportunity to talk about the situation if she desires. Review care of the client suspected of being abused and the test-taking strategies for answering communication questions if you had difficulty with this question.

Tip for the Beginning Nursing Student: Physical abuse is a form of violence. If abuse occurs, the priority is to treat any physical injuries sustained. Next it is important to provide support and a safe environment for the victim. The nurse should use therapeutic communication techniques to communicate with the client. Therapeutic communication techniques promote and encourage the client to communicate and share his or her feelings with the nurse. You will learn about therapeutic communication techniques in your fundamentals of nursing course. In addition, you will learn about violence and abuse in your mental health nursing course.

References

Fortinash, K., & Holoday-Worret, P. (2008). *Psychiatric mental health nursing* (4th ed., p. 485). St. Louis: Mosby.

Varcarolis, E., Carlson, V., & Shoemaker, N. (2006). *Foundations of psychiatric mental health nursing* (5th ed., p. 509). Philadelphia: Saunders.

---

70. A mental health client is angry after an argument on the telephone with her son and tells the nurse about her conversation. Which statement by the nurse would be therapeutic?

Answer: 1

Rationale: Option 1 provides an opportunity for the client to further share and discuss feelings. Option 2 is a stereotypical comment. Options 3 and 4 seem to console the client, but they indicate that the nurse has taken "a side" in the argument, which is nontherapeutic.

1 "You seem quite upset."

2 "All mothers have arguments with their children."

3 "You need to focus your energy on building your strength and getting better."

4 "That is not very kind of your son. Does he not realize that you are trying to recuperate from surgery?"

Level of Cognitive Ability: Application
Client Needs: Psychosocial Integrity
Integrated Process: Communication and Documentation
Content Area: Mental Health

Test-Taking Strategy: Use therapeutic communication techniques. Remember to address the client's concerns or feelings and elicit further information from the client. This will direct you to option 1. Review therapeutic communication techniques and the test-taking strategies for answering communication questions if you had difficulty with this question.

Tip for the Beginning Nursing Student: Therapeutic communication techniques promote and encourage the client to communicate and share his or her feelings with the nurse. Nontherapeutic communication techniques block the communication process and are not methods that the nurse would use when caring for a client. You will learn about therapeutic and nontherapeutic communication techniques in your fundamentals of nursing course and in your mental health nursing course.

References
deWit, S. (2009). *Medical-surgical nursing: Concepts & practice* (p. 9). St. Louis: Saunders.
Varcarolis, E., Carlson, V., & Shoemaker, N. (2006). *Foundations of psychiatric mental health nursing* (5th ed., pp. 185-190). Philadelphia: Saunders.

---

71. A mental health nurse is performing an admission interview with a depressed client who has suicidal ideation. Following the interview which nursing intervention is carried out first?

1 Develop a plan of activities for the client.

2 Provide the client with diversional activities.

3 Isolate the client from other clients in the nursing unit.

4 Communicate the client's risk for suicide to all team members.

Level of Cognitive Ability: Application
Client Needs: Safe and Effective Care Environment
Integrated Process: Nursing Process/ Implementation
Content Area: Mental Health

Answer: 4

Rationale: The first priority intervention for the suicidal individual is to communicate the risk for suicide to all team members. The plan of activities (options 1 and 2) would take second priority. Client isolation is inappropriate. The client should be placed on 1:1 supervision if he or she is suicidal.

Test-Taking Strategy: Note the strategic word *first*. Eliminate options 1 and 2 first because they are comparable or alike. From the remaining options the priority item is communication to other members of the health care team, with the ultimate aim to increase client safety. Review care of the client with suicidal ideation and the test-taking strategies for answering prioritizing questions if you had difficulty with this question.

Tip for the Beginning Nursing Student: Suicidal ideation means that the client is having thoughts about self-inflicted death. All suicidal behavior is serious and requires the nurse's immediate attention and highest priority care. You will learn about suicide and the several interventions for the care of a client experiencing suicidal ideation in your mental health nursing course.

References
Keltner, N., Schwecke, L., & Bostro, C. (2007). *Psychiatric nursing* (5th ed., pp. 56-57). St. Louis: Mosby.
Varcarolis, E., Carlson, V., & Shoemaker, N. (2006). *Foundations of psychiatric mental health nursing* (5th ed., p. 481). Philadelphia: Saunders.

72. A client has received electroconvulsive therapy (ECT) for the treatment of major depression. The nurse implements which of the following activities first in the posttreatment area when the client awakens?

1 Discusses the treatment
2 Encourages the client to eat
3 Monitors the client's vital signs
4 Provides frequent reassurance to the client

Level of Cognitive Ability: Application
Client Needs: Physiological Integrity
Integrated Process: Nursing Process/ Implementation
Content Area: Mental Health

Answer: 3

Rationale: The nurse first monitors vital signs and then reviews the ECT treatment with the client. The nursing interventions outlined in options 1, 2, and 4 follow accordingly. In addition, the nurse would assess for the return of a gag reflex before encouraging the client to eat.

Test-Taking Strategy: Note the strategic word *first.* Use the ABCs—airway, breathing, and circulation—to direct you to option 3. Review care of the client receiving electroconvulsive therapy and the test-taking strategies for answering prioritizing questions if you had difficulty with this question.

Tip for the Beginning Nursing Student: Depression is a state of sadness or grief and can range from mild and moderate states to severe states. ECT is a treatment in which a tonic-clonic (grand mal) seizure is artificially induced in an anesthetized client by passing an electrical current through electrodes applied to the client's head. A primary indication for using ECT is major depression. Because the client has been anesthetized and experienced an artificially induced seizure, monitoring vital signs is a priority. You will learn about major depression and ECT in your mental health nursing course.

References

Fortinash, K., & Holoday-Worret, P. (2008). *Psychiatric mental health nursing* (4th ed., p. 536). St. Louis: Mosby.
Linton, A. (2007). *Introduction to medical-surgical nursing* (4th ed., p. 1257). Philadelphia: Saunders.

73. A nurse is developing a plan of care for a client with mania and formulates a nursing diagnosis of *Disturbed thought processes.* Which activity related to this nursing diagnosis would the nurse provide for the client initially?

1 Writing
2 Playing cards with another client
3 Playing checkers with another client
4 Playing a board game with another client

Level of Cognitive Ability: Application
Client Needs: Psychosocial Integrity
Integrated Process: Nursing Process/ Planning
Content Area: Mental Health

Answer: 1

Rationale: When the client is manic, solitary activities requiring a short attention span or mild physical exertion activities, such as writing, painting, finger-painting, woodworking, or walks with the staff, are best initially. Solitary activities minimize stimuli, and mild physical activities release tension constructively. When less manic, the client may join one or two other clients in quiet nonstimulating activities. Competitive games should be avoided because they can stimulate aggression and cause increased psychomotor activity.

Test-Taking Strategy: Note that options 2, 3, and 4 are comparable or alike in that they all involve activities with another individual. Option 1 is the only solitary activity that will minimize stimuli. Review care of the manic client and the various test-taking strategies if you had difficulty with this question.

Tip for the Beginning Nursing Student: Mania is a component of bipolar disorder and is characterized by an elevated, expansive, or irritable mood. The client lacks judgment in anticipating consequences and exhibits disturbed thought processes, pressured speech, flight of ideas, distractibility, inflated self-esteem, and hypersexuality. You will learn about caring for the client with mania in your mental health nursing course.

References

Keltner, N., Schwecke, L., & Bostro, C. (2007). *Psychiatric nursing* (5th ed., pp. 373-374). St. Louis: Mosby.

Varcarolis, E., Carlson, V., & Shoemaker, N. (2006). *Foundations of psychiatric mental health nursing* (5th ed., p. 369). Philadelphia: Saunders.

---

74. A client who has been raped arrives at the emergency department. Which of these observations would be most important for the nurse to consider when planning the immediate care for the client?

1 The victim states that "she feels numb."

2 The victim states that she "feels like it did not happen."

3 The victim states that she knows the rapist well; in fact they had been dating for several weeks.

4 The victim states that the rapist knows where she lives and that "He will kill me if I tell anyone about the rape."

Level of Cognitive Ability: Application
Client Needs: Safe and Effective Care Environment
Integrated Process: Nursing Process/ Planning
Content Area: Mental Health

Answer: 4

Rationale: The nurse's primary concern is to provide for safety. The priority statement by the victim is that the rapist will kill her. The victim who states that she *feels like it did not happen* or that she *feels numb* is most likely in the denial stage, which can be a helpful defense mechanism for the client. The fact that the rapist and the victim knew each other is a common phenomenon; in many situations of abuse, the victim does know the rapist.

Test-Taking Strategy: Note the strategic words *most important* and *immediate.* Eliminate options 1 and 2 first because they are comparable or alike. From the remaining options use Maslow's Hierarchy of Needs theory. Option 4 is concerned with safety. Review care of the rape victim and the test-taking strategies for answering prioritizing questions if you had difficulty with this question.

Tip for the Beginning Nursing Student: Rape is the forced act of sexual intercourse with another person without that person's consent. Safety of the client is a primary concern. In addition, nonjudgmental listening and psychological support are essential. Physical evidence may need to be obtained if the victim chooses to take legal action against the perpetrator. You will learn about the many important nursing interventions in the care of a client who has been raped in your mental health nursing course.

References

Keltner, N., Schwecke, L., & Bostro, C. (2007) *Psychiatric nursing* (5th ed., pp. 610-611). St. Louis: Mosby.

Varcarolis, E., Carlson, V., & Shoemaker, N. (2006). *Foundations of psychiatric mental health nursing* (5th ed., pp. 496, 533). Philadelphia: Saunders.

---

75. A client says to the nurse, "Ever since my wife passed on, my life is empty and has no meaning." The appropriate nursing response is which of the following?

1 "Your life has no meaning?"

2 "Most people who lose a loved one feel empty."

Answer: 1

Rationale: In option 1 the nurse uses the therapeutic technique of restating. In this technique the nurse explores more thoroughly topics that are significant to the client. Option 2 generalizes and does not focus on the client. Option 3 focuses on the client's children rather than on the client's feelings. Option 4 avoids the client's feelings.

3 "What would your children think if they knew how you felt?"

4 "Let's talk about the positive things that you have in your life."

Level of Cognitive Ability: Application
Client Needs: Psychosocial Integrity
Integrated Process: Communication and Documentation
Content Area: Mental Health

Test-Taking Strategy: Note the strategic word *appropriate*, and use therapeutic communication techniques. Eliminate options 3 and 4 first because they are comparable or alike and do not focus on the client's feelings. Next eliminate option 2 because it is a generalized statement and stereotypes the client. Option 1 uses the therapeutic technique of restating. Review therapeutic communication techniques and the test-taking strategies for answering communication questions if you had difficulty with this question.

Tip for the Beginning Nursing Student: Therapeutic communication techniques promote and encourage the client to communicate and share his or her feelings with the nurse. Nontherapeutic communication techniques block the communication process and are not methods that the nurse would use when caring for a client. You will learn about therapeutic and nontherapeutic communication techniques in your fundamentals of nursing course and in your mental health nursing course.

References
Fortinash, K., & Holoday-Worret, P. (2008). *Psychiatric mental health nursing* (4th ed., pp. 69-73, 601-602). St. Louis: Mosby.
Varcarolis, E., Carlson, V., & Shoemaker, N. (2006). *Foundations of psychiatric mental health nursing* (5th ed., pp. 185-190, 616-617). Philadelphia: Saunders.

---

76. A nurse is having a conversation with a client hospitalized in a mental health unit. The client says to the nurse, "I work in a factory doing piece work, and I am very competitive with the people with whom I work." The appropriate nursing response is which of the following?

1 "Do you find that your fellow employees are competitive also?"

2 "When you are being paid by piece work then you need to be competitive."

3 "In other words, you seem to be saying that you try to do better than your fellow employees."

4 "Why are you competitive? After all, you get paid based on the amount of work that you do, not your fellow employees."

Level of Cognitive Ability: Application
Client Needs: Psychosocial Integrity
Integrated Process: Communication and Documentation
Content Area: Mental Health

Answer: 3
Rationale: Option 3 uses the therapeutic technique of paraphrasing. In paraphrasing the nurse restates in different words what the client has said to confirm an understanding of what has been said. Option 1 focuses on fellow employees and not the client. In option 2 the nurse agrees with the client. In option 4 the nurse uses the word *why*, which can make the client feel defensive and often implies criticism.

Test-Taking Strategy: Note the strategic word *appropriate*, and use therapeutic communication techniques. Eliminate option 1 first because it does not focus on the client. Next eliminate option 4 because the nurse uses the word *why*. From the remaining options eliminate option 2 because the nurse agrees with the client. In addition, option 3 uses the therapeutic technique of paraphrasing. Review therapeutic communication techniques and the test-taking strategies for answering communication questions if you had difficulty with this question.

Tip for the Beginning Nursing Student: Therapeutic communication techniques promote and encourage the client to communicate and share his or her feelings with the nurse. Nontherapeutic communication techniques block the communication process and are not methods that the nurse would use when caring for a client. You will learn about therapeutic and nontherapeutic communication techniques in your fundamentals of nursing course and in your mental health nursing course.

References

Keltner, N., Schwecke, L., & Bostro, C. (2007). *Psychiatric nursing* (5th ed., pp. 90-91). St. Louis: Mosby.

Linton, A. (2007). *Introduction to medical-surgical nursing* (4th ed., p. 42). Philadelphia: Saunders.

Varcarolis, E., Carlson, V., & Shoemaker, N. (2006). *Foundations of psychiatric mental health nursing* (5th ed., pp. 185-190, 202). Philadelphia: Saunders.

---

77. A client receiving therapy at a mental health clinic says to the nurse, "When I have a stressful day at work and when my boss 'is on my case all day' I go home and take my frustrations out on my children." The appropriate response to the client is which of the following?

  1 "Let's talk about some other ways that you can handle your frustrations."

  2 "Why do you do this? Can you think of another way to take out your frustrations?"

  3 "Is there some place that you can go after work to relieve your frustrations before going home?"

  4 "The only way to take out your frustrations is to join a health care center that provides equipment for weight-lifting and boxing."

Level of Cognitive Ability: Application
Client Needs: Psychosocial Integrity
Integrated Process: Communication and Documentation
Content Area: Mental Health

Answer: 1

Rationale: The nursing response in option 1 provides the client the opportunity to problem-solve. Option 2 uses the word *why*, which can make the client feel defensive and often implies criticism. Option 3 avoids the fact that the client needs to deal with the subject, namely, taking her frustrations out on her children. Option 4 is incorrect because physical activity is not the only way to relieve frustrations. In addition, this may not be appropriate for this client.

Test-Taking Strategy: Note the strategic word *appropriate,* and use therapeutic communication techniques. Eliminate option 2 because of the word *why.* Next eliminate option 4 because of the close-ended word *only.* From the remaining options, note that option 2 is comparable or alike to option 3 and that option 1 provides the client the opportunity to problem-solve. Review therapeutic communication techniques and the test-taking strategies for answering communication questions if you had difficulty with this question.

Tip for the Beginning Nursing Student: Therapeutic communication techniques promote and encourage the client to communicate and share his or her feelings with the nurse. Nontherapeutic communication techniques block the communication process and are not methods that the nurse would use when caring for a client. You will learn about therapeutic and nontherapeutic communication techniques in your fundamentals of nursing course and in your mental health nursing course.

References

deWit, S. (2009). *Medical-surgical nursing: Concepts & practice* (pp. 9, 1101). St. Louis: Saunders.

Varcarolis, E., Carlson, V., & Shoemaker, N. (2006). *Foundations of psychiatric mental health nursing* (5th ed., pp. 185-190, 204). Philadelphia: Saunders.

---

78. A female client who is hospitalized in the mental health unit for treatment of depression says to a female nurse, "Women always get put down. It is as if we are useless members of society." The

Answer: 1

Rationale: In option 1 the nurse uses the therapeutic technique of focusing and encourages the client to verbalize and expand on her feelings. In option 2 the nurse disagrees with the client. In option 3 the nurse provides an opinion; in addition, this option uses the close-ended word *never.* In appropriate nursing response is which of the following?

1 "Tell me how you feel as a woman."

2 "Think about it. That is no longer true in today's society."

3 "I never let anyone make me feel as though I am useless!"

4 "Yes, that does happen to women but it does not mean that women have to stand for that kind of treatment."

Level of Cognitive Ability: Application
Client Needs: Psychosocial Integrity
Integrated Process: Communication and Documentation
Content Area: Mental Health

option 4 the nurse agrees with the client and then takes a forceful stance with regard to how the client would deal with these feelings.

Test-Taking Strategy: Note the strategic word *appropriate*, and use therapeutic communication techniques. Eliminate option 3 first because of the close-ended word *never*. In addition, in this option the nurse provides an opinion, which is nontherapeutic. Next eliminate options 2 and 4. In option 4 the nurse agrees with the client, and in option 2 the nurse disagrees with the client. Review therapeutic communication techniques and the test-taking strategies for answering communication questions if you had difficulty with this question.

Tip for the Beginning Nursing Student: Depression is a state of sadness or grief and can range from mild and moderate states to severe states. Therapeutic communication techniques promote and encourage the client to communicate and share his or her feelings with the nurse. Nontherapeutic communication techniques block the communication process and are not methods that the nurse would use when caring for a client. You will learn about therapeutic and nontherapeutic communication techniques in your fundamentals of nursing course and about depression in your mental health nursing course.

References

Keltner, N., Schwecke, L., & Bostro, C. (2007). *Psychiatric nursing* (5th ed., pp. 90-91, 375). St. Louis: Mosby.

Varcarolis, E., Carlson, V., & Shoemaker, N. (2006). *Foundations of psychiatric mental health nursing* (5th ed., pp. 185-190, 335). Philadelphia: Saunders.

---

79. A nurse employed in a mental health unit is meeting with a client for the first time. Which nursing statement would be appropriate to initiate the conversation?

1 "Are you feeling sad?"

2 "What would you like to discuss?"

3 "Have you ever been admitted to a mental health facility?"

4 "Have psychiatric medications ever been prescribed for you?"

Level of Cognitive Ability: Application
Client Needs: Psychosocial Integrity
Integrated Process: Communication and Documentation
Content Area: Mental Health

Answer: 2

Rationale: The nursing statement in option 2 is an open-ended question that encourages conversation because it requires more than a one-word answer. In options 1, 3, and 4 the nurse attempts to obtain information from the client; however, these statements are close ended in that the client can respond by a *yes* or *no* response. They do not encourage discussion.

Test-Taking Strategy: Note the strategic word *appropriate*, and use therapeutic communication techniques. Eliminate options 1, 3, and 4 because they are comparable or alike and all are close-ended questions. Review therapeutic communication techniques and the test-taking strategies for answering communication questions if you had difficulty with this question.

Tip for the Beginning Nursing Student: Therapeutic communication techniques promote and encourage the client to communicate and share his or her feelings with the nurse. Nontherapeutic communication techniques block the communication process and are not methods that the nurse would use when caring for a client. You will learn about therapeutic and nontherapeutic communication techniques in your fundamentals of nursing course and in your mental health nursing course.

References

Linton, A. (2007). *Introduction to medical-surgical nursing* (4th ed., pp. 1242-1243). Philadelphia: Saunders.

Keltner, N., Schwecke, L., & Bostro, C. (2007). *Psychiatric nursing* (5th ed., pp. 90-91). St. Louis: Mosby.

Varcarolis, E., Carlson, V., & Shoemaker, N. (2006). *Foundations of psychiatric mental health nursing* (5th ed., pp. 78, 185-190). Philadelphia: Saunders.

---

80. An emergency department nurse suspects that a female client is a victim of physical abuse. The nurse makes which appropriate statement to the client?

   1 "If your boyfriend is physically abusing you, you can get a restraining order."

   2 "That bruise looks very sore. I do not know how a man can do that to a woman."

   3 "You have a huge bruise on your back. How often does your boyfriend hit you?"

   4 "I sometimes see women who have been hurt by their boyfriends. Did anyone hit you?"

Level of Cognitive Ability: Application
Client Needs: Psychosocial Integrity
Integrated Process: Communication and Documentation
Content Area: Mental Health

Answer: 4

Rationale: Women must be asked in a caring and nonthreatening manner about violence in their lives. Options 1 and 3 are confrontational, and option 1 is based on the nurse's assumption that the client wants a restraining order. Option 2 is a judgmental statement on the nurse's part. The nurse must avoid judgment of the victim or suspected victim's situation. It can take a great deal of time for a woman to admit that there is, in fact, abuse occurring, and the nurse must avoid becoming another controller in the woman's life. Only option 4 allows the client the option of rejecting or accepting further intervention because the nurse is making an indirect, general statement to which the client can answer *yes* or *no.*

Test-Taking Strategy: Use therapeutic communication techniques, and note that the client may be a victim of violence. Eliminate options 1 and 3 first because they are comparable or alike and are both confrontational statements. Next eliminate option 2 because it is a judgmental statement. Also note that option 4 is a general statement. Review therapeutic communication techniques and the test-taking strategies for answering communication questions if you had difficulty with this question.

Tip for the Beginning Nursing Student: Physical abuse is a form of violence. If abuse occurs, the priority is to treat any physical injuries sustained. Next it is important to provide support and a safe environment for the victim. The nurse should use therapeutic communication techniques to communicate with the client. Therapeutic communication techniques promote and encourage the client to communicate and share his or her feelings with the nurse. Nontherapeutic communication techniques block the communication process and are not methods that the nurse would use when caring for a client. You will learn about therapeutic and nontherapeutic communication techniques in your fundamentals of nursing course. In addition, you will learn about violence and abuse in your mental health nursing course.

References

deWit, S. (2009). *Medical-surgical nursing: Concepts & practice* (p. 9). St. Louis: Saunders.

Fortinash, K., & Holoday-Worret, P. (2008). *Psychiatric mental health nursing* (4th ed., p. 491). St. Louis: Mosby.

Varcarolis, E., Carlson, V., & Shoemaker, N. (2006). *Foundations of psychiatric mental health nursing* (5th ed., pp. 185-190, 510). Philadelphia: Saunders.

---

81. Choose the department statements that indicate the use of a therapeutic communication technique. Select all that apply.

☐ **1** "I would not worry about that."

☐ **2** "You'll do just fine. You'll see."

☐ **3** "What would you like to discuss?"

☐ **4** "Can you describe your feelings?"

☐ **5** "Can you tell me what the voices are saying?"

☐ **6** "Let's not talk about that now, and let's focus on some other issues."

Level of Cognitive Ability: Application
Client Needs: Psychosocial Integrity
Integrated Process: Communication and Documentation
Content Area: Mental Health

Answer: 3, 4, 5

Rationale: The nursing statement "What would you like to discuss?" is therapeutic and an open-ended question that invites the client to share personal feelings. The nursing statements "Can you describe your feelings?" and "Can you tell me what the voices are saying?" are therapeutic and focused statements that are exploratory. The nursing statements "I would not worry about that" and "You'll do just fine. You'll see" are nontherapeutic and provide false reassurance. The statement "Let's not talk about that now, and let's focus on some other issues" avoids a client's feelings and concerns.

Test-Taking Strategy: Read each nursing statement and focus on the subject—use of therapeutic communication techniques. Recalling the therapeutic and nontherapeutic techniques will assist in answering the question. Review therapeutic communication techniques and the test-taking strategies for answering communication questions if you had difficulty with this question.

Tip for the Beginning Nursing Student: Therapeutic communication techniques promote and encourage the client to communicate and share his or her feelings with the nurse. Nontherapeutic communication techniques block the communication process and are not methods that the nurse would use when caring for a client. You will learn about therapeutic and nontherapeutic communication techniques in your fundamentals of nursing course and in your mental health nursing course.

References

Keltner, N., Schwecke, L., & Bostro, C. (2007). *Psychiatric nursing* (5th ed. pp. 90-91). St. Louis: Mosby.

Varcarolis, E., Carlson, V., & Shoemaker, N. (2006). *Foundations of psychiatric mental health nursing* (5th ed., pp. 185-186). Philadelphia: Saunders.

---

82. A psychiatrist prescribes aripiprazole (Abilify) for a client with a diagnosis of schizophrenia. Which of the following nursing interventions would be therapeutic?

1 Administer the medication only after meals.

Answer: 3

Rationale: Aripiprazole is an antipsychotic agent that may be referred to as a dopamine system stabilizer (DSS). Because antipsychotics cause sedation, bedtime dosing helps to promote sleep while decreasing daytime drowsiness. Aripiprazole may be administered with or without food and is well absorbed both in the presence or absence of food. It is not necessary for the client to increase his or

2 Advise the client to limit his alcohol intake to one drink each day.

3 Instruct the client that the medication may cause sedation and should be taken at bedtime.

4 Advise the client to increase his usual exercise pattern threefold to help with medication absorption.

Level of Cognitive Ability: Application
Client Needs: Physiological Integrity
Integrated Process: Teaching and Learning
Content Area: Mental Health

her usual exercise pattern to assist in absorption of the medication. Alcohol is avoided, not limited.

Test-Taking Strategy: Noting that the client has schizophrenia will assist in determining that the medication is an antipsychotic. Eliminate option 1 because of the close-ended word *only*. Eliminate option 2 by recalling that alcohol intake is avoided, not limited. From the remaining options eliminate option 4 because of the words *increase his usual exercise pattern threefold*. Review aripiprazole and the test-taking strategies for answering pharmacology questions if you had difficulty with this question.

Tip for the Beginning Nursing Student: Schizophrenia is a psychotic disorder characterized by gross distortion of reality, disturbances of language and communication, withdrawal from social interactions, and disorganization and fragmentation of thoughts. Antipsychotic medication is administered to control the delusions and hallucinations that the client experiences. You will learn about schizophrenia and its treatment in your mental health nursing course.

Reference

Lehne, R. (2007). *Pharmacology for nursing care* (6th ed., p. 326). Philadelphia: Saunders.

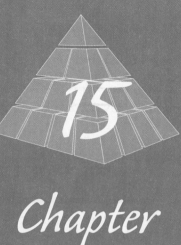

Chapter 15

Maternity Questions

83. A nurse is performing a postpartum fundal assessment and notes that the client's uterus feels soft and spongy. Which nursing action is most appropriate initially?
1 Notify the physician.
2 Massage the fundus gently.
3 Encourage the mother to ambulate.
4 Document fundal position and consistency and height.

Level of Cognitive Ability: Application
Client Needs: Physiological Integrity
Integrated Process: Nursing Process/
  Implementation
Content Area: Maternity

Answer: 2

Rationale: If the uterus feels soft and spongy (boggy), it should be massaged gently, observing for increased vaginal bleeding or clots. Option 3 is inappropriate at this time. The nurse should document fundal position, consistency, and height and the need to perform fundal massage, along with the client's response to the intervention. The physician is notified if uterine massage is not helpful.

Test-Taking Strategy: Note the strategic words *most appropriate initially.* Note the relationship of the data in the question (soft and spongy) and the data in the correct option (massage the fundus gently). Review nursing interventions related to this occurrence and the various test-taking strategies if you had difficulty with this question.

Tip for the Beginning Nursing Student: The postpartum period is the time following delivery of a newborn. During this time the nurse needs to check the new mother's fundus for firmness. If the fundus is soft and boggy (and not firm as it should be), the nurse would massage the fundus gently. You will learn about the postpartum period and associated nursing interventions in your maternity nursing course when you study postpartum assessments.

References
Leifer, G. (2008). *Maternity nursing: An introductory text* (10th ed., p. 227). Philadelphia: Saunders.
Murray, S., & McKinney, E. (2006). *Foundations of maternal-newborn nursing* (4th ed., p. 410). Philadelphia: Saunders.

84. A client arrives at the prenatal clinic for the first prenatal assessment. She tells the nurse that the first day of her last menstrual period (LMP) was August 19, 2011. Using Nägele's rule, the nurse determines the estimated date of delivery as:
1 May 12, 2012
2 May 26, 2012
3 June 12, 2012
4 June 26, 2012

Level of Cognitive Ability:
   Comprehension
Client Needs: Physiological Integrity
Integrated Process: Nursing Process/
   Assessment/Data Collection
Content Area: Maternity

Answer: 2
Rationale: Accurate use of Nägele's rule requires that the woman have a regular 28-day menstrual cycle. Add 7 days to the first day of the LMP, subtract 3 months, and then add 1 year to that date if it is appropriate to change it to the next year. First day of the LMP is August 19, 2011; add 7 days: August 26, 2011; subtract 3 months: May 26, 2011; add 1 year: May 26, 2012.

Test-Taking Strategy: Use Nägele's rule to answer this question, but use caution when following the steps to determine the estimated date of delivery. Read all options carefully, noting the dates and years in the options before selecting an option. Review Nägele's rule and the various test-taking strategies if you had difficulty with this question.

Tip for the Beginning Nursing Student: Nägele's rule is a method of determining the date of delivery for a client who is pregnant. Determining the date of delivery requires knowing the date of the LMP and then using the rule to determine the delivery date. This is a simple way to determine the date, and memorizing the rule will assist you in determining a client's delivery date. You will learn about Nägele's rule and how to use the rule to determine the delivery date in your maternity nursing course when you study prenatal assessment procedures.

References
Leifer, G. (2008). *Maternity nursing: An introductory text* (10th ed., p. 42). Philadelphia: Saunders.
Murray, S., & McKinney, E. (2006). *Foundations of maternal-newborn nursing* (4th ed., p. 793). Philadelphia: Saunders.

85. A nurse is monitoring a client who is receiving magnesium sulfate for preeclampsia and is assessing the client every 30 minutes. Which of the following findings would indicate a need to immediately report the findings?
1 Urinary output of 20 mL
2 Deep tendon reflexes of 2+
3 Respirations of 10 breaths/ minute
4 Fetal heart rate (FHR) of 116 beats/min

Level of Cognitive Ability: Analysis
Client Needs: Physiological Integrity
Integrated Process: Nursing Process/
   Implementation
Content Area: Maternity

Answer: 3
Rationale: The acceptable criterion for urine output is at least 30 mL/hour. The amount of urine output identified in option 1 is adequate (20 mL of urine in 30 minutes). Deep tendon reflexes of 2+ are normal. Magnesium sulfate depresses the respiratory rate. If the rate is less than 12 breaths/minute, continuation of the medication needs to be reassessed. The FHR is within normal limits for a resting fetus.

Test-Taking Strategy: Note the strategic words *need to immediately report the findings.* Select the option that indicates an abnormal finding that requires further intervention. Recalling the normal respiratory rate will direct you to option 3. Review the findings in preeclampsia, the effects of magnesium sulfate, and the various test-taking strategies if you had difficulty with this question.

Tip for the Beginning Nursing Student: Preeclampsia is an abnormal condition of pregnancy characterized by the onset of acute hypertension after week 24 of pregnancy. The classic signs include hypertension, proteinuria (protein in the urine), and edema (swelling). One concern is that preeclampsia can progress to eclampsia (seizures). Preeclampsia is treated with magnesium sulfate to prevent its progression to eclampsia. The nurse needs to monitor clients receiving this medication closely because of its many adverse effects and the risk of toxicity. One primary concern is that magnesium sulfate depresses respirations; therefore the nurse monitors the client's respiratory status closely. You will learn about this medication and important nursing interventions when it is administered in a pharmacology course or in your maternity nursing course when you study high-risk conditions in pregnancy.

References
Leifer, G. (2008). *Maternity nursing: An introductory text* (10th ed., p. 259). Philadelphia: Saunders.
Murray, S., & McKinney, E. (2006). *Foundations of maternal-newborn nursing* (4th ed., p. 646). Philadelphia: Saunders.

---

86. A nurse receives report at the beginning of the shift about a client with an intrauterine fetal demise. On assessment of the client, the nurse expects to note which of the following?
1 Intractable vomiting and dehydration
2 Elevated blood pressure, proteinuria, and edema
3 Uterine size greater than expected for gestational age
4 Regression of pregnancy symptoms and absence of fetal heart tones

Level of Cognitive Ability: Analysis
Client Needs: Physiological Integrity
Integrated Process: Nursing Process/ Assessment/Data Collection
Content Area: Maternity

Answer: 4
Rationale: Symptoms of a fetal demise include decreased fetal movement, unchanged or decreased fundal height, and absent fetal heart tones. In addition, many symptoms of the pregnancy may diminish, such as breast size and tenderness. Option 1 is associated with hyperemesis gravidarum. Option 2 is associated with preeclampsia.

Test-Taking Strategy: Focus on the subject, *intrauterine fetal demise.* Note the relationship between the subject and option 4. Recalling that fetal demise means fetal death will direct you to option 4. Review the signs associated with fetal demise and the various test-taking strategies if you had difficulty with this question.

Tip for the Beginning Nursing Student: Fetal demise refers to the intrauterine death of a fetus. If this occurs, fetal movement and heart tones would be absent. Hyperemesis gravidarum is an abnormal condition of pregnancy characterized by protracted vomiting, weight loss, and fluid and electrolyte imbalance. Preeclampsia is an abnormal condition of pregnancy characterized by the onset of acute hypertension after week 24 of pregnancy. The classic signs include hypertension, proteinuria (protein in the urine), and edema (swelling). You will learn about these complications of pregnancy in your maternity nursing course.

References
Leifer, G. (2008). *Maternity nursing: An introductory text* (10th ed., p. 255). Philadelphia: Saunders.
Murray, S., & McKinney, E. (2006). *Foundations of maternal-newborn nursing* (4th ed., p. 626). Philadelphia: Saunders.

87. Immediately following the delivery of a newborn infant, the nurse prepares to assist in the delivery of the placenta. The appropriate action to deliver the placenta is to:

1 Pull on the umbilical cord.

2 Instruct the mother to push during a uterine contraction.

3 Place traction on the umbilical cord and pull on the placenta as it enters the vaginal canal.

4 Separate the placenta from the uterine wall using the forceps, and then allow the placenta to deliver spontaneously.

Level of Cognitive Ability: Application
Client Needs: Physiological Integrity
Integrated Process: Nursing Process/ Implementation
Content Area: Maternity

Answer: 2

Rationale: After the placenta separates, the mother is instructed to push during a uterine contraction. Pulling on the umbilical cord or placing traction on the umbilical cord may cause it to break, making the placenta harder to deliver. The placenta is not separated from the uterine wall using forceps. This may result in bleeding.

Test-Taking Strategy: Eliminate option 1 because of the word *pull* and option 3 because of the word *traction*. From the remaining options eliminate option 4 by recalling that the placenta is attached to the uterine wall and unnatural separation will result in bleeding. Review the procedure for placental delivery and the various test-taking strategies if you had difficulty with this question.

Tip for the Beginning Nursing Student: The placenta is a fetal structure that provides nourishment to and removes wastes from the developing fetus. After the delivery of the baby, the placenta separates from the uterine wall and is delivered. You will learn about the purpose of the placenta and its delivery in your maternity nursing course.

References
Leifer, G. (2008). *Maternity nursing: An introductory text* (10th ed., pp. 97-98). Philadelphia: Saunders.
Murray, S., & McKinney, E. (2006). *Foundations of maternal-newborn nursing* (4th ed., p. 258). Philadelphia: Saunders.

88. A client tells the nurse that she is really worried about knowing how to care for her first-born child. The nurse formulates which nursing diagnosis for this client?

1 *Ineffective coping*

2 *Deficient knowledge*

3 *Complicated grieving*

4 *Situational low self-esteem*

Level of Cognitive Ability: Analysis
Client Needs: Health Promotion and Maintenance
Integrated Process: Nursing Process/ Planning
Content Area: Maternity

Answer: 2

Rationale: Deficient knowledge indicates a lack of information or psychomotor skill concerning a skill, condition, or treatment. This nursing diagnosis best describes the situation presented in the question. *Ineffective coping* implies that the person is unable to manage stressors adequately. *Complicated grieving* implies prolonged unresolved grief leading to detrimental activities. *Situational low self-esteem* represents temporary negative feelings about self in response to an event.

Test-Taking Strategy: When a question asks to identify a nursing diagnosis, focus on the information in the question. Option 2 will focus on the mother's concern about *knowing how to care for her first-born child.* Review the defining characteristics of *Deficient knowledge* and the various test-taking strategies if you had difficulty with this question.

Tip for the Beginning Nursing Student: Teaching is an important nursing responsibility. It is common for a new mother to be concerned about how to care for her newborn. The nurse needs to alleviate fears and concerns by providing the mother with opportunities to care for the newborn after delivery while hospitalized. You will learn about therapeutic measures to alleviate these concerns and fears and the important points to teach the mother about caring for her newborn in your maternity nursing course.

References
Leifer, G. (2008). *Maternity nursing: An introductory text* (10th ed., pp. 242-243). Philadelphia: Saunders.
Murray, S., & McKinney, E. (2006). *Foundations of maternal-newborn nursing* (4th ed., pp. 433, 933-934). Philadelphia: Saunders.

89. A nurse is monitoring the status of a client in labor who is experiencing hypotonic uterine dysfunction. The nurse interprets that which finding would be least consistent with this type of dysfunctional labor?
1 Contractions weaken during the active stage of labor.
2 Contractions become inefficient or stop during the active stage of labor.
3 The client initially makes normal progress into the active stage of labor, and then contractions weaken.
4 The client is having painful and frequent contractions that are ineffective in causing cervical dilation or effacement to progress.

Level of Cognitive Ability: Analysis
Client Needs: Physiological Integrity
Integrated Process: Nursing Process/ Assessment/Data Collection
Content Area: Maternity

Answer: 4
Rationale: In hypotonic uterine dysfunction the client initially makes normal progress into the active stage of labor and then contractions weaken, become inefficient, or stop. Option 4 is characteristic of hypertonic uterine dysfunction.

Test-Taking Strategy: Note the strategic words *least consistent*. These words indicate a negative event query and that you need to identify the option that is not characteristic of hypotonic uterine dysfunction. Noting that options 1, 2 and 3 are comparable or alike and noting the word *hypotonic* in the question will direct you to option 4. Review the manifestations of hypotonic uterine dysfunction and the various test-taking strategies if you had difficulty with this question.

Tip for the Beginning Nursing Student: A contraction is a rhythmic tightening of the musculature of the upper uterus that begins as mild tightening and progresses to strong tightening late in labor. Contractions decrease the size of the uterus and squeeze the fetus through the birth canal. Normal labor contractions are coordinated, involuntary, and intermittent. You will learn about contractions and the labor process in your maternity nursing course.

References
Leifer, G. (2008). *Maternity nursing: An introductory text* (10th ed., pp. 283-284). Philadelphia: Saunders.
Murray, S., & McKinney, E. (2006). *Foundations of maternal-newborn nursing* (4th ed., pp. 698-700). Philadelphia: Saunders.

90. A client has just experienced a precipitate labor. The nurse notes that the mother is lying quietly in bed and is avoiding physical contact with her newborn infant. The nurse appropriately:
1 Contacts the physician
2 Requests a psychiatric consult
3 Provides support to the mother
4 Encourages the mother to breast-feed the infant

Level of Cognitive Ability: Application
Client Needs: Psychosocial Integrity

Answer: 3
Rationale: Precipitate labor is defined as labor that lasts less than 3 hours from the onset of contractions to the time of birth. After a precipitate labor the mother may need help to process what has happened and time to assimilate it all. The mother may be exhausted, in pain, stunned by the rapid nature of the delivery, or simply following cultural norms. Providing support to the mother is the most appropriate and therapeutic action by the nurse. Options 1 and 2 are comparable or alike and do not enhance the therapeutic relationship. Option 4 is an appropriate nursing intervention, but the question does not indicate whether the mother is going to be breast-feeding.

Integrated Process: Caring
Content Area: Maternity

Test-Taking Strategy: Eliminate options 1 and 2 first because they are comparable or alike. From the remaining options note that no data indicate that the mother is going to breast-feed. This will direct you to option 3. Review care of the client following precipitate labor and the various test-taking strategies if you had difficulty with this question.

Tip for the Beginning Nursing Student: The total duration of normal labor differs for women who have never given birth and for those who have previously given birth by the vaginal route. Normal labor consists of four stages. In the first stage, which normally lasts 6 to 10 hours, effacement and dilation occur. The second stage involves expulsion of the fetus and normally lasts 20 to 60 minutes. Stage three involves separation of the placenta and usually takes 5 to 30 minutes. Stage four, which lasts 1 to 4 hours after delivery, is the time for physical recovery and newborn bonding. You will learn about the normal labor process and the stages of labor in your maternity nursing course.

References

Leifer, G. (2007). *Introduction to maternity and pediatric nursing* (5th ed., p. 192). Philadelphia: Saunders.

Murray, S., & McKinney, E. (2006). *Foundations of maternal-newborn nursing* (4th ed., p. 706). Philadelphia: Saunders.

---

91. A pregnant client experienced a uterine rupture with subsequent fetal death. After ensuring that the client is physiologically stable, the nurse uses which of the following approaches as the best first step to support the client psychologically?

1 Avoids talking about the dead fetus

2 Assesses how the client perceived the event

3 Asks the client and husband about plans for future pregnancies

4 Suggests that family members see and hold the dead infant if they wish

Level of Cognitive Ability: Application
Client Needs: Psychosocial Integrity
Integrated Process: Caring
Content Area: Maternity

Answer: 2

Rationale: Because of anesthesia, anxiety, and the experience of a sudden catastrophic event, the client may well have experienced a decreased ability to take in and process information. The nurse should first assess the client's perception of the event before deciding how to intervene. Option 4 may be helpful but not as a first step. Options 1 and 3 are not helpful because they are not therapeutic. Option 1 avoids the subject, and option 3 deals with subjects the client may not be ready to face.

Test-Taking Strategy: Use the steps of the nursing process, remembering that assessment/data collection comes first. This will direct you to option 2. Review care of the pregnant client who experienced a crisis and the various test-taking strategies if you had difficulty with this question.

Tip for the Beginning Nursing Student: Uterine rupture results when a tear in the wall of the uterus occurs because the uterine wall cannot stand the pressure placed against it from the growing fetus. Uterine rupture is a rare condition associated with previous uterine surgery, such as a cesarean birth or surgery to remove fibroids. If the placenta is involved, the fetus is often dead. You will learn about the complications of pregnancy and uterine rupture in your maternity nursing course.

References

Leifer, G. (2007). *Introduction to maternity and pediatric nursing* (5th ed., pp. 195-196). Philadelphia: Saunders.

Murray, S., & McKinney, E. (2006). *Foundations of maternal-newborn nursing* (4th ed., pp. 726-727). Philadelphia: Saunders.

---

92. A pregnant client with a suspected diagnosis of placenta previa arrives at the health care clinic for an examination. The nurse prepares the client for the examination and tells the client that which of the following will be deferred until the diagnosis is confirmed?

1 Abdominal ultrasound
2 Vital sign measurement
3 Urine testing for glucose
4 Vaginal speculum examination

Level of Cognitive Ability: Application
Client Needs: Physiological Integrity
Integrated Process: Nursing Process/
   Implementation
Content Area: Maternity

Answer: 4

Rationale: The placenta is implanted low in the uterus in placenta previa, and a vaginal speculum examination could cause disruption of the placenta and initiate severe hemorrhage. The abdominal ultrasound is used to confirm the diagnosis of placenta previa. There is no reason to defer urine testing or vital sign measurement.

Test-Taking Strategy: Note the strategic word *deferred*, and focus on the client's suspected diagnosis. Recalling that in this condition the placenta is implanted low in the uterus and that the client is at risk for hemorrhage will direct you to option 4. Review nursing care of the client with placenta previa and the various test-taking strategies if you had difficulty with this question.

Tip for the Beginning Nursing Student: The placenta is a fetal structure that provides nourishment to and removes wastes from the developing fetus. It is normally implanted in the upper uterine area. In placenta previa the placenta is implanted low in the uterus near the presenting part. Disruption of the placenta can cause severe hemorrhage and compromises fetal status. Therefore any activity or procedure that could disrupt the placenta is avoided. You will learn about placenta previa and the risks associated with it in your maternity nursing course.

References

Leifer, G. (2007). *Introduction to maternity and pediatric nursing* (5th ed., p. 89). Philadelphia: Saunders.

Murray, S., & McKinney, E. (2006). *Foundations of maternal-newborn nursing* (4th ed., p. 632). Philadelphia: Saunders.

---

93. A nurse is preparing to perform an assessment on a client with placenta previa and plans to assess which of the following first?

1 The fetal heart rate (FHR)
2 The client's temperature
3 The client's compliance with activity limitations
4 The client's understanding of the treatment for placenta previa

Level of Cognitive Ability: Application
Client Needs: Physiological Integrity
Integrated Process: Nursing Process/
   Assessment/Data Collection
Content Area: Maternity

Answer: 1

Rationale: A primary concern with placenta previa is fetal injury related to potentially decreased placental perfusion. Although all the options may be assessed, assessing the FHR is the priority.

Test-Taking Strategy: Note the strategic word *first* and that options 3 and 4 are comparable or alike and therefore can be eliminated. Also use the ABCs—airway, breathing, and circulation—to direct you to option 1. Review care of the client with placenta previa and the test-taking strategies for answering prioritizing questions if you had difficulty with this question.

Tip for the Beginning Nursing Student: Placenta previa is an abnormal condition in which the placenta is implanted low in the uterus near the presenting part. A primary concern when a client has placenta previa is disruption of the placenta leading to severe hemorrhage and a compromised fetal status. Both the mother and fetus are monitored closely. Any activity or procedure that could disrupt the placenta, such as a vaginal examination, is avoided. You will learn about placenta previa and the risks associated with it in your maternity nursing course.

References

Leifer, G. (2007). *Introduction to maternity and pediatric nursing* (5th ed., p. 89). Philadelphia: Saunders.

Murray, S., & McKinney, E. (2006). *Foundations of maternal-newborn nursing* (4th ed., p. 632). Philadelphia: Saunders.

---

94. A nurse is preparing to perform fundal massage on a client with uterine atony. The nurse performs this procedure by:
  1 Placing one hand just above the symphysis pubis and pushing on the uterus in a vertical direction
  2 Placing one hand just below the symphysis pubis and massaging the fundus in a horizontal motion
  3 Placing one hand just below the symphysis pubis and massaging the fundus in a circular motion
  4 Placing one hand just above the symphysis pubis and gently but firmly massaging the fundus in a circular motion

Level of Cognitive Ability: Application
Client Needs: Physiological Integrity
Integrated Process: Nursing Process/ Implementation
Content Area: Maternity

Answer: 4

Rationale: When performing fundal massage, one hand is placed just above the symphysis pubis to support the lower uterine segment while the fundus is gently but firmly massaged in a circular motion. Pushing on an uncontracted uterus could invert the uterus and cause massive hemorrhage.

Test-Taking Strategy: Eliminate option 1 first because of the word *pushing* and recalling that pushing on an uncontracted uterus could invert the uterus and cause massive hemorrhage. Next visualize the anatomy of the uterus. Eliminate options 2 and 3 because the hand is not placed below the symphysis pubis. If you had difficulty with this question, review the procedure for fundal massage and the various test-taking strategies.

Tip for the Beginning Nursing Student: Uterine atony refers to a lack of uterine muscle tone and can result in bleeding. Bleeding occurs because the uterine muscle fibers fail to contract firmly around the blood vessels when the placenta separates. A soft or "boggy" feel when the fundus of the uterus is located is one manifestation of uterine atony. Fundal massage is performed to contract the uterus when uterine atony is present. You will learn about uterine atony, its manifestations, and uterine massage in your maternity nursing course.

References

Leifer, G. (2008). *Maternity nursing: An introductory text* (10th ed., p. 338). Philadelphia: Saunders.

Murray, S., & McKinney, E. (2006). *Foundations of maternal-newborn nursing* (4th ed., p. 735). Philadelphia: Saunders.

---

95. A woman is seen in the prenatal clinic with morning sickness. The nurse will tell the client, as a self-care measure, to eat:
  1 Five or six small meals per day
  2 Gas-forming foods only during the afternoon hours

Answer: 1

Rationale: Morning sickness is common during the first trimester of pregnancy and is associated with increased levels of human chorionic gonadotropin (hCG) and changes in carbohydrate metabolism. It most often occurs on arising although a few women experience it throughout the day. Several self-care measures can be implemented to prevent

3 A high-protein and high-fat snack before getting out of bed
4 Fried foods only during the afternoon and early evening hours

Level of Cognitive Ability: Application
Client Needs: Health Promotion and Maintenance
Integrated Process: Teaching and Learning
Content Area: Maternity

or alleviate morning sickness. These include avoiding an empty or overloaded stomach; not smoking; eating a dry carbohydrate food item such as a dry cracker or toast before getting out of bed; eating five or six small meals per day; and avoiding fried, odorous, greasy, gas-forming, or spicy foods.

Test-Taking Strategy: Focus on the subject of the question—morning sickness. Eliminate options 2 and 4 first because of the close-ended word *only.* From the remaining options eliminate option 3 because of the word *fat.* Review measures to prevent or alleviate morning sickness and the various test-taking strategies if you had difficulty with this question.

Tip for the Beginning Nursing Student: Morning sickness is nausea and vomiting that occur during pregnancy. It is called morning sickness because the symptoms are more acute in the morning (although it can occur at any time of the day). This is a common discomfort of pregnancy and is usually temporary. You will learn about morning sickness and the measures to alleviate it in your maternity nursing course.

References

Leifer, G. (2007). *Introduction to maternity and pediatric nursing* (5th ed., pp. 48, 79). Philadelphia: Saunders.
Murray, S., & McKinney, E. (2006). *Foundations of maternal-newborn nursing* (4th ed., pp. 136-137). Philadelphia: Saunders.

---

96. A client in the third trimester of pregnancy seen in the clinic is experiencing urinary frequency. Which of the following self-care measures will the nurse provide to the client?
1 Perform Kegel exercises.
2 Avoid fluid intake after 6:00 PM.
3 Avoid emptying the bladder frequently.
4 Sip on small amounts of fluids during the day restricting intake to 1000 mL.

Level of Cognitive Ability: Application
Client Needs: Health Promotion and Maintenance
Integrated Process: Teaching and Learning
Content Area: Maternity

Answer: 1
Rationale: Urinary frequency may occur in the first trimester and then again late in the third trimester because of the pressure placed on the bladder by the enlarged uterus. Self-care measures for urinary frequency include emptying the bladder frequently (every 2 hours), drinking at least 2000 mL of fluid per day, limiting fluid intake before bedtime (not avoiding fluid intake), performing Kegel exercises to strengthen the perineal muscles, and wearing a perineal pad. Options 2, 3, and 4 are incorrect and could lead to urinary stasis (option 3) and fluid volume deficit (options 2 and 4).

Test-Taking Strategy: Eliminate options 2 and 4 first because they are comparable or alike and could lead to fluid volume deficit. Eliminate option 3 next because it does not make sense to avoid emptying the bladder frequently. This action could lead to urinary stasis and cause discomfort. Review measures that will assist with the discomfort of urinary frequency and the various test-taking strategies if you had difficulty with this question.

Tip for the Beginning Nursing Student: Urinary frequency is a common discomfort of pregnancy and usually occurs during the first trimester of pregnancy and near term. This is a temporary condition and Kegel exercises help to maintain bladder control. Kegel exercises involve contracting muscles around the vagina, holding tightly for 10 seconds, and then relaxing for 10 seconds. Thirty contraction-relaxation cycles should be done each day. You will learn about urinary frequency as a common discomfort of pregnancy and about Kegel exercises in your maternity nursing course.

References
Leifer, G. (2007). *Introduction to maternity and pediatric nursing* (5th ed., p. 49). Philadelphia: Saunders.
Leifer, G. (2008). *Maternity nursing: An introductory text* (10th ed., p. 68). Philadelphia: Saunders.
Murray, S., & McKinney, E. (2006). *Foundations of maternal-newborn nursing* (4th ed., pp. 125, 140). Philadelphia: Saunders.
Wong, D., Perry, S., Hockenberry, M., Lowdermilk, D., & Wilson, D. (2006). *Maternal-child nursing care* (3rd ed., p. 288). St. Louis: Mosby.

---

97. A client seen in the prenatal clinic is experiencing ankle edema. The nurse assesses the client and notes that the edema is nonpitting, the client's blood pressure is within normal limits, and proteinuria is not present. The nurse provides home care instructions to the client and tells the client to:

1 Restrict fluid intake.
2 Avoid exercising until the edema subsides.
3 Rest periodically with the legs and hips elevated.
4 Stop wearing the support stockings prescribed by the obstetrician.

Level of Cognitive Ability: Application
Client Needs: Health Promotion and Maintenance
Integrated Process: Teaching and Learning
Content Area: Maternity

Answer: 3

Rationale: Ankle edema is common in the third trimester of pregnancy and is caused by decreased venous return from the feet because of gravity. It is a minor discomfort; and as long as the edema is nonpitting and hypertension and proteinuria are not present, it is not a cause for concern. Self-care measures include resting periodically with the legs and hips elevated; wearing supportive stockings or hose; drinking ample amounts of fluid; partaking in moderate exercise; and avoiding standing in one position or place for long periods.

Test-Taking Strategy: Eliminate option 1 first because of the word *restrict*. Restricting fluids can be detrimental to the fetus. Next eliminate option 4 because the nurse would not tell a client to ignore the obstetrician's prescription. From the remaining options use principles related to the effects of gravity to direct you to option 3. Review the measures to alleviate ankle edema and the various test-taking strategies if you had difficulty with this question.

Tip for the Beginning Nursing Student: Edema refers to swelling from the accumulation of excess fluid in body tissues. Edema can occur during pregnancy because the weight of the uterus compresses the veins of the pelvis delaying venous return. Edema of the feet and ankles is most noticeable at the end of the day. Dependent edema is insignificant, but if edema of the face or hands occurs, the client should be further assessed for developing complications of pregnancy. You will learn about dependent edema that occurs during pregnancy in your maternity nursing course.

References
Leifer, G. (2008). *Maternity nursing: An introductory text* (10th ed., p. 69). Philadelphia: Saunders.
Wong, D., Perry, S., Hockenberry, M., Lowdermilk, D., & Wilson, D. (2006). *Maternal-child nursing care* (3rd ed., p. 288). St. Louis: Mosby.

98. The nurse provides instructions to a prenatal client with heartburn about measures to alleviate the discomfort. Which statement by the client indicates a need for further instructions?
1 "I need to lie down after eating."
2 "I need to eat small, frequent meals."
3 "I need to avoid fatty or spicy foods."
4 "I need to drink approximately 2000 mL of fluid per day."

Level of Cognitive Ability: Analysis
Client Needs: Health Promotion and Maintenance
Integrated Process: Teaching and Learning
Content Area: Maternity

Answer: 1
Rationale: Heartburn is associated with regurgitation of gastric acid contents into the esophagus. Self-care measures for heartburn include eating small, frequent meals; avoiding fatty or spicy foods; remaining upright for 30 minutes after eating; and drinking approximately 2000 mL of fluid per day.

Test-Taking Strategy: Note the strategic words *need for further instructions.* These words indicate a negative event query and that you need to select the option that indicates an incorrect client statement. Recalling that heartburn is associated with regurgitation of gastric acid contents into the esophagus will direct you to option 1. Review measures to relieve or prevent heartburn and the various test-taking strategies if you had difficulty with this question.

Tip for the Beginning Nursing Student: Heartburn is described as an acute burning sensation in the epigastric and sternal regions. During pregnancy it normally occurs as a result of diminished gastric motility, displacement of the stomach by the enlarging uterus, and relaxation of the lower esophageal sphincter. You will learn about heartburn as a discomfort of pregnancy and the measures to prevent or alleviate it in your maternity nursing course.

References
Leifer, G. (2008). *Maternity nursing: An introductory text* (10th ed., p. 68). Philadelphia: Saunders.
Wong, D., Perry, S., Hockenberry, M., Lowdermilk, D., & Wilson, D. (2006). *Maternal-child nursing care* (3rd ed., p. 286). St. Louis: Mosby.

99. A nurse is performing an assessment on a client who is at 38 weeks' gestation and notes that the fetal heart rate (FHR) is 174 beats/min. Based on this finding, the most appropriate nursing action would be to:
1 Notify the physician.
2 Document the finding.
3 Check the mother's heart rate.
4 Tell the client that the FHR is normal.

Level of Cognitive Ability: Application
Client Needs: Physiological Integrity
Integrated Process: Nursing Process/ Implementation
Content Area: Maternity

Answer: 1
Rationale: The FHR should be 110 to 160 beats/min at term. Since the FHR is elevated from the normal range, the nurse would notify the physician. The FHR would be documented, but option 1 is the most appropriate action. Options 3 and 4 are inappropriate actions based on the data in the question.

Test-Taking Strategy: Note the strategic words *most appropriate.* Focus on the FHR noted in the question. Recalling that the normal FHR should be 110 to 160 beats/min at term will direct you to option 1. Remember that an abnormal finding noted in the pregnant client needs to be reported to the physician. Review the normal FHR and the test-taking strategies related to physician notification if you had difficulty with this question.

Tip for the Beginning Nursing Student: FHR monitoring is an important part of maternal assessment during pregnancy. The nurse usually uses a Doppler device to auscultate the FHR, which creates an electronic sound based on movements. You will learn about the procedures for monitoring the FHR in your maternity nursing course.

References

Leifer, G. (2008). *Maternity nursing: An introductory text* (10th ed., p. 115). Philadelphia: Saunders.

Murray, S., & McKinney, E. (2006). *Foundations of maternal-newborn nursing* (4th ed., p. 127). Philadelphia: Saunders.

---

100. A nurse is assessing a client in the fourth stage of labor and notes that the uterine fundus is firmly contracted and is midline at the level of the umbilicus. Based on this finding, the nurse would appropriately:

1 Record the findings.
2 Massage the fundus.
3 Contact the physician.
4 Assist the mother to void.

Level of Cognitive Ability: Application
Client Needs: Physiological Integrity
Integrated Process: Nursing Process/ Implementation
Content Area: Maternity

Answer: 1

Rationale: In the postpartum period the nurse assesses for uterine atony and checks the consistency and location of the uterine fundus. The uterine fundus should be firmly contracted, at or near the level of the umbilicus, and midline. Therefore the nurse would record the findings. Since the finding is normal, options 2, 3, and 4 are not necessary. The nurse would massage the uterine fundus if it was soft and boggy. The physician would be contacted if the client experienced excessive bleeding. A full bladder may cause a displaced fundus and one that is above the level of the umbilicus.

Test-Taking Strategy: Use the process of elimination, and focus on the data in the question. Recalling the normal location and consistency of the fundus will direct you to option 1. Review the expected postpartum findings if you had difficulty with this question.

Tip for the Beginning Nursing Student: Involution is a retrogressive change in the uterus to its nonpregnant size. In the fourth stage of labor (1 to 4 hours following delivery), the nurse monitors the location of the uterine fundus to determine whether involution is progressing normally. Immediately after delivery the fundus can be palpated midway between the symphysis pubis and the umbilicus. Within a few hours the fundus rises to the level of the umbilicus and should remain at this level for 24 hours. After 24 hours the fundus descends by approximately 1 cm/day. You will learn about involution and assessment of the location of the uterine fundus in your maternity nursing course.

References

Leifer, G. (2008). *Maternity nursing: An introductory text* (10th ed., p. 100). Philadelphia: Saunders.

Wong, D., Perry, S., Hockenberry, M., Lowdermilk, D., & Wilson, D. (2006). *Maternal-child nursing care* (3rd ed., p. 600). St. Louis: Mosby.

---

101. A home care nurse is visiting a postpartum client. The nurse reviews the information in the client's medical record and performs an assessment on the client. The nurse would suspect endometritis if which of the following is noted?

1 Breast engorgement
2 Fever beginning 3 days postpartum

Answer: 2

Rationale: Fever on the third or fourth day postpartum should raise concerns about possible endometritis until proven otherwise. The woman with endometritis normally presents with a temperature over 100.4° F. Breast engorgement is a normal response and is not associated with endometritis. The white blood cell count of a postpartum woman is normally increased. Thus this method of detecting infection is not of great value in the postpartum period. Lochia rubra on the second day postpartum is a normal finding.

3 Slightly elevated white blood cell count

4 Lochia rubra on the second day postpartum

Level of Cognitive Ability: Analysis
Client Needs: Physiological Integrity
Integrated Process: Nursing Process/ Assessment/Data Collection
Content Area: Maternity

Test-Taking Strategy: Focus on the subject—suspected endometritis. Use medical terminology to recall that -*itis* indicates inflammation or infection. This will assist in eliminating options 1 and 4. From the remaining options noting the word *slightly* in option 3 will assist in eliminating this option. Also note that options 1, 3, and 4 are comparable or alike in that they are normal postpartum findings. Review the signs of endometritis and the various test-taking strategies if you had difficulty with this question.

Tip for the Beginning Nursing Student: Endometritis is an inflammation of the endometrium or decidua and is usually caused by a bacterial infection. It occurs most frequently after childbirth or abortion and is associated with the use of an intrauterine device. Conservative treatment includes rest, antibiotics, pain medication, and adequate fluid intake. You will learn about endometritis in your maternity nursing course when you study postpartum disorders.

References

Leifer, G. (2008). *Maternity nursing: An introductory text* (10th ed., p. 344). Philadelphia: Saunders.

Murray, S., & McKinney, E. (2006). *Foundations of maternal-newborn nursing* (4th ed., pp. 747-748). Philadelphia: Saunders.

---

102. A client in the second trimester of pregnancy is admitted to the maternity unit with a diagnosis of abruptio placentae. The nurse expects to note which clinical manifestation associated with this disorder?
1 Nontender uterus
2 Uterine hypertonicity
3 Painless vaginal bleeding
4 Soft, relaxed uterus with normal tone

Level of Cognitive Ability: Analysis
Client Needs: Physiological Integrity
Integrated Process: Nursing Process/ Assessment/Data Collection
Content Area: Maternity

Answer: 2

Rationale: In abruptio placentae, abdominal pain, uterine tenderness, and uterine hypertonicity are present. Uterine tenderness accompanies placental abruption, especially with a central abruption in which blood becomes trapped behind the placenta. The abdomen will feel hard and board-like on palpation as the blood penetrates the myometrium and causes uterine irritability. Excessive uterine activity with poor relaxation between contractions is present. Observation of the fetal monitoring often reveals increased uterine resting tone, caused by failure of the uterus to relax in an attempt to constrict blood vessels and control bleeding. Painless, bright red vaginal bleeding; a soft, relaxed uterus with normal tone; and a nontender uterus are signs of placenta previa.

Test-Taking Strategy: Eliminate options 1 and 3 first because they are comparable or alike. From the remaining options note that option 2 indicates a sign opposite to the sign in option 4. This provides a clue that one of these options is the correct one. Recalling the signs of abruptio placentae will direct you to option 2. Review these signs and the various test-taking strategies if you had difficulty with this question.

Tip for the Beginning Nursing Student: In abruptio placentae the normally implanted placenta separates before the fetus is born. The major concerns for the mother are bleeding, shock, and clotting abnormalities. The major concerns for the fetus are blood loss, anoxia, preterm birth, and fetal death. Placenta previa is an abnormal condition in which the placenta is implanted low in the uterus near the presenting part. A primary concern when a client has placenta previa is disruption of the placenta leading to severe hemorrhage and a compromised fetal status. You will learn about these complications of pregnancy in your maternity nursing course.

References

Leifer, G. (2008). *Maternity nursing: An introductory text* (10th ed., pp. 253-254). Philadelphia: Saunders.

Murray, S., & McKinney, E. (2006). *Foundations of maternal-newborn nursing* (4th ed., pp. 634-636). Philadelphia: Saunders.

---

103. A nurse is performing an assessment on a client with severe preeclampsia. Which sign would indicate an improvement in the client's condition?
   1 Protein in the urine is trace.
   2 Blood urea nitrogen is 40 mg/dL.
   3 Blood pressure is 148/102 mm Hg.
   4 Client complains of abdominal pain.

Level of Cognitive Ability: Analysis
Client Needs: Physiological Integrity
Integrated Process: Nursing Process/ Evaluation
Content Area: Maternity

Answer: 1
Rationale: Preeclampsia is considered mild when the diastolic blood pressure does not exceed 100 mm Hg; proteinuria is no more than 500 mg/day (trace to 1+), and symptoms such as headache, visual disturbances, or abdominal pain are absent. In addition, signs of kidney or liver involvement are absent. An elevated blood urea nitrogen level indicates the presence of kidney damage as a result of preeclampsia.

Test-Taking Strategy: Use the process of elimination, noting the strategic words *severe preeclampsia* and *improvement in the client's condition*. Note the strategic word *trace* in option 1. This is the only option that does not indicate severe preeclampsia. Review the signs of mild and severe preeclampsia, the signs that indicate improvement, and the various test-taking strategies if you had difficulty with this question.

Tip for the Beginning Nursing Student: Preeclampsia is an abnormal condition of pregnancy characterized by the onset of acute hypertension after week 24 of gestation. Manifestations include hypertension, proteinuria, and edema (swelling). If preeclampsia is untreated, it can lead to serious complications, such as premature separation of the placenta or eclampsia (seizures). You will learn about preeclampsia, its manifestations, and its treatment in your maternity nursing course.

References

Leifer, G. (2008). *Maternity nursing: An introductory text* (10th ed., p. 258). Philadelphia: Saunders.

Murray, S., & McKinney, E. (2006). *Foundations of maternal-newborn nursing* (4th ed., p. 644). Philadelphia: Saunders.

---

104. Artificial rupture of the membranes is done to induce labor in a client. Following this procedure the nurse immediately:
   1 Checks the fetal heart rate (FHR)

Answer: 1
Rationale: Artificial rupture of the membranes may be done to augment or induce labor or to facilitate placement of internal monitors when fetal status indicates the need for some form of direct assessment. Because the umbilical cord can prolapse when the membranes rupture, the FHR

2 Cleans the client's perineal area

3 Places the client in a comfortable position

4 Tells the client that a wet feeling in the perineal area is normal and expected

Level of Cognitive Ability: Application
Client Needs: Physiological Integrity
Integrated Process: Nursing Process/ Implementation
Content Area: Maternity

and fetal pattern should be monitored immediately and for several minutes following the procedure to ascertain fetal well-being. Although options 2, 3, and 4 are appropriate they are not the priority concern. In addition, in the pre-procedure period (rather than post-procedure period), the client should be told that a wet feeling in the perineal area is normal and expected.

Test-Taking Strategy: Use the ABCs—airway, breathing, and circulation—to direct you to option 1. Also use of the steps of the nursing process will direct you to option 1 because it is the only option that addresses assessment/ data collection. Review care of the client following artificial rupture of the membranes and the test-taking strategies for answering prioritizing questions if you had difficulty with this question.

Tip for the Beginning Nursing Student: Artificial rupture of the membranes is also known as amniotomy and is done to stimulate labor. In this procedure, performed by the physician or nurse-midwife, a disposable plastic hook is inserted through the cervix to the amniotic membranes and a hole is made to allow the amniotic fluid to drain. Major risks associated with amniotomy include prolapse of the umbilical cord, infection, and abruptio placentae (abnormal separation of the placenta from the uterine wall). You will learn about the procedure for performing amniotomy in your maternity nursing course.

References

Leifer, G. (2008). *Maternity nursing: An introductory text* (10th ed., p. 288). Philadelphia: Saunders.

Murray, S., & McKinney, E. (2006). *Foundations of maternal-newborn nursing* (4th ed., pp. 281-282). Philadelphia: Saunders.

---

105. A client in labor tells the nurse that she suddenly has a wet feeling in the vaginal area. The nurse quickly checks the client and notes a large amount of bright red blood. The nurse would immediately:

1 Notify the obstetrician.

2 Insert an intravenous catheter.

3 Prepare to perform a vaginal examination.

4 Prepare the client for an emergency cesarean birth.

Level of Cognitive Ability: Application
Client Needs: Physiological Integrity
Integrated Process: Nursing Process/ Implementation
Content Area: Maternity

Answer: 1

Rationale: Vaginal bleeding (bright red, dark red, or in an amount in excess of that expected during normal cervical dilation) requires immediate notification of the obstetrician. This finding indicates an emergency situation and could have occurred as a result of placenta previa or placental separation. Although the nurse will prepare the client for an emergency cesarean delivery and insert an intravenous catheter, these are not the immediate actions. A vaginal examination is not performed on a pregnant client who is bleeding vaginally.

Test-Taking Strategy: Note the strategic word *immediately*, and focus on the data in the question. Noting the words *large amount of bright red blood* will direct you to option 1. Remember that when an emergency situation is presented in the question, it is likely that the correct option will be to notify the health care provider. Review care of the client in labor and the test-taking strategies for answering prioritizing questions and those related to contacting the health care provider if you had difficulty with this question.

Tip for the Beginning Nursing Student: Vaginal bleeding during pregnancy is always a concern. Two conditions that can cause vaginal bleeding are abruptio placentae and placenta previa. In abruptio placentae the normally implanted placenta separates before the fetus is born. Placenta previa is an abnormal condition in which the placenta is implanted low in the uterus near the presenting part. You will learn about the causes of bleeding during pregnancy and the immediate interventions if bleeding occurs in your maternity nursing course.

References

Leifer, G. (2008). *Maternity nursing: An introductory text* (10th ed., pp. 97-98). Philadelphia: Saunders.

Murray, S., & McKinney, E. (2006). *Foundations of maternal-newborn nursing* (4th ed., pp. 632-633). Philadelphia: Saunders.

---

106. While caring for a client in labor, the nurse suspects an umbilical cord prolapse. The nurse would immediately:

1 Set up for an emergency cesarean delivery.

2 Adjust the bed to Trendelenburg's position.

3 Encourage the woman to push with each contraction.

4 Calmly reassure the woman and her partner that all possible measures are being taken.

Level of Cognitive Ability: Application
Client Needs: Physiological Integrity
Integrated Process: Nursing Process/
   Implementation
Content Area: Maternity

Answer: 2

Rationale: Adjusting the bed into Trendelenburg's position (mattress flat, foot of bed elevated) uses gravity to reverse the direction of the pressure, keeping the presenting part off the umbilical cord. In addition, the knee-chest or modified Sims' position can be used. Pushing with contractions is contraindicated because it will push the presenting part against the cord. Not all prolapsed cords require a cesarean delivery. The nurse would reassure the woman and her partner after placing the woman in Trendelenburg's position.

Test-Taking Strategy: Note the strategic word *immediately*, and visualize the situation. Eliminate option 4 first using Maslow's Hierarchy of Needs theory because it does not address a physiological need. From the remaining options, select the option that addresses the physiological safety of the primary client (the fetus). Also remember that, in a prioritizing question if repositioning is indicated in one of the options, that option may be the correct one. Review immediate interventions for umbilical cord prolapse and the test-taking strategies for answering prioritizing questions if you had difficulty with this question.

Tip for the Beginning Nursing Student: A prolapsed umbilical cord refers to a condition in which the umbilical cord slips down after the amniotic membranes rupture, subjecting it to compression between the fetus and pelvis. This is a serious occurrence because it causes interruption in blood flow, and thus oxygenation, through the cord to the fetus and is potentially fatal. You will learn about prolapsed umbilical cord and the immediate interventions in your maternity nursing course.

References

Leifer, G. (2007). *Introduction to maternity and pediatric nursing* (5th ed., p. 194). Philadelphia: Saunders.

Murray, S., & McKinney, E. (2006). *Foundations of maternal-newborn nursing* (4th ed., p. 725). Philadelphia: Saunders.

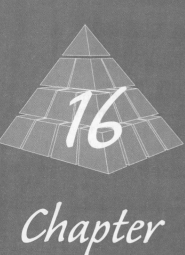

16

Chapter

Child Health Questions

107. A nurse at a playground witnesses a child fall off a swing. The nurse rushes to the child and suspects that he has a broken right leg. The nurse takes which priority action?
1 Immobilizes the leg
2 Calls for an ambulance
3 Removes the child's shoes
4 Tells the child that everything will be fine

Level of Cognitive Ability: Application
Client Needs: Physiological Integrity
Integrated Process: Nursing Process/ Implementation
Content Area: Child Health

Answer: 1

Rationale: When a fracture is suspected, the area is immobilized and splinted before the victim is moved. Shoes are not removed because this action can cause increased trauma. Emergency help is called for, and the nurse should remain with the child and provide realistic reassurance. Telling the child that everything will be fine is nontherapeutic.

Test-Taking Strategy: Note the strategic word *priority*. Focusing on the subject—a broken right leg—will direct you to option 1. When a fracture is suspected, remember to immobilize and splint that area. Review care of the victim with a fracture and the various test-taking strategies if you had difficulty with this question.

Tip for the Beginning Nursing Student: A fracture is a break or disruption in a bone's continuity and generally occurs when traumatic or excessive force is placed on a bone. The signs and symptoms will vary depending on the location, type, and cause of injury but generally include pain at the site of injury, immobility or decreased range of motion, deformity, and edema. You will learn about fractures and the immediate interventions in your pediatrics nursing course when you study musculoskeletal disorders.

References
Christensen, B., & Kockrow, E. (2006). *Foundations of nursing* (5th ed., p. 764). St. Louis: Mosby.
Wong, D., Perry, S., Hockenberry, M., Lowdermilk, D., & Wilson, D. (2006). *Maternal-child nursing care* (3rd ed., p. 1809). St. Louis: Mosby.

108. A newborn infant with a diagnosis of subdural hematoma is admitted to the newborn nursery. The nurse does which of the following to assess for the major symptom associated with subdural hematoma?
1 Monitors the urine for blood
2 Monitors the urinary output pattern
3 Tests for contractures of the extremities
4 Tests for equality of extremities when stimulating reflexes

Level of Cognitive Ability: Analysis
Client Needs: Physiological Integrity
Integrated Process: Nursing Process/ Assessment/Data Collection
Content Area: Child Health

Answer: 4
Rationale: A subdural hematoma can cause pressure on a specific area of the cerebral tissue. Especially if the infant is actively bleeding, this can cause changes in the stimuli responses in the extremities on the opposite side of the body. Option 3 is incorrect because contractures would not occur this soon after delivery. Options 1 and 2 are incorrect. An infant, after delivery, would normally be incontinent of urine. Blood in the urine would indicate abdominal trauma and not be a result of the subdural hematoma.

Test-Taking Strategy: Note the strategic words *major symptom.* Eliminate options 1 and 2 first because they are comparable or alike. Next focus on the infant's condition— subdural hematoma—and recall that this condition is a neurological disorder. Remember that the method of checking for complications and active bleeding into the cranial cavity would be a neurological assessment. Checking newborn reflexes is a neurological assessment. Although contractures of extremities could occur as residual effects, they would not occur immediately; therefore eliminate option 3. Review the signs of subdural hematoma in the newborn infant and the various test-taking strategies if you had difficulty with this question.

Tip for the Beginning Nursing Student: A subdural hematoma is an accumulation of blood in the subdural space and is usually caused by an injury. It can be acute with rapid bleeding or subacute with the accumulation of blood occurring over a longer period. Because the accumulation of blood is in the cranial cavity, neurological assessment and monitoring for signs of increased intracranial pressure are a priority. You will learn about subdural hematomas in your medical-surgical nursing course and in your pediatrics (child health) nursing course when you study neurological disorders.

Reference
Wong, D., Perry, S., Hockenberry, M., Lowdermilk, D., & Wilson, D. (2006). *Maternal-child nursing care* (3rd ed., p. 832). St. Louis: Mosby.

109. A nurse is reviewing the record of an infant admitted to the newborn nursery. The nurse notes that the physician has documented bladder exstrophy. On assessment of the infant, the nurse expects to note which of the following?
1 Undescended or hidden testes
2 Urinary bladder on the outside of the body
3 Opening of the urethral meatus on the ventral side of the glans penis

Answer: 2
Rationale: Bladder exstrophy is a congenital anomaly characterized by the extrusion of the urinary bladder to the outside of the body through a defect in the lower abdominal wall. Option 1 describes cryptorchidism, option 3 describes epispadias, and option 4 describes hypospadias.

Test-Taking Strategy: Note the relationship between the prefix in the name of the disorder, *ex-*, and the word *outside* in option 2. Review this disorder and the various test-taking strategies if you had difficulty with this question.

Tip for the Beginning Nursing Student: Bladder exstrophy is a congenital anomaly. In the newborn infant the nurse

4 Opening of the urethral meatus below the normal placement on the glans penis

Level of Cognitive Ability: Analysis
Client Needs: Physiological Integrity
Integrated Process: Nursing Process/Assessment/Data Collection
Content Area: Child Health

would note the extrusion of the urinary bladder to the outside of the body. This occurs as a result of a defect in the lower abdominal wall. The nurse would institute measures as prescribed to protect the urinary bladder and prevent injury to the bladder mucosa. Surgical intervention will be planned to correct the condition. You will learn about this congenital anomaly in your maternity nursing course when you study newborn disorders.

Reference
Wong, D., Perry, S., Hockenberry, M., Lowdermilk, D., & Wilson, D. (2006). *Maternal-child nursing care* (3rd ed., p. 863). St. Louis: Mosby.

---

110. A nurse notes that a child with Hirschsprung's disease who is scheduled for surgery has a nursing diagnosis of *Deficient fluid volume.* The nurse plans to implement which intervention to stabilize the child's hydration status before surgery?
  1 Monitor daily weight.
  2 Monitor intake and output.
  3 Administer tap water enemas.
  4 Administer intravenous fluids and electrolytes.

Level of Cognitive Ability: Application
Client Needs: Physiological Integrity
Integrated Process: Nursing Process/Planning
Content Area: Child Health

Answer: 4
Rationale: A child is stabilized with intravenous fluids and electrolytes before surgical management of the aganglionic portion of the bowel. Measurement of daily weight and intake and output assesses hydration status. Tap water enemas will alter the child's hydration status further.

Test-Taking Strategy: Focus on the subject—to stabilize the child's hydration status. Eliminate options 1 and 2 because they are assessments rather than interventions. Eliminate option 3 because it will further cause a *Deficient fluid volume.* Option 4 addresses stabilization. Review care to the child with Hirschsprung's disease and the various test-taking strategies if you had difficulty with this question.

Tip for the Beginning Nursing Student: Hirschsprung's disease is also known as congenital aganglionosis or megacolon and is the result of an absence of ganglion cells in the rectum and, to varying degrees, upward in the colon. Constipation, signs of bowel obstruction, abdominal pain and distention, vomiting, and failure to thrive are manifestations. You will learn about Hirschsprung's disease in your pediatrics nursing course when you study gastrointestinal disorders.

References
Leifer, G. (2007). *Introduction to maternity and pediatric nursing* (5th ed., p. 639). Philadelphia: Saunders.
Wong, D., Perry, S., Hockenberry, M., Lowdermilk, D., & Wilson, D. (2006). *Maternal-child nursing care* (3rd ed., p. 1506). St. Louis: Mosby.

---

111. A nurse provides home care instructions to the parents of a toddler newly diagnosed with hemophilia. Which statement by the parents indicates a need for further instructions?
  1 "We need to pad crib rails and table corners."
  2 "If our child has any discomfort, it is acceptable to give him aspirin."

Answer: 2
Rationale: In the child with hemophilia, bleeding is a priority concern. Therefore measures are implemented to prevent this occurrence. The parents are instructed about dental hygiene measures, such as using a soft-bristled, small toothbrush. The environment should be made as safe as possible, and the parents are instructed to pad crib side rails and table corners to prevent injury. The child should wear a Medic-Alert bracelet for identification of the disorder. Neither aspirin nor aspirin-containing compounds should be used, primarily because of their antiplatelet

3 "We need to obtain a medical identification bracelet for our child."
4 "We need to have our child use a soft-bristled, small toothbrush for dental hygiene."

Level of Cognitive Ability: Analysis
Client Needs: Safe and Effective Care Environment
Integrated Process: Teaching and Learning
Content Area: Child Health

properties. Acetaminophen (Tylenol) can be used for discomfort if needed.

Test-Taking Strategy: Note the strategic words *a need for further instructions.* These indicate a negative event query and the need to find the option that indicates an incorrect parental statement. Recalling that bleeding is the priority concern and that aspirin has antiplatelet properties will direct you to option 2. Review discharge teaching points for a child with hemophilia and the test-taking strategies for answering negative event query questions if you had difficulty with this question.

Tip for the Beginning Nursing Student: Hemophilia is a hereditary bleeding disorder characterized by a deficiency of one of the factors necessary for the coagulation of blood. The severity of the disorder varies with the extent of the deficiency. Nursing care focuses on preventing bleeding and providing a safe environment. You will learn about hemophilia in your pediatrics nursing course when you study hematological disorders.

References
Price, D., & Gwin, J. (2008). *Pediatric nursing: An introductory text* (10th ed., p. 247). St. Louis: Saunders.
Wong, D., Perry, S., Hockenberry, M., Lowdermilk, D., & Wilson, D. (2006). *Maternal-child nursing care* (3rd ed., pp. 1615-1616). St. Louis: Mosby.

112. The nurse is preparing to care for a pediatric client with an intravenous solution infusing. The nurse ensures that which item is in place to prevent fluid overload in this client?
1 Armboard
2 Infusion pump
3 Macrodrip infusion set
4 Large-bore intravenous catheter

Level of Cognitive Ability: Application
Client Needs: Safe and Effective Care Environment
Integrated Process: Nursing Process/Implementation
Content Area: Child Health

Answer: 2
Rationale: The most effective means of preventing irregularities in volume infusion for the pediatric client is the use of an infusion pump. This prevents both overhydration and underhydration. A small-bore catheter and a microdrip infusion set, rather than a macrodrip set, are used in the pediatric client An armboard may be helpful in certain instances to minimize movement of the extremity with the catheter, but it is not the most effective means for regulating intravenous flow.

Test-Taking Strategy: Focus on the subject—to prevent fluid overload. The only item in the options that will accomplish this is option 2. Use of an infusion pump will assist in preventing fluid overload. Review care of the pediatric client receiving an intravenous infusion and the various test-taking strategies if you had difficulty with this question.

Tip for the Beginning Nursing Student: When a child (or adult) is receiving fluids by the intravenous route (through a vein), the nurse needs to monitor the client and infusion closely to ensure that the fluid is infusing at the prescribed rate. If the fluid infuses too rapidly, serious complications can occur from the excess fluid. An infusion pump, which controls the amount of fluid infusing, should be used to administer intravenous fluids to a pediatric client. An important point to remember, however, is that the infusion pump (as with any device or machine) can fail or work improperly, so the nurse needs to monitor the child closely during intravenous infusion, even if an infusion pump is used. You will learn about the administration of intravenous fluids to the child in your pediatrics nursing course.

References

Leifer, G. (2007). *Introduction to maternity and pediatric nursing* (5th ed., p. 622). Philadelphia: Saunders.

Wong, D., Perry, S., Hockenberry, M., Lowdermilk, D., & Wilson, D. (2006). *Maternal-child nursing care* (3rd ed., pp. 1405-1406). St. Louis: Mosby.

---

113. A mother tells the clinic nurse that she does not want her child to receive any immunizations because she has heard that they cause serious illnesses. The nurse makes which appropriate statement to the mother?

1 "Are you afraid your child is going to die from the injection?"

2 "Why are you afraid? Children are immunized every day without a problem."

3 "There will be a slight discomfort at the time of the injection, but that is all that will happen."

4 "I can see you are very concerned about your child. What do you think might happen after an immunization is given?"

Level of Cognitive Ability: Application
Client Needs: Psychosocial Integrity
Integrated Process: Communication and Documentation
Content Area: Child Health

Answer: 4

Rationale: Option 4 acknowledges the mother's concern, which provides an opportunity for the mother to respond to the nurse's open-ended question. Options 1, 2, and 3 are nontherapeutic. Option 1 attempts to verify an assumption not supported in the question. Option 2 can make the mother feel defensive, devalues the mother's feelings, and requires an explanation from the mother. Option 3 provides false reassurance.

Test-Taking Strategy: Use therapeutic communication techniques. The correct option demonstrates empathy and helps the mother focus on specific fears so that the nurse can clarify information. Remember to focus on the client's feelings. Review therapeutic communication techniques and the test-taking strategies for answering communication questions if you had difficulty with this question.

Tip for the Beginning Nursing Student: An immunization is a procedure in which resistance to an infectious disease is induced. A schedule of various types of immunizations needs to be followed to prevent infectious childhood diseases. In addition, all states require immunizations for children enrolled in licensed child care programs and school. You will learn about the administration of immunizations and the immunization schedule in your pediatrics nursing course when you study communicable diseases.

References

deWit, S. (2009). *Medical-surgical nursing: Concepts & practice.* (p. 9). St. Louis: Saunders.

Price, D., & Gwin, J. (2008). *Pediatric nursing: An introductory text* (10th ed., p. 129). St. Louis: Saunders.

Wong, D., Perry, S., Hockenberry, M., Lowdermilk, D., & Wilson, D. (2006). *Maternal-child nursing care* (3rd ed., pp. 1062-1064). St. Louis: Mosby.

---

114. A child with hemophilia is brought into the emergency room after being hit on the neck with a baseball. The nurse should immediately check the child for:

1 Headache
2 Slurred speech

Answer: 3

Rationale: Trauma to the neck may cause bleeding into the tissues of the neck, which may compromise the airway. Hematuria is a symptom of hemophilia, although it is not associated with neck injury. Headache and slurred speech are associated with head trauma and are not the priority in this situation.

3 Airway obstruction
4 Spontaneous hematuria

Level of Cognitive Ability: Application
Client Needs: Physiological Integrity
Integrated Process: Nursing Process/
   Assessment/Data Collection
Content Area: Child Health

Test-Taking Strategy: Note the strategic word *immediately.* Use the ABCs—airway, breathing, and circulation. Airway assessment is always a first priority. This directs you to option 3. Review care of the child with hemophilia and the test-taking strategies for answering prioritizing questions if you had difficulty with this question.

Tip for the Beginning Nursing Student: Hemophilia is a hereditary bleeding disorder characterized by a deficiency of one of the factors necessary for the coagulation of blood. The severity of the disorder varies with the extent of the deficiency. Bleeding is always a concern if the child is injured. You will learn about hemophilia in your pediatrics nursing course when you study hematological disorders.

References

Hockenberry, M., & Wilson, D. (2007). *Nursing care of infants and children* (8th ed., pp. 1537, 1540). St. Louis: Mosby.

Price, D., & Gwin, J. (2008). *Pediatric nursing: An introductory text* (10th ed., p. 246). St. Louis: Saunders.

---

115. A 4-year-old child is admitted to the hospital for surgery. The nurse asks the parents which priority question to identify the adequacy of support for the child's psychosocial needs?
  1 "What are your child's favorite toys?"
  2 "What signs and symptoms has your child been having?"
  3 "Will a family member be able to stay with the child most of the time?"
  4 "How much do you know about the surgery and its expected outcome?"

Level of Cognitive Ability: Application
Client Needs: Psychosocial Integrity
Integrated Process: Nursing Process/
   Assessment/Data Collection
Content Area: Child Health

Answer: 3

Rationale: Separation from family is the most stressful aspect of hospitalization in young children. A primary goal is to prevent separation from family in children under the age of 5 years. Identifying support and the ability of family members to stay with the child takes priority over favorite toys or diversional activities. Options 2 and 4 relate to physiological needs.

Test-Taking Strategy: Focus on the subject—*adequacy of support and the child's psychosocial needs.* Options 2 and 4 relate to physiological needs so eliminate these options. From the remaining options, use Maslow's Hierarchy of Needs theory to select the security issue instead of the diversional activity. Review psychosocial needs of a 4-year-old child and the test-taking strategies for answering prioritization questions if you had difficulty with this question.

Tip for the Beginning Nursing Student: Hospitalization can be a stressful experience for the child, who can experience separation anxiety. How a child reacts to the experience depends on a number of factors, including age, cognitive development, preparation for the experience, coping skills, cultural influences, and previous experience with the health care system. You will learn about the stressors associated with hospitalization of the child in your pediatrics nursing course.

References

Hockenberry, M., & Wilson, D. (2007). *Nursing care of infants and children* (8th ed., pp. 511, 1047-1048). St. Louis: Mosby

Price, D., & Gwin, J. (2008). *Pediatric nursing: An introductory text* (10th ed., p. 25). St. Louis: Saunders.

116. A nurse is assessing a child who has just returned from surgery in a hip spica cast. Which of the following outcomes is the priority?
  1 The hips are abducted.
  2 Circulation is adequate.
  3 The child is on the right side.
  4 The head of the bed is elevated.

Level of Cognitive Ability: Analysis
Client Needs: Physiological Integrity
Integrated Process: Nursing Process/
  Evaluation
Content Area: Child Health

Answer: 2
Rationale: The priority concern during the first few hours after a cast is applied is swelling, which may cause the cast to act as a tourniquet and constrict circulation. Therefore circulatory assessment is a high priority. Elevating the head of a bed of a child in a hip spica cast causes discomfort. Using pillows to abduct the hips is not necessary because a hip spica cast immobilizes the hip and knee. Turning the child side to side at least every 2 hours is important because it allows the body cast to dry evenly and prevents complications related to immobility; however, it is not a higher priority than checking circulation.

Test-Taking Strategy: Note the strategic word *priority*. Use the ABCs—airway, breathing, and circulation. Option 2 reflects circulation. Review care of the child in a hip spica cast and the test-taking strategies for answering prioritizing questions if you had difficulty with this question.

Tip for the Beginning Nursing Student: A hip spica cast is an orthopedic cast that is applied to immobilize part or all of the body trunk and part or all of the lower extremities. It is used to treat various fractures, such as fractures of the hip or femur, and to correct a hip deformity. It may be used to treat developmental dysplasia of the hip, a condition in which the head of the femur is improperly seated in the acetabulum of the pelvis. You will learn about a hip spica cast and other types of casts in your pediatrics nursing course when you study musculoskeletal disorders.

References
Hockenberry, M., & Wilson, D. (2007). *Nursing care of infants and children* (8th ed., p. 1757). St. Louis: Mosby.
Price, D., & Gwin, J. (2008). *Pediatric nursing: An introductory text* (10th ed., pp. 108-109). St. Louis: Saunders.

117. The parents of a newborn infant diagnosed with esophageal atresia ask the nurse to explain the diagnosis. The nurse tells the parents that in this condition:
  1 Gastric contents regurgitate back into the esophagus.
  2 The esophagus terminates before it reaches the stomach.
  3 A portion of the stomach protrudes through part of the diaphragm.
  4 Abdominal contents herniate through an opening of the diaphragm.

Level of Cognitive Ability: Application
Client Needs: Physiological Integrity

Answer: 2
Rationale: Esophageal atresia and tracheoesophageal fistula (TEF) are congenital malformations in which the esophagus terminates before it reaches the stomach and/ or a fistula is present that forms an unnatural connection with the trachea. Option 1 describes gastroesophageal reflux. Option 3 describes a hiatal hernia. Option 4 describes a congenital diaphragmatic hernia.

Test-Taking Strategy: Focus on the diagnosis—esophageal atresia. Note the relationship between the word *atresia* and option 2. Review the characteristics of esophageal atresia and the various test-taking strategies if you had difficulty with this question.

Tip for the Beginning Nursing Student: Esophageal atresia is a congenital malformation in which the esophagus terminates before it reaches the stomach. It can cause

Integrated Process: Nursing Process/
Implementation
Content Area: Child Health

respiratory distress secondary to the aspiration of saliva and any oral fluids that may be given to the infant before being diagnosed with the disorder. Some manifestations of the disorder include excessive oral secretions, abdominal distention, and vomiting. Surgical repair will need to be done to correct the condition. You will learn about esophageal atresia in your pediatrics nursing course when you study gastrointestinal disorders.

References

Leifer, G. (2008). *Maternity nursing: An introductory text* (10th ed., p. 324). Philadelphia: Saunders.

Murray, S., & McKinney, E. (2006). *Foundations of maternal-newborn nursing* (4th ed., pp. 824-825). Philadelphia: Saunders.

---

118. A mother brings her child to the emergency room because he said that dirt flew into his eye during softball practice. The nurse takes which action first?
1 Assesses vision
2 Removes the dirt
3 Places ice on the eye
4 Irrigates the eye with sterile saline

Level of Cognitive Ability: Application
Client Needs: Physiological Integrity
Integrated Process: Nursing Process/
Implementation
Content Area: Child Health

Answer: 1

Rationale: If a surface foreign body injury occurs to the eye, the nurse would first assess visual acuity. The eye will then be assessed for corneal abrasions, followed by irrigating the eye with sterile normal saline to gently remove the particles. There is no reason to place ice on the eye. Placing ice on the eye would be done if the client sustained an eye contusion.

Test-Taking Strategy: Note the strategic word *first*, and use the steps of the nursing process. Option 1 is the only option that relates to assessment/data collection. Options 2, 3, and 4 relate to implementation. Review content related to initial treatment of various eye injuries and the various test-taking strategies if you had difficulty with this question.

Tip for the Beginning Nursing Student: Interventions to treat an eye injury are based on the type of injury that occurred. If a contusion (blow) to the eye occurred, the nurse would immediately place ice on the eye. If a substance splashed into the eye, the immediate intervention is to flush (irrigate) the eye. If dirt flew into the eye, the nurse would assess vision and check for the presence of the dirt substances and corneal abrasions before irrigating the eye. You will learn about interventions for treating various eye injuries in your pediatrics nursing course and in your medical-surgical nursing course when you study eye disorders.

References

deWit, S. (2009). *Medical-surgical nursing: Concepts & practice* (pp. 640-641). St. Louis: Saunders.

Hockenberry, M., & Wilson, D. (2007). *Nursing care of infants and children* (8th ed., pp. 1011-1012). St. Louis: Mosby.

119. A nurse is assessing a child with increased intracranial pressure who has been exhibiting decorticate posturing. On assessment the nurse notes extension of the upper and lower extremities with internal rotation of the upper arms, wrists, knees, and feet. The nurse determines that the child's condition:

1 Is unchanged
2 Has improved
3 Indicates decreased intracranial pressure
4 Indicates a deterioration in neurological function

Level of Cognitive Ability: Analysis
Client Needs: Physiological Integrity
Integrated Process: Nursing Process/ Assessment/Data Collection
Content Area: Child Health

Answer: 4
Rationale: In decorticate posturing the nurse would note flexion of the upper extremities and extension of the lower extremities. In decerebrate posturing the nurse would note extension of the upper and lower extremities with internal rotation of the upper arms, wrists, knees, and feet. The progression from decorticate to decerebrate posturing usually indicates deteriorating neurological function and warrants physician notification. Options 1, 2, and 3 are inaccurate interpretations.

Test-Taking Strategy: Eliminate options 2 and 3 first because they are comparable or alike. From the remaining options, recalling the significance of decerebrate posturing will direct you to option 4. Review the significance of posturing and the various test-taking strategies if you had difficulty with this question.

Tip for the Beginning Nursing Student: Posture is the position of the body and is determined and maintained by coordination of the muscles that move the limbs and a sense of balance. Abnormal postures occur in neurological disorders, such as head injuries, and in conditions that cause increased intracranial pressure. These types of posturing include decorticate, decerebrate, and flaccid. The presence of abnormal posturing needs to be reported to the physician. You will learn about posturing when you study neurological disorders in your pediatrics nursing course and in your medical-surgical nursing course.

References
Hockenberry, M., & Wilson, D. (2007). *Nursing care of infants and children* (8th ed., p. 1622). St. Louis: Mosby.
Price, D., & Gwin, J. (2008). *Pediatric nursing: An introductory text* (10th ed., pp. 211, 213). St. Louis: Saunders.

120. A nurse is reviewing the assessment findings and laboratory results of a child diagnosed with new-onset glomerulonephritis. Which of the following findings would the nurse most likely expect to note?

1 Hypotension
2 Tea-colored urine
3 Low serum potassium
4 Elevated creatinine levels

Level of Cognitive Ability: Analysis
Client Needs: Physiological Integrity
Integrated Process: Nursing Process/ Assessment/Data Collection
Content Area: Child Health

Answer: 2
Rationale: Gross hematuria resulting in dark brown or smoky, tea-colored urine is a classic symptom of glomerulonephritis. Hypertension is also a common finding in glomerulonephritis. Blood urea nitrogen levels and creatinine levels are elevated only when there is an 80% decrease in glomerular filtration rate and renal insufficiency is severe. A high potassium level results from inadequate glomerular filtration.

Test-Taking Strategy: Note that the child is experiencing a renal disorder, and note the strategic words *new-onset* and *most likely.* Recalling that the creatinine level is elevated only when there is an 80% decrease in glomerular filtration rate will assist in eliminating option 4. Next eliminate options 1 and 3 knowing that hypertension rather than hypotension and hyperkalemia rather than hypokalemia will occur in this renal disorder. Review the clinical manifestations associated with glomerulonephritis and the various test-taking strategies if you had difficulty with this question.

Tip for the Beginning Nursing Student: Glomerulonephritis is a kidney disorder characterized by an inflammatory injury in the glomerulus. It is characterized by proteinuria, hematuria, decreased urine production, and edema (swelling). Acute poststreptococcal glomerulonephritis is the most common type and occurs as an immune reaction to a group A beta-hemolytic streptococcal infection of the throat. You will learn about glomerulonephritis when you study renal disorders in your pediatrics nursing course.

References

Hockenberry, M., & Wilson, D. (2007). *Nursing care of infants and children* (8th ed., p. 1244). St. Louis: Mosby.

Price, D., & Gwin, J. (2008). *Pediatric nursing: An introductory text* (10th ed., p. 258). St. Louis: Saunders.

---

121. A child newly diagnosed with type 1 diabetes mellitus who is receiving insulin suddenly experiences signs of a hypoglycemic reaction. The nurse would immediately give the child:
  1 1 teaspoon of sugar
  2 1 teaspoon of honey
  3 ½ cup of diet cola
  4 8 oz of skim milk

Level of Cognitive Ability: Application
Client Needs: Physiological Integrity
Integrated Process: Nursing Process/ Implementation
Content Area: Child Health

Answer: 4

Rationale: Hypoglycemia is immediately treated with 15 g of carbohydrate. Glucose tablets or glucose gel may be administered. Other items used to treat hypoglycemia include ½ cup of fruit juice, ½ cup of regular (nondiet) soft drink, 8 oz of skim milk, 6 to 10 hard candies, 4 cubes or 4 teaspoons of sugar, 6 saltines, 3 graham crackers, or 1 tablespoon of honey or syrup. The items in options 1, 2, and 3 would not adequately treat hypoglycemia.

Test-Taking Strategy: Eliminate options 1 and 2 first because they are comparable or alike. From the remaining options, select option 4 because a diet cola does not contain the amount of carbohydrate needed to treat hypoglycemia. Review the treatment measures for hypoglycemia and the various test-taking strategies if you had difficulty with this question.

Tip for the Beginning Nursing Student: Diabetes mellitus is a disorder of carbohydrate, fat, and protein metabolism that is primarily the result of a deficiency or complete lack of insulin secretion by the beta cells of the pancreas or resistance to insulin. Hypoglycemia (a low blood glucose level) is a complication and is characterized by symptoms such as weakness, headache, hunger, and visual disturbances. It is immediately treated with 15 g of carbohydrate. It is important to recognize the signs and symptoms of hypoglycemia and how to treat it. You will learn about diabetes mellitus and its complications in your pediatrics nursing course and in your medical-surgical nursing course when you study endocrine disorders.

References

Hockenberry, M., & Wilson, D. (2007). *Nursing care of infants and children* (8th ed., p. 1414). St. Louis: Mosby.

Price, D., & Gwin, J. (2008). *Pediatric nursing: An introductory text* (10th ed., p. 298). St. Louis: Saunders.

122. A clinic nurse has provided instructions to the mother of a child with a urinary tract infection. Which statement by the mother indicates a need for further instructions?
 1 "I should increase my child's fluid intake."
 2 "I should not use bubble baths with my child."
 3 "I should wipe my child from front to back after urination or a bowel movement."
 4 "I should encourage my child to hold the urine and to urinate at least four times each day."

Level of Cognitive Ability: Analysis
Client Needs: Health Promotion and Maintenance
Integrated Process: Teaching and Learning
Content Area: Child Health

Answer: 4
Rationale: Fluid intake including water should be encouraged. Bubble baths are avoided secondary to possible urethral irritation. The parents should be taught to wipe the child from front to back after urination or a bowel movement to avoid moving bacteria from the anus to the urethra. The child should be encouraged to avoid holding urine and to urinate at least four times per day and should be told that the bladder should be emptied with each void to avoid residual urine.

Test-Taking Strategy: Note the strategic words *need for further instructions*. These words indicate a negative event query and the need to look for the incorrect statement. Careful reading of the options and applying principles related to prevention of urinary tract infections will direct you to option 4. Review client instructions related to a urinary tract infection and the various test-taking strategies if you had difficulty with this question.

Tip for the Beginning Nursing Student: A urinary tract infection is an infection of one or more structures in the urinary system. The infection is usually characterized by urinary frequency, burning pain with urinating, fever, back pain, and possible blood or pus in the urine. A sterile urine specimen is collected to check for the bacteria causing the infection and to determine treatment. Several measures can be taken to prevent and treat a urinary tract infection. You will learn about urinary tract infections in your pediatrics nursing course and in your medical-surgical nursing course when you study renal disorders.

References
Hockenberry, M., & Wilson, D. (2007). *Nursing care of infants and children* (8th ed., pp. 1237-1239, 1241). St. Louis: Mosby.
Price, D., & Gwin, J. (2008). *Pediatric nursing: An introductory text* (10th ed., pp. 256-257). St. Louis: Saunders.

123. A nurse is monitoring a newborn of a mother with diabetes mellitus. The nurse determines that the newborn is at risk for which of the following?
 1 Hypercalcemia
 2 Hyperglycemia
 3 Hypobilirubinemia
 4 Respiratory distress syndrome

Level of Cognitive Ability: Analysis
Client Needs: Physiological Integrity
Integrated Process: Nursing Process/ Assessment/Data Collection
Content Area: Child Health

Answer: 4
Rationale: The major neonatal complications of preexisting diabetes mellitus in the mother are hypoglycemia, hypocalcemia, hypomagnesemia, hyperbilirubinemia, and polycythemia. Congenital anomalies, macrosomia, birth trauma, perinatal asphyxia, respiratory distress syndrome, and cardiomyopathy are also problems seen in newborns of a diabetic mother.

Test-Taking Strategy: Focusing on the mother's diagnosis will assist in eliminating option 2. From the remaining options it is necessary to know the complications of the newborn of a mother with diabetes mellitus. Review the complications associated with the newborn of the mother with diabetes mellitus and the various test-taking strategies if you had difficulty with this question.

Tip for the Beginning Nursing Student: It is important to know the effects of maternal diabetes on the newborn. Respiratory distress syndrome is an acute lung disease caused by a deficiency of pulmonary surfactant. Fetal hyperinsulinemia retards cortisol production, which is necessary for surfactant production. It is characterized by airless alveoli, inelastic lungs, a respiration rate greater than 60 breaths/minute, nasal flaring, retractions, grunting, and edema. You will learn about the effects of maternal diabetes on the newborn in your pediatrics nursing course and in your maternity nursing course.

References
Leifer, G. (2008). *Maternity nursing: An introductory text* (10th ed., pp. 331-332). Philadelphia: Saunders.

Wong, D., Perry, S., Hockenberry, M., Lowdermilk, D., & Wilson, D. (2006). *Maternal-child nursing care* (3rd ed., pp. 822-823). St. Louis: Mosby.

---

124. A 16-year-old client who underwent emergency surgery for a ruptured appendix refuses to allow the nurse to change the abdominal dressing, saying, "Go away. There is nothing wrong with this dressing." Which of the following nursing responses would be best?

1 "Please do not be upset with me. I am just doing my job."

2 "I promise to do this really quickly, and then I will leave you alone."

3 "You can refuse the dressing change at this time, but your friends cannot visit you until it is done."

4 "I will draw the curtain and expose only the area on your abdomen that is needed. Can I go ahead with that?"

Level of Cognitive Ability: Application
Client Needs: Health Promotion and Maintenance
Integrated Process: Communication and Documentation
Content Area: Child Health

Answer: 4

Rationale: The primary developmental need of the hospitalized adolescent is maintenance of privacy, modesty, and control. The correct option strives to meet these needs. Options 1 and 2 do not address the client's concerns, and option 3 contains a threat.

Test-Taking Strategy: Note the strategic words *16-year-old client.* Remember the developmental needs of the adolescent when answering this question. Also use therapeutic communication techniques. Option 4 is the only one that focuses on client's feelings and needs. Review therapeutic communication techniques and the test-taking strategies for answering communication questions if you had difficulty with this question.

Tip for the Beginning Nursing Student: Adolescence is a time of transition from childhood to adulthood and is characterized by biological and psychological changes, including the appearance of secondary sex characteristics. The adolescent is very aware of the body changes that are taking place, and the nurse needs to respect the adolescent's need for body privacy. Many other growth and development changes also take place during the adolescent period, which you will learn about in your pediatrics nursing course.

References
Potter, P., & Perry, A. (2009) *Fundamentals of nursing* (7th ed., pp. 352-357). St. Louis: Mosby.

Price, D., & Gwin, J. (2008). *Pediatric nursing: An introductory text* (10th ed., p. 327). St. Louis: Saunders.

Wong, D., Perry, S., Hockenberry, M., Lowdermilk, D., & Wilson, D. (2006). *Maternal-child nursing care* (3rd ed., p. 1192). St. Louis: Mosby.

125. A nurse is caring for a child who sustained a head injury from a fall. The nurse avoids which of the following in the care of the child?

1 Restrict oral fluids.
2 Elevate the head of the bed.
3 Coughing and deep breathing.
4 Perform neurological assessments.

Level of Cognitive Ability: Application
Client Needs: Physiological Integrity
Integrated Process: Nursing Process/
  Implementation
Content Area: Child Health

Answer: 3

Rationale: A child with a head injury is at risk for increased intracranial pressure (ICP). Elevating the head of the bed decreases fluid retention in cerebral tissue and promotes drainage. Fluids may be restricted to reduce the chance of fluid overload and resultant increased ICP. Hypoxia and Valsalva's maneuver associated with coughing both acutely elevate ICP. Neurological assessments should be performed to monitor for increased ICP.

Test-Taking Strategy: Note the strategic word *avoids*, and recall that a head injury places the child at risk for increased ICP. From this point identify the option that would cause an increase in the ICP. This will direct you to option 3. Review care of the child who sustained a head injury and the various test-taking strategies if you had difficulty with this question.

Tip for the Beginning Nursing Student: A head injury results from trauma to the head from any mechanical force to the scalp, skull, meninges, or brain. A primary concern when a child sustains a head injury is resultant pressure in the brain from swelling. This is known as increased ICP. If this occurs, structures within the cranium are compressed, which can result in serious neurological complications. You will learn about head injuries and increased ICP in your pediatrics nursing course when you study neurological disorders.

References
Hockenberry, M., & Wilson, D. (2007). *Nursing care of infants and children* (8th ed., pp. 1631-1632). St. Louis: Mosby.

Price, D., & Gwin, J. (2008). *Pediatric nursing: An introductory text* (10th ed., pp. 211-212). St. Louis: Saunders.

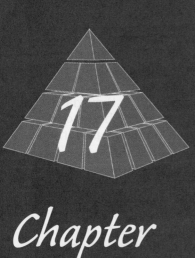

17

Chapter

Pharmacology Questions

126. A nurse is instructing a client about quinapril hydrochloride (Accupril). The nurse tells the client:

1 To take the medication with food only
2 To rise slowly from a lying to a sitting position
3 To discontinue the medication if nausea occurs
4 That a therapeutic effect will be seen immediately

Level of Cognitive Ability: Application
Client Needs: Physiological Integrity
Integrated Process: Teaching and Learning
Content Area: Pharmacology

Answer: 2

Rationale: Quinapril hydrochloride is an angiotensin-converting enzyme (ACE) inhibitor used in the treatment of hypertension. The client should be instructed to rise slowly from a lying to a sitting position and to permit the legs to dangle from the bed momentarily before standing to reduce the hypotensive effect. The medication may be given without regard to food. The client should be instructed to drink a noncaffinated carbonated beverage and eat crackers or dry toast if nauseous. A full therapeutic effect may occur in 1 to 2 weeks.

Test-Taking Strategy: Eliminate option 1 because of the close-ended word *only* and option 4 because of the word *immediately.* Next focus on the name of the medication, and recall that most ACE inhibitor medication names end with the letters *-pril* and that these medications are used to treat hypertension. This will direct you to option 2. Review this medication and the test-taking strategies for answering pharmacology questions if you had difficulty with this question.

Tip for the Beginning Nursing Student: Hypertension refers to an elevated blood pressure and is a known cardiovascular risk factor. ACE inhibitor medications are one class of medications used to treat hypertension. Because medication used to treat hypertension lowers the blood pressure, lightheadedness and dizziness can occur. Therefore it is important for the nurse to teach the client safety measures. You will learn about ACE inhibitors in your pharmacology course and in your medical-surgical nursing course when you study cardiovascular disorders.

Reference
Hodgson, B., & Kizior, R. (2009). *Saunders nursing drug handbook 2009* (p. 988). Philadelphia: Saunders.

127. The nurse notes that a client is receiving ganciclovir sodium (Cytovene). The nurse suspects that the client is receiving this medication for the treatment of:
1 Pancreatitis
2 Urolithiasis
3 Nephrotic syndrome
4 Cytomegalovirus retinitis

Level of Cognitive Ability: Analysis
Client Needs: Physiological Integrity
Integrated Process: Nursing Process/ Assessment/Data Collection
Content Area: Pharmacology

Answer: 4
Rationale: Ganciclovir sodium is an antiviral medication used to treat cytomegalovirus (CMV) retinitis in immuno-compromised clients and CMV gastrointestinal infections and pneumonitis; it is also used to prevent CMV disease in transplant clients. It is not used to treat pancreatitis, urolithiasis, or nephrotic syndrome.

Test-Taking Strategy: Focus on the name of the medication. Recalling that most antiviral medications names contain the letters *vir* will direct you to option 4. Review this medication and the test-taking strategies for answering pharmacology questions if you had difficulty with this question.

Tip for the Beginning Nursing Student: Cytomegalovirus retinitis is an infection of the retina caused by a herpes type of virus. Pancreatitis is an inflammatory condition of the pancreas that can be acute or chronic. Urolithiasis refers to the presence of calculi (stones) in the urinary system. Nephrotic syndrome is an abnormal condition of the kidney characterized by marked proteinuria, hypoalbuminemia, and edema. You will learn about cytomegalovirus retinitis, pancreatitis, and urolithiasis in your medical-surgical nursing course and about nephrotic syndrome in your pediatric nursing course.

Reference
Hodgson, B., & Kizior, R. (2009). *Saunders nursing drug handbook 2009* (p. 528). Philadelphia: Saunders.

---

128. A nurse is planning to teach a client how to mix regular and NPH insulin in the same syringe. Which of the following instructions is included in the plan of care?
1 Take all air out of the bottle before mixing.
2 Draw up the regular insulin first into the syringe.
3 Keep both bottles stored in the refrigerator for 1 month.
4 Shake the NPH insulin bottle in the hands before mixing.

Level of Cognitive Ability: Application
Client Needs: Physiological Integrity
Integrated Process: Nursing Process/ Planning
Content Area: Pharmacology

Answer: 2
Rationale: Before mixing different types of insulin, the bottle should be rotated for at least 1 minute between both hands. This resuspends the insulin and helps warm the medication. The nurse should not shake the bottles. Shaking causes foaming and bubbles to form, which may trap particles of insulin and alter the dosage. Insulin may be maintained at room temperature. Additional bottles of insulin should be stored in the refrigerator for future use. Regular insulin is drawn up before NPH insulin. Air does not need to be removed from the insulin bottle.

Test-Taking Strategy: Visualize the procedure as you carefully read each option. When answering questions that relate to mixing insulin remember the letters *RN*—draw the *r*egular insulin into the syringe before the *N*PH insulin. Review the procedures for administering insulin and the test-taking strategies for answering pharmacology questions if you had difficulty with this question.

Tip for the Beginning Nursing Student: Insulin is a medication used to treat diabetes mellitus, a disorder of fat, carbohydrate, and protein metabolism. Regular insulin is short-acting insulin, and NPH is an intermediate-acting insulin. When both types of insulin are prescribed they can be mixed together in one syringe so that only one injection is necessary. There is a specific procedure for mixing these types of insulin, which you will learn when you learn about injections and when you study pharmacology.

References
Lehne, R. (2007). *Pharmacology for nursing care* (6th ed., p. 670). Philadelphia: Saunders.

Lewis, S., Heitkemper, M., Dirksen, S., & Bucher, L. (2007). *Medical-surgical nursing: Assessment and management of clinical problems* (7th ed., p. 1262). St. Louis: Mosby.

---

129. A client has been taking lansoprazole (Prevacid). The nurse monitors the client for the relief of which of the following symptoms?
1 Diarrhea
2 Heartburn
3 Flatulence
4 Constipation

Level of Cognitive Ability: Analysis
Client Needs: Physiological Integrity
Integrated Process: Nursing Process/ Evaluation
Content Area: Pharmacology

Answer: 2
Rationale: Lansoprazole is a gastric pump inhibitor (proton pump inhibitor). Its intended effect is relief of gastric irritation pain, often referred to as heartburn. The medication does not improve constipation, diarrhea, or flatulence.

Test-Taking Strategy: Focus on the strategic words *relief of*. Note the name of the medication, and recall that most proton pump inhibitor medication names end with the letters *-zole*. This will direct you to option 2. Review this medication and the test-taking strategies for answering pharmacology questions if you had difficulty with this question.

Tip for the Beginning Nursing Student: Heartburn is a painful burning sensation in the esophagus. It is usually caused by the reflux of gastric acid into the esophagus. Proton pump inhibitors are one type of medication used to treat heartburn. You will learn about heartburn when you study gastrointestinal disorders in your medical-surgical nursing course and about proton pump inhibitors when you study pharmacology.

Reference
Hodgson, B., & Kizior, R. (2009). *Saunders nursing drug handbook 2009* (p. 660). Philadelphia: Saunders.

---

130. A client is taking amiloride hydrochloride (Midamor) daily. The nurse tells the client to take the dose:
1 At bedtime
2 On an empty stomach
3 Between lunch and dinner
4 In the morning with breakfast

Level of Cognitive Ability: Application
Client Needs: Physiological Integrity
Integrated Process: Teaching and Learning
Content Area: Pharmacology

Answer: 4
Rationale: Amiloride is a potassium-sparing diuretic used to treat edema or hypertension. A daily dose should be taken in the morning to avoid nocturia. The dose should be taken with food to increase bioavailability.

Test-Taking Strategy: Eliminate options 1, 2, and 3 because they are comparable or alike in that they all indicate taking the medication dose without food. Review this medication and the test-taking strategies for answering pharmacology questions if you had difficulty with this question.

Tip for the Beginning Nursing Student: Edema is the abnormal accumulation of fluid in body tissues. Hypertension refers to an elevated blood pressure and is a known cardiovascular risk factor. Potassium-sparing diuretics are one class of medications used to treat edema or hypertension. Only a few medications are potassium sparing, and amiloride is one of them. A concern with potassium-sparing diuretics is that the client retains potassium, which can lead to hyperkalemia (a high potassium level). Therefore the nurse monitors the client for signs of hyperkalemia. You will learn about potassium-sparing diuretics when you study pharmacology.

References
Hodgson, B., & Kizior, R. (2009). *Saunders nursing drug handbook 2009* (p. 53). Philadelphia: Saunders.
Lehne, R. (2007). *Pharmacology for nursing care* (6th ed., p. 447). Philadelphia: Saunders.

---

131. A nurse is caring for a client with a diagnosis of rheumatoid arthritis who is receiving aspirin (acetylsalicylic acid, ASA) 5 g orally daily. The nurse recognizes which of the following as an adverse effect related to the medication?
1 Tinnitus
2 Joint pain
3 Urinary retention
4 Difficulty voiding

Level of Cognitive Ability: Analysis
Client Needs: Physiological Integrity
Integrated Process: Nursing Process/ Assessment/Data Collection
Content Area: Pharmacology

Answer: 1
Rationale: Aspirin is a nonsteroidal anti-inflammatory drug. Adverse effects include gastrointestinal bleeding or gastric mucosal lesions, ringing in the ears (tinnitus), or generalized pruritus. Headache, dizziness, flushing, tachycardia, hyperventilation, sweating, and thirst are also adverse effects. Options 2, 3, and 4 are incorrect. In addition, aspirin is administered to the client with rheumatoid arthritis to relieve joint pain.

Test-Taking Strategy: Focus on the subject—*an adverse effect.* Eliminate options 3 and 4 first because they are comparable or alike. Next eliminate option 2 because aspirin is administered to relieve joint pain. Last, remembering that aspirin can cause gastrointestinal disturbances and ototoxicity will direct you to the correct option. Review aspirin and the test-taking strategies for pharmacology questions if you had difficulty with this question.

Tip for the Beginning Nursing Student: Arthritis is an inflammatory condition of the joints characterized by pain, swelling, heat, redness, and limitation of movement. It can affect the client's ability to perform activities of daily living and result in debilitation. Arthritis can occur in childhood or adulthood. Large doses of aspirin may be administered to alleviate the joint pain. However, aspirin can cause gastrointestinal bleeding, ringing in the ears (tinnitus), or generalized pruritus. You will learn about the effects of aspirin when you study pharmacology and will learn about arthritis in your pediatrics and medical-surgical nursing courses.

Reference
Hodgson, B., & Kizior, R. (2009). *Saunders nursing drug handbook 2009* (p. 95). Philadelphia: Saunders.

132. A nurse is preparing a plan of care for a client who is receiving meperidine hydrochloride (Demerol) for pain. The nurse includes in the plan of care to monitor for which adverse effect of this medication?
1 Nausea
2 Sedation
3 Flushed face
4 Skeletal muscle flaccidity

Level of Cognitive Ability: Application
Client Needs: Physiological Integrity
Integrated Process: Nursing Process/ Planning
Content Area: Pharmacology

Answer: 4
Rationale: Frequent side effects of this medication include sedation, decreased blood pressure, diaphoresis, flushed face, dizziness, nausea, vomiting, and constipation. Adverse effects include respiratory depression; skeletal muscle flaccidity; cold and clammy skin; cyanosis; and extreme somnolence progressing to convulsions, stupor, and coma.

Test-Taking Strategy: Note the strategic words *adverse effect,* and recall that this medication is an opiate analgesic. Recalling that an adverse effect is more severe than a side effect and is always an undesirable effect will direct you to option 4. Review the adverse effects of meperidine hydrochloride and the test-taking strategies for answering pharmacology questions if you had difficulty with this question.

Tip for the Beginning Nursing Student: Meperidine hydrochloride (Demerol) is an opiate analgesic that is used to alleviate pain that occurs in many types of disorders. Because it is an opiate analgesic it will cause skeletal muscle flaccidity, which can place the client at risk for injury. Another critical adverse effect of opiate analgesics is that they cause respiratory depression so assessment of respiratory status is an important part of your nursing interventions. You will learn about this medication and other opiate analgesics in a pharmacology course or in your medical-surgical nursing course.

Reference
Hodgson, B., & Kizior, R. (2009). *Saunders nursing drug handbook 2009* (p. 727). Philadelphia: Saunders.

133. Theophylline (Theo-24) is prescribed for a client with bronchial asthma. The nurse provides dietary instructions to the client and tells the client to avoid consuming which item?
1 Iced tea
2 Lemonade
3 Orange juice
4 Tomato juice

Level of Cognitive Ability: Application
Client Needs: Physiological Integrity
Integrated Process: Teaching and Learning
Content Area: Pharmacology

Answer: 1
Rationale: The client is instructed to avoid the use of products that contain caffeine, such as cola, coffee, tea, and chocolate because caffeine could lead to an increased incidence of cardiovascular and central nervous system side effects of the medication. The items in options 2, 3, and 4 are acceptable to consume.

Test-Taking Strategy: Recall that medication names that end with the letters -*line* are xanthine bronchodilators and that these medications can cause cardiovascular and central nervous system side effects. Also, eliminate options 2, 3, and 4 because they are comparable or alike in that they are fruit drinks. Review the items to be avoided by a client taking a xanthine bronchodilator and the test-taking strategies for answering pharmacology questions if you had difficulty with this question.

Tip for the Beginning Nursing Student: Theophylline (Theo-24) is a xanthine bronchodilator that dilates bronchial airways and pulmonary blood vessels and is used to treat respiratory disorders, such as bronchial asthma, bronchitis, emphysema, chronic obstructive pulmonary disease, or bronchospasm. An important point to remember is that these medications can cause cardiovascular and central nervous system side effects, particularly if taken with caffeine-containing products. Therefore an important teaching point is to tell the client to avoid caffeine-containing products. In addition, another important intervention is to monitor the client for changes in the cardiovascular or central nervous system. You will learn about this medication in a pharmacology course or in your medical-surgical nursing course when you study respiratory disorders.

Reference
Hodgson, B., & Kizior, R. (2009). *Saunders nursing drug handbook 2009* (p. 1122). Philadelphia: Saunders.

---

134. The nurse is providing instructions to a client about the medication lithium carbonate (Lithobid) that has been prescribed for acute mania. The nurse tells the client that:

1 Foods that contain salt need to be avoided.
2 Medication blood levels need to be checked yearly.
3 Blurred vision needs to be reported to the physician.
4 Vomiting and diarrhea are expected effects of the medication.

Level of Cognitive Ability: Application
Client Needs: Physiological Integrity
Integrated Process: Teaching and Learning
Content Area: Pharmacology

Answer: 3
Rationale: Because therapeutic and toxic dosage ranges are so close, lithium blood levels must be monitored closely (every 3 or 4 days at the initiation of therapy and then every 1 to 2 months). The client should be instructed to notify the physician if excessive diarrhea, vomiting, blurred vision, or other signs of toxicity occur. A normal diet and normal salt and fluid intake (1500 to 3000 mL per day of fluid) should be maintained because lithium decreases sodium reabsorption in the renal tubules, which could cause sodium depletion. A low sodium intake causes an increase in lithium retention and could lead to toxicity.

Test-Taking Strategy: Recall the action of this medication and that toxicity is a concern with its use. This will direct you to option 3. Also eliminate options 1, 2, and 4 because of the words *avoided, yearly,* and *are expected,* respectively, in these options. Review the client teaching points related to the administration of this medication and the test-taking strategies for answering pharmacology questions if you had difficulty with this question.

Tip for the Beginning Nursing Student: Lithium carbonate (Lithobid) is an antimanic and antidepressant medication used to treat the manic phase of bipolar disease, which is a manic-depressive disorder. A primary concern when administering this medication is the risk for toxicity. Therefore monitoring blood levels for toxicity is important. For long-term control a therapeutic serum lithium level ranges between 0.5 and 1.3 mEq/L. The client is taught about the importance of monitoring follow-up blood levels, diet and fluid requirements, and the signs and symptoms of toxicity. You will learn about this medication in a pharmacology course or in your psychiatric/mental health nursing course.

Reference
Hodgson, B., & Kizior, R. (2009). *Saunders nursing drug handbook 2009* (p. 693). Philadelphia: Saunders.

135. Allopurinol (Zyloprim) has been prescribed for a client with gout, and the nurse provides instructions to the client about the medication. The nurse tells the client that this medication has been prescribed to:

1 Relieve pain
2 Maintain dilute urine
3 Reduce the uric acid level in the body
4 Reduce the need to consume large amounts of fluid

Level of Cognitive Ability: Application
Client Needs: Physiological Integrity
Integrated Process: Teaching and Learning
Content Area: Pharmacology

Answer: 3
Rationale: Allopurinol (Zyloprim) is used in the treatment of gout to decrease uric acid production. Options 1, 2, and 4 are not actions of the medication. Clients taking allopurinol are encouraged to drink at least 10 to 12 eight-oz glasses of water per day to aid in uric acid excretion. Although the urine may become dilute as a result of increased fluid intake, dilute urine is not an action of the medication. This medication does not relieve pain.

Test-Taking Strategy: Note that the question identifies the client's diagnosis. Recalling the pathophysiology associated with this disorder will direct you to option 3. Review the action of this medication and test-taking strategies for answering pharmacology questions if you had difficulty with this question.

Tip for the Beginning Nursing Student: Gout is a disease associated with an inborn error of metabolism that increases the production or interferes with excretion of uric acid. The excess uric acid is converted to urate crystals and deposits in joints and other tissues. The great toe is a common site for the accumulation of urate crystals. This condition can cause exceedingly painful swelling of the joint. Medication to decrease uric acid production is an important component of treatment. You will learn about this medication in a pharmacology course or in your medical-surgical nursing course.

References
Hodgson, B., & Kizior, R. (2009). *Saunders nursing drug handbook 2009* (p. 36). Philadelphia: Saunders.
Mosby. (2006). *Mosby's dictionary of medicine, nursing & health professions.* (7th ed., p. 825). St. Louis: Mosby.

136. A client with bulimia nervosa was started on fluoxetine hydrochloride (Prozac) 10 mg daily 3 days ago. The client calls the clinic and reports that she is experiencing nausea after taking the medication. The nurse would appropriately instruct the client to:

1 Contact the physician.
2 Take the medication with milk.
3 Lie down for 30 minutes after taking the medication.
4 Stop the medication until a different medication can be prescribed.

Level of Cognitive Ability: Application
Client Needs: Physiological Integrity

Answer: 2
Rationale: Fluoxetine hydrochloride (Prozac) is an antidepressant, antiobsessional agent, and antibulimic. The client who experiences gastrointestinal distress should be instructed to take the medication with food or milk. Although nausea may be a sign of toxicity (overdosage), this client has only been taking the medication for 3 days and overdosage is not likely to occur in this short period. Therefore it is not necessary to contact the physician. Lying down for 30 minutes after taking the medication is not the best measure to alleviate the client's complaint. The nurse would not instruct a client to stop a medication.

Test-Taking Strategy: Focus on the information in the question and note that the client has been taking the medication for 3 days. Eliminate option 4 using general guidelines related to medication administration. From the remaining options, noting that the client began taking the medication 3 days ago will direct you to option 2. Review

Integrated Process: Nursing Process/
Implementation
Content Area: Pharmacology

this medication and the test-taking strategies for answering pharmacology questions if you had difficulty with this question.

Tip for the Beginning Nursing Student: Bulimia nervosa is an eating disorder that is characterized by craving for food, often resulting in episodes of continuous eating followed by purging, depression, and self-deprivation. Treatment consists of measures to improve nourishment and therapy to overcome the underlying emotional conflicts leading to the disorder. You will learn about this medication and this disorder in a pharmacology course or in your psychiatric/mental health course when you study eating disorders.

Reference

Hodgson, B., & Kizior, R. (2009). *Saunders nursing drug handbook 2009* (p. 495). Philadelphia: Saunders.

---

137. A nurse is caring for a client with a diagnosis of venous thrombosis in the left lower leg who is receiving heparin sodium by continuous intravenous (IV) infusion. The nurse monitors the client for which adverse effect of this therapy?
  1 Nausea
  2 Dark urine
  3 Left calf tenderness
  4 Increased blood pressure

Level of Cognitive Ability: Application
Client Needs: Physiological Integrity
Integrated Process: Nursing Process/
Assessment/Data Collection
Content Area: Pharmacology

Answer: 2

Rationale: The client who receives heparin sodium is at risk for bleeding. The nurse monitors for signs of bleeding, which include bleeding from the gums, ecchymoses on the skin, red or dark urine, black or red stools, and body fluids that test positive for occult blood. Tenderness is likely to be noted in the area of the thrombosis. Increased blood pressure and nausea are not signs of an adverse effect of the medication.

Test-Taking Strategy: Note the strategic words *adverse effect.* Focus on the name of the medication and the client's diagnosis. Recalling the manifestations of venous thrombosis will assist in eliminating option 3. Next, recalling that this medication is an anticoagulant will direct you to option 2 from the remaining options. Review this medication and the test-taking strategies for answering pharmacology questions if you had difficulty with this question.

Tip for the Beginning Nursing Student: Venous thrombosis is also known as phlebothrombosis and is an abnormal condition in which a clot forms within a vein. It is usually caused by hemostasis, hypercoagulability, or occlusion. A concern with this disorder is that the clot will break free from the vein and travel to the lungs causing a pulmonary embolus, which can be life threatening. Therefore heparin sodium is administered to prevent further extension of the existing clot or new clot formation. You will learn about this medication and this disorder in a pharmacology course or in your medical-surgical nursing course when you study cardiovascular disorders.

Reference

Hodgson, B., & Kizior, R. (2009). *Saunders nursing drug handbook 2009* (p. 566). Philadelphia: Saunders.

138. A postoperative client has an order to begin short-term therapy with enoxaparin (Lovenox). The nurse explains to the client that this medication is being ordered to:
1 Prevent pain
2 Relieve back spasms
3 Increase energy levels
4 Reduce the risk of deep vein thrombosis

Level of Cognitive Ability: Application
Client Needs: Physiological Integrity
Integrated Process: Nursing Process/
  Implementation
Content Area: Pharmacology

Answer: 4
Rationale: Enoxaparin (Lovenox) is an anticoagulant that is administered to prevent deep vein thrombosis and thromboembolism in selected clients, such as postoperative clients following hip or knee replacement therapy. It is not used to prevent pain, relieve back spasms, or increase energy levels.

Test-Taking Strategy: Focus on the subject—an intended medication effect. Noting the word *postoperative* in the question will assist in eliminating options 2 and 3. From the remaining options, recalling that this medication is an anticoagulant will direct you to option 4. Review this medication and the test-taking strategies for answering pharmacology questions if you had difficulty with this question.

Tip for the Beginning Nursing Student: Deep vein thrombosis is a disorder involving a thrombus in one of the deep veins in the body. Thromboembolism is a condition is which a blood vessel is obstructed by a clot carried in the blood-stream from its site of formation. These are potentially life-threatening disorders, and treatment includes bedrest and the use of anticoagulant medications. Enoxaparin (Lovenox) is a medication that will prevent deep vein thrombosis and thromboembolism and is prescribed for clients at risk for the development of these disorders. You will learn about this medication and these disorders in a pharmacology course or in your medical-surgical nursing course when you study cardiovascular disorders.

Reference
Hodgson, B., & Kizior, R. (2009). *Saunders nursing drug handbook 2009* (p. 413). Philadelphia: Saunders.

139. A clinic nurse notes that a client is taking metoprolol (Lopressor). The nurse performs which assessment to determine medication effectiveness?
1 Takes the client's temperature
2 Takes the client's blood pressure
3 Checks the client's peripheral pulses
4 Checks the client's eyes for peripheral vision

Level of Cognitive Ability: Analysis
Client Needs: Physiological Integrity
Integrated Process: Nursing Process/
  Assessment/Data Collection
Content Area: Pharmacology

Answer: 2
Rationale: Metoprolol (Lopressor) is a β-blocker that is used to treat mild to moderate hypertension. Therefore to determine medication effectiveness the nurse would monitor the client's blood pressure. Options 1, 3, and 4 are unrelated to the medication effectiveness.

Test-Taking Strategy: Note the subject—to determine medication effectiveness. Recalling that medication names that end with the letters *-lol* are β-blockers and that β-blockers are used to treat hypertension will direct you to option 2. Review this medication and the test-taking strategies for answering pharmacology questions if you had difficulty with this question.

Tip for the Beginning Nursing Student: Metoprolol (Lopressor) is a medication that is primarily used to treat hypertension. A priority nursing intervention when a medication with antihypertensive effects is administered is to monitor the client's blood pressure. Additional important interventions include client teaching related to safety because of the hypotensive effects of the medication. One important point to teach the client is to rise slowly from a lying to sitting position and to permit the legs to dangle from the bed momentarily before standing. You will learn about this medication in a pharmacology course or in your medical-surgical nursing course when you study cardiovascular disorders.

Reference
Hodgson, B., & Kizior, R. (2009). *Saunders nursing drug handbook 2009* (p. 757). Philadelphia: Saunders.

---

140. Betaxolol (Betoptic) eye drops have been prescribed for a client for the treatment of glaucoma. The nurse tells the client that it is important to return to the clinic for monitoring for:
    1 Hypotension
    2 Hyperglycemia
    3 The presence of Trousseau's sign
    4 The presence of a positive Homans' sign

Level of Cognitive Ability: Application
Client Needs: Physiological Integrity
Integrated Process: Nursing Process/ Implementation
Content Area: Pharmacology

Answer: 1

Rationale: Betaxolol (Betoptic) is an antiglaucoma medication and a β-blocker. Systemic effects of the medication include hypotension manifested as dizziness, nausea, diaphoresis, headache, fatigue, constipation, and diarrhea. Nursing interventions include monitoring the blood pressure for hypotension and assessing the pulse for strength, weakness, irregularities, and bradycardia. This medication may mask the symptoms of hypoglycemia and prolong the hypoglycemic effect in the client taking insulin or oral hypoglycemics. The presence of Homans' or Trousseau's sign is unrelated to the use of this medication. A positive Homans' sign indicates the presence of deep vein thrombosis. A positive Trousseau's sign indicates a calcium imbalance.

Test-Taking Strategy: Remember that β-blocker medication names end with the letters *-lol,* and recall that β-blockers are used to treat hypertension. Also use the ABCs—airway, breathing, and circulation—to direct you to option 1. Review this medication and the test-taking strategies for answering pharmacology questions if you had difficulty with this question.

Tip for the Beginning Nursing Student: Glaucoma is an abnormal eye disorder characterized by elevated pressure within the eye. It is caused by the obstruction of the outflow of aqueous humor. If untreated, it will result in complete and permanent blindness. Medication therapy is extremely important to keep the intraocular pressure within the normal range of 10 to 21 mm Hg, and the client needs to be instructed about the importance of the medication. You will learn about this medication and this disorder in a pharmacology course or in your medical-surgical nursing course when you study eye disorders.

Reference
Hodgson, B., & Kizior, R. (2009). *Saunders nursing drug handbook 2009* (p. 130). Philadelphia: Saunders.

141. Bupropion (Wellbutrin) is pre-scribed for a client to treat an anxiety disorder. The nurse tells the client that which of the following is a common side effect of the medication?
1 Diarrhea
2 Dry mouth
3 Weight gain
4 Slowed pulse rate

Level of Cognitive Ability: Application
Client Needs: Physiological Integrity
Integrated Process: Nursing Process/ Implementation
Content Area: Pharmacology

Answer: 2
Rationale: Bupropion (Wellbutrin) is an antianxiety medi-cation. Common side effects include agitation, headache, dry mouth, constipation, weight loss, gastrointestinal upset, dizziness, tremors, insomnia, blurred vision, and tachycardia. Options 1, 3, and 4 are not side effects of this medication.

Test-Taking Strategy: Focus on the subject—a common side effect. Noting the words *to treat an anxiety disorder* will assist in determining that the medication is an antianxiety medication. Recall that dry mouth can occur with the use of some antianxiety medications. Review the side effects of this medication and the test-taking strategies for answering pharmacology questions if you had difficulty with this question.

Tip for the Beginning Nursing Student: Anxiety is the anticipation of danger or dread accompanied by restless-ness, tension, tachycardia, and breathing difficulty. In an anxiety disorder the primary characteristic is anxiety ranging from mild to severe states. Antianxiety medications are a component of therapy for anxiety disorders. You will learn about these medications and this disorder in a phar-macology course or in your psychiatric/mental health nursing course when you study anxiety disorders.

Reference
Hodgson, B., & Kizior, R. (2009). *Saunders nursing drug handbook 2009* (p. 160). Philadelphia: Saunders.

142. A nurse is caring for a client with systemic candidiasis who is receiving amphotericin B (Fungi-zone) intravenously. The nurse does which of the following during administration of the medication to monitor for an adverse effect?
1 Monitors urinary output
2 Checks peripheral pulses
3 Monitors for hypothermia
4 Checks the neurological status

Level of Cognitive Ability: Application
Client Needs: Physiological Integrity
Integrated Process: Nursing Process/ Implementation
Content Area: Pharmacology

Answer: 1
Rationale: Amphotericin B (Fungizone) is an antifungal medication and can cause toxicity, which can produce symptoms during administration, such as chills, fever, headache, vomiting, and impaired renal function. The med-ication is also very irritating to the IV site, commonly causing thrombophlebitis. The nurse administering this medication watches for signs of these problems. Options 2, 3, and 4 are not specifically related to the administration of this medication.

Test-Taking Strategy: Note the strategic words *adverse effect.* Also note the name of the medication *Fungiz*one. This will assist in determining that the medication is an anti-fungal medication. Recalling that nephrotoxicity can occur with the use of this medication will direct you to option 1. Review the adverse effects of this medication and the test-taking strategies for answering pharmacology questions if you had difficulty with this question.

Tip for the Beginning Nursing Student: Candidiasis is an infection caused by a species of *Candida,* usually *Candida albicans.* It usually occurs in a local area, such as the oral cavity, but can also occur in other areas. Treatment includes oral and topical administration of antifungal infections if candidiasis occurs locally. If it becomes a systemic infection, IV antifungal medications are prescribed. One adverse effect of antifungal medications administered intravenously is nephrotoxicity (destruction to the kidney cells). You will learn about these medications and this disorder in a pharmacology course or in your medical-surgical nursing course when you study infectious disorders.

Reference

Gahart, B., & Nazareno, A. (2009). *Intravenous medications* (25th ed., p. 102). St. Louis: Mosby.

---

143. A nurse is reviewing the laboratory results of a client receiving intravenous (IV) chemotherapy. The nurse initiates neutropenic precautions if which of the following laboratory results is noted?
    1 Clotting time of 10 minutes
    2 Ammonia level of 20 mg/dL
    3 Platelet count of 100,000 cells/mm^3
    4 White blood cell (WBC) count of 2000 cells/mm^3

Level of Cognitive Ability: Application
Client Needs: Physiological Integrity
Integrated Process: Nursing Process/ Implementation
Content Area: Pharmacology

Answer: 4

Rationale: The normal WBC count is 5000 to 10,000 cells/ mm^3. When the WBC count drops, neutropenic precautions need to be implemented. These include protective isolation measures to protect the client from infection. Bleeding precautions need to be initiated when the platelet count drops. Bleeding precautions include avoiding all trauma, such as rectal temperatures or injections. The normal platelet count is 150,000 to 450,000 cells/mm^3. The normal clotting time is 8 to 15 minutes. The normal ammonia value is 15 to 45 mg/dL.

Test-Taking Strategy: Eliminate options 1 and 2 first because they identify normal laboratory values. To select between the remaining options, note that the client is receiving chemotherapy and focus on the words *neutropenic precautions*. Correlate a low WBC count with the need for neutropenic precautions and a low platelet count with the need for bleeding precautions. Review the interventions associated with caring for the client receiving chemotherapy and the test-taking strategies for answering pharmacology questions.

Tip for the Beginning Nursing Student: Neutropenia is an abnormal decrease in the number of neutrophils in the blood. This can occur in conditions such as acute leukemia, infection, and chronic splenomegaly and in the client receiving chemotherapy because chemotherapy destroys normal cells in addition to cancer cells. When neutropenia occurs, the client is at risk for developing an infection and the nurse needs to implement measures to protect the client from infection, such as strict handwashing, wearing protective clothing when caring for the client, and keeping fresh fruits and flowers and standing water out of the client's room because these items harbor bacteria. The nurse would also restrict visits with the client from anyone who is ill. You will learn about this medication and neutropenic precautions in a pharmacology course or in your medical-surgical nursing course when you study oncologic disorders.

References

Lehne, R. (2007). *Pharmacology for nursing care* (6th ed., p. 1151). Philadelphia: Saunders.

Linton, A., & Maebius, N. (2007). *Introduction to medical-surgical nursing* (4th ed., p. 604). Philadelphia: Saunders.

---

144. A nurse is providing instructions to a client who is taking codeine sulfate. The nurse tells the client to:
1 Decrease fluid intake.
2 Change positions slowly.
3 Maintain a low-fiber diet.
4 Limit the intake of alcoholic beverages.

Level of Cognitive Ability: Application
Client Needs: Physiological Integrity
Integrated Process: Teaching and Learning
Content Area: Pharmacology

Answer: 2

Rationale: Codeine sulfate is an opioid analgesic. The medication can cause constipation, and the client is instructed to increase fluid intake and maintain a high-fiber diet. Alcohol intake is avoided not limited. The medication can cause drowsiness, lightheadedness, and hypotension; and the client is instructed to change positions slowly to prevent orthostatic hypotension.

Test-Taking Strategy: Eliminate option 4 first using general pharmacology guidelines and recalling that alcohol is avoided not limited. From the remaining options, recalling that codeine sulfate can cause constipation will eliminate options 1 and 3. If you had difficulty with this question, review nursing measures related to the administration of codeine sulfate and the test-taking strategies for answering pharmacology questions.

Tip for the Beginning Nursing Student: Codeine sulfate is an opioid analgesic that is used primarily to treat pain. Opioid analgesics can cause many side effects, including drowsiness, lightheadedness, and hypotension. Therefore client safety is a concern with the use of opioid analgesics. Because of this concern, nursing interventions with the use of opioid analgesics focus on implementing measures that protect the client from injury and teaching the client measures to prevent injury. You will learn about this medication and this disorder in a pharmacology course or in your medical-surgical nursing course when you study pain management.

Reference

Hodgson, B., & Kizior, R. (2009). *Saunders nursing drug handbook 2009* (p. 278). Philadelphia: Saunders.

---

145. A client is receiving diazepam (Valium) to treat painful muscle spasms. The nurse monitors the client for which frequent side effect of the medication?
1 Ataxia
2 Diarrhea
3 Nervousness
4 Hypertension

Answer: 1

Rationale: Valium is a centrally acting skeletal muscle relaxant. Incoordination (ataxia), fatigue, and drowsiness are frequent side effects. Occasional side effects include slurred speech, orthostatic hypotension, headache, hypoactivity, constipation, nausea, and blurred vision.

Test-Taking Strategy: Note the name of the medication, *diazepam.* Recalling that some benzodiazepine medication

Level of Cognitive Ability: Analysis
Client Needs: Physiological Integrity
Integrated Process: Nursing Process/
   Assessment/Data Collection
Content Area: Pharmacology

names end with the letters -*pam* will assist in answering the question. Also noting that the medication is used for muscle spasms will direct you to think that this medication relaxes muscles. The only option that directly relates to this medication action is option 1. Review the action and side effects of this medication and the test-taking strategies for answering pharmacology questions if you had difficulty with this question.

Tip for the Beginning Nursing Student: Muscle spasms are involuntary contractions or twitching that occurs in a muscle. These can be quite painful for the client, and one component of therapy is to treat the spasms with a centrally acting skeletal muscle relaxant. Because the medication is centrally acting, it can cause incoordination. This places the client at risk for injury so nursing interventions focus on implementing measures to protect the client from injury. You will learn about this medication in a pharmacology course or in your medical-surgical nursing course when you study musculoskeletal disorders.

Reference
Hodgson, B., & Kizior, R. (2009). *Saunders nursing drug handbook 2009* (pp. 346-347). Philadelphia: Saunders.

---

146. A nurse is preparing to administer medications to a hospitalized client and notes that the client takes levothyroxine (Synthroid) daily. The nurse suspects that the client has a history of:
   1 Hypotension
   2 Hypertension
   3 Hypothyroidism
   4 Hyperthyroidism

Level of Cognitive Ability: Analysis
Client Needs: Physiological Integrity
Integrated Process: Nursing Process/
   Assessment/Data Collection
Content Area: Pharmacology

Answer: 3
Rationale: Levothyroxine is a synthetic thyroid hormone used to treat hypothyroidism. It is not used to treat hypotension, hypertension, or hyperthyroidism.

Test-Taking Strategy: Focus on the name of the medication. Recalling that most thyroid medications contain the letters *thy* in their name will assist in eliminating options 1 and 2. From the remaining options eliminate option 4 because it would be harmful to administer thyroid to a client who is in a hyperthyroid state. Review levothyroxine (Synthroid) and the test-taking strategies for answering pharmacology questions if you had difficulty with this question.

Tip for the Beginning Nursing Student: Hypothyroidism is a condition characterized by decreased activity of the thyroid gland resulting in slowing of the body's metabolic processes. Treatment includes thyroid replacement therapy with thyroid medication. You will learn about this medication when you study pharmacology and will learn about hypothyroidism when you study endocrine disorders in your medical-surgical nursing course.

Reference
Hodgson, B., & Kizior, R. (2009). *Saunders nursing drug handbook 2009* (p. 682). Philadelphia: Saunders.

147. A nurse checks the serum digoxin level for a client who is taking digoxin (Lanoxin) and notes that the result is 1.5 ng/mL. Which action will the nurse take based on this laboratory result?
1 Notify the physician.
2 Withhold the next scheduled dose of digoxin.
3 Place the report in the client's medical record.
4 Obtain another serum digoxin level to verify the results.

Level of Cognitive Ability: Application
Client Needs: Physiological Integrity
Integrated Process: Nursing Process/ Implementation
Content Area: Pharmacology

Answer: 3

Rationale: The normal therapeutic range for digoxin is from 0.5 to 2 ng/mL. A value of 1.5 ng/mL is within therapeutic range; therefore the nurse would most appropriately place the report in the client's medical record. Options 1, 2, and 4 are unnecessary actions.

Test-Taking Strategy: Note the strategic words *result is 1.5 ng/mL.* Recalling that the normal therapeutic range for digoxin is from 0.5 to 2 ng/mL will direct you to option 3. Review this therapeutic serum level and the various test-taking strategies if you had difficulty with this question.

Tip for the Beginning Nursing Student: Digoxin is a cardiac glycoside used to manage and treat heart failure, control atrial fibrillation, and treat and prevent atrial tachycardia. A concern with the medication is that it can cause toxicity, and an important nursing responsibility is to monitor for signs of toxicity. Before administering this medication the nurse checks the client's apical heart rate and if the rate is below 60 beats/min the nurse withholds the medication, collects additional client data, and contacts the physician for further orders. Some manifestations of digoxin toxicity include gastrointestinal disturbances and ocular disturbances. You will learn about this medication when you study pharmacology and when you study cardiovascular disorders in your medical-surgical nursing course.

References
Hodgson, B., & Kizior, R. (2009). *Saunders nursing drug handbook 2009* (p. 356). Philadelphia: Saunders.
Linton, A., & Maebius, N. (2007). *Introduction to medical-surgical nursing* (4th ed., p. 642). Philadelphia: Saunders.

148. A client with acute renal failure has been treated with sodium polystyrene sulfonate (Kayexalate) by mouth. The nurse would evaluate this therapy as effective if which of the following values was noted on follow-up laboratory testing?
1 Calcium 9.8 mg/dL
2 Sodium 142 mEq/L
3 Potassium 4.9 mEq/L
4 Phosphorus 3.9 mg/dL

Level of Cognitive Ability: Analysis
Client Needs: Physiological Integrity
Integrated Process: Nursing Process/ Evaluation
Content Area: Pharmacology

Answer: 3

Rationale: Of all the electrolyte imbalances that accompany renal failure, hyperkalemia is the most dangerous because it can lead to cardiac dysrhythmias and death. If the potassium level rises too high, sodium polystyrene sulfonate (Kayexalate) may be administered to cause excretion of potassium through the gastrointestinal tract. Each electrolyte level noted in the options falls within the normal reference range for that electrolyte. The potassium level, however, is measured following administration of this medication to note the extent of its effectiveness.

Test-Taking Strategy: Note the name of the medication, and use medical terminology *(Kayexalate = K[potassium]ex [excrete]).* Note the relationship between the medication name and option 3. Review this medication and the test-taking strategies for answering pharmacology questions if you had difficulty with this question.

Tip for the Beginning Nursing Student: Renal failure is the inability of the kidneys to excrete wastes, concentrate urine, and maintain electrolyte balance. Acute renal failure is characterized by the rapid accumulation of wastes in the blood. Many electrolyte imbalances can occur in renal failure because the kidneys are unable to maintain electrolyte balance. Sodium polystyrene sulfonate (Kayexalate) is an antihyperkalemic medication used to treat high potassium levels. You will learn about this medication in a pharmacology course or in your medical-surgical nursing course when you study kidney disorders.

References

Christensen, B., & Kockrow, E. (2006). *Adult health nursing* (5th ed., p. 502). St. Louis: Mosby.

Hodgson, B., & Kizior, R. (2009). *Saunders nursing drug handbook 2009* (pp. 1067-1068). Philadelphia: Saunders.

Monahan, F., Sands, J., Marek, J., Neighbors, M., & Green, C. (2007). *Phipps' medical-surgical nursing: Health and illness perspectives* (8th ed., p. 1016). St. Louis: Mosby.

---

149. A nurse notes that the physician has prescribed sulfasalazine (Azulfidine) for a client. The nurse checks the nursing history form in the client's medical record for documentation of an allergy to which of the following?
1 Shellfish
2 Strawberries
3 Sulfonamides
4 Acetaminophen (Tylenol)

Level of Cognitive Ability: Analysis
Client Needs: Physiological Integrity
Integrated Process: Nursing Process/ Assessment/Data Collection
Content Area: Pharmacology

Answer: 3
Rationale: The client who has been prescribed sulfasalazine should be checked for a history of allergy to either sulfonamides or salicylates because the chemical compositions of sulfasalazine and these medications are similar. The other options are incorrect.

Test-Taking Strategy: Focus on the subject—history of allergy. Note the relationship of *sulfasalazine* in the question and *sulfonamides* in the correct option. Review this medication and the test-taking strategies for answering pharmacology questions if you had difficulty with this question.

Tip for the Beginning Nursing Student: Sulfasalazine (Azulfidine) is sulfonamide and an anti-inflammatory medication that is used to treat a variety of conditions. An important point to remember about this medication is that it is important to ask the client about allergies to sulfonamides or salicylates, such as aspirin, before administration. In addition, before administering any medication it is always important to ask the client about allergies. You will learn about this medication in a pharmacology course or in your medical-surgical nursing course.

Reference

Hodgson, B., & Kizior, R. (2009). *Saunders nursing drug handbook 2009* (p. 1083). Philadelphia: Saunders.

---

150. A client with a diagnosis of sepsis is receiving tobramycin (Tobrex). The nurse realizes that the client is responding well to the medication therapy if which of the following laboratory results is noted?

Answer: 1
Rationale: Tobramycin is an antibiotic (aminoglycoside) that causes nephrotoxicity and ototoxicity. The medication is effective if the WBC count drops back into the normal range and the kidney function remains normal. Option 2 indicates an abnormal WBC count, and options 3 and 4 are unrelated to the use of this medication.

1 White blood cell (WBC) count of 8000 cells/mm^3 and creatinine level of 0.9 mg/dL
2 WBC count of 15,000 cells/mm^3 and a blood urea nitrogen (BUN) of 38 mg/dL
3 Sodium of 140 mEq/L and potassium of 3.9 mEq/L
4 Sodium of 145 mEq/L and chloride of 106 mEq/L

Level of Cognitive Ability: Analysis
Client Needs: Physiological Integrity
Integrated Process: Nursing Process/ Evaluation
Content Area: Pharmacology

Test-Taking Strategy: Noting the client's diagnosis will assist in determining that this medication is an antibiotic. This will assist in eliminating options 3 and 4. To select correctly from the remaining options, focus on the words *the client is responding well.* Option 1 is the option that identifies normal laboratory values. Review this medication, normal laboratory values, and the various test-taking strategies if you had difficulty with this question.

Tip for the Beginning Nursing Student: Sepsis refers to a systemic infection that can occur as a result of a localized or other type of infection in the body. This serious infection needs to be treated aggressively with antibiotics, and usually blood cultures are done to determine the antibiotic of choice. Tobramycin (Tobrex) is an antibiotic (aminoglycoside) that may be used to treat sepsis. As with many antibiotics, it causes nephrotoxicity and ototoxicity. The normal WBC count ranges from 5000 to 10,000 cells/mm^3. The normal creatinine level ranges from 0.6 to 1.3 mg/dL. The normal blood urea nitrogen ranges from 8 to 25 mg/dL. The normal potassium level ranges from 3.5 to 5.1 mEq/L. The normal sodium level ranges from 135 to 145 mEq/L. The normal chloride level ranges from 98 to 107 mEq/L. You will learn about antibiotics in a pharmacology course or in your medical-surgical nursing course when you study infections and immune disorders.

Reference
Hodgson, B., & Kizior, R. (2009). *Saunders nursing drug handbook 2009* (p. 1146). Philadelphia: Saunders.

18
Chapter

Delegating/ Prioritizing Questions

151. A client is being admitted to the neurological unit from the emergency department with a diagnosis of a cervical (C4) spinal cord injury. Which assessment would the nurse perform first when admitting the client to the nursing unit?

1 Listen to breath sounds.
2 Check peripheral pulses.
3 Check for muscle flaccidity.
4 Assess extremity muscle strength.

Level of Cognitive Ability: Application
Client Needs: Physiological Integrity
Integrated Process: Nursing Process/ Assessment/Data Collection
Content Area: Delegating/Prioritizing

Answer: 1

Rationale: Because compromise of respiration is a leading cause of death in cervical cord injury, respiratory assessment is the highest priority. Assessment of peripheral pulses and muscle strength can be done after adequate oxygenation is ensured.

Test-Taking Strategy: Eliminate options 3 and 4 first because they are comparable or alike. Next use the ABCs— airway, breathing, and circulation—to direct you to option 1. Remember that a cord injury, particularly at the level of C4, can affect respiratory status. Breath sounds will be diminished if respiratory muscles are weakened or paralyzed. Review priority care of the client with a C4 spinal cord injury and the test-taking strategies for answering prioritizing questions if you had difficulty with this question.

Tip for the Beginning Nursing Student: A spinal cord injury is caused by a traumatic disruption of the spinal cord occurring from a car accident or another type of violent impact. It is often associated with extensive musculoskeletal injury. Where the injury occurred in the spinal cord (level of injury) will determine the effect on the client. A major concern with a cervical spinal cord injury is respiratory status. You will learn about spinal cord injuries and the important nursing interventions in your medical-surgical nursing course when you study neurological disorders.

References

deWit, S. (2009). *Medical-surgical nursing: Concepts & practice* (p. 552). St. Louis: Saunders.

Ignatavicius, D., & Workman, M. (2010). *Medical-surgical nursing: Patient-centered collaborative care* (6th ed., p. 993). Philadelphia: Saunders.

152. A nurse notes redness, warmth, and a purulent drainage at the insertion site of a central venous catheter in a client receiving parenteral nutrition (PN). The nurse takes which priority action?
1 Notifies the physician
2 Changes the intravenous tubing
3 Slows the rate of infusion of the PN
4 Calls the pharmacy for a new bag of PN solution

Level of Cognitive Ability: Application
Client Needs: Physiological Integrity
Integrated Process: Nursing Process/ Implementation
Content Area: Delegating/Prioritizing

Answer: 1
Rationale: Redness, warmth, and purulent drainage are signs of an infection. Infections of a central venous catheter site can lead to septicemia; therefore the physician needs to be notified. The nurse would not adjust the rate of an intravenous solution without a specific order to do so. In addition, this action is unrelated to the client's complication. Although the nurse may change the intravenous tubing and hang a new bag of PN solution, these are not priority actions.

Test-Taking Strategy: Note the strategic word *priority.* Also note the words *redness, warmth, and a purulent drainage,* and recall that these signs indicate infection. Recalling that infections of a central venous catheter site can lead to septicemia (a life-threatening condition) will direct you to option 1. If you had difficulty with this question, review nursing interventions related to complications of PN and the test-taking strategies related to notifying the physician.

Tip for the Beginning Nursing Student: Parenteral nutrition involves the administration of nutrients by a route other than orally and is usually administered intravenously. It is administered by means of an intravenous catheter through a central vein, such as the subclavian vein. The tip of the catheter normally rests in the superior vena cava. This type of catheter is known as a central venous catheter, and meticulous nursing care is required in the care of the catheter and catheter site to prevent infection. You will learn about PN and central venous catheters in your medical-surgical nursing course.

References
deWit, S. (2009). *Medical-surgical nursing: Concepts & practice* (p. 62). St. Louis: Saunders.
Ignatavicius, D., & Workman, M. (2010). *Medical-surgical nursing: Patient-centered collaborative care* (6th ed., p. 911). Philadelphia: Saunders.

---

153. A client is brought to the emergency department by emergency medical services after having seriously lacerated both wrists. The nurse would first:
1 Assess and treat the wound sites.
2 Perform a psychosocial assessment.
3 Contact the crisis intervention team.
4 Encourage the client to talk about his feelings.

Level of Cognitive Ability: Application
Client Needs: Physiological Integrity

Answer: 1
Rationale: The initial action when a client has attempted suicide is to assess and treat any injuries. Although options 2, 3, and 4 may be appropriate at some point, the initial action would be to treat the wounds.

Test-Taking Strategy: Use Maslow's Hierarchy of Needs theory to prioritize. Physiological needs come first. Option 1 is the only one that addresses a physiological need. Options 2, 3, and 4 address psychosocial needs. Review initial care to the client who has attempted suicide and the test-taking strategies for answering prioritizing questions if you had difficulty with this question.

Tip for the Beginning Nursing Student: Suicide is the intentional taking of one's own life. A suicide attempt is an

Integrated Process: Nursing Process/
Implementation
Content Area: Delegating/Prioritizing

act taken by a client to intentionally take one's own life. If a client has attempted suicide, it is extremely important to assess the injuries as a result of the suicide attempt. Other very important interventions include one-to-one supervision of the client and other therapy. You will learn about the concepts related to suicide and the important nursing interventions for a client at risk for self-harm in your psychiatric/mental health nursing course.

References

Linton, A., & Maebius, N. (2007). *Introduction to medical-surgical nursing* (4th ed., p. 1262). Philadelphia: Saunders.

Monahan, F., Sands, J., Marek, J., Neighbors, M., & Green, C. (2007). *Phipps' medical-surgical nursing: Health and illness perspectives* (8th ed., p. 175). St. Louis: Mosby.

---

154. A nurse develops a plan of care for a client receiving a chemotherapy treatment with intravenous bleomycin sulfate (Blenoxane). The nurse documents which priority intervention in the plan?
   1 Monitor for dyspnea.
   2 Monitor for alopecia.
   3 Monitor for anorexia.
   4 Change the client's position every 2 hours.

Level of Cognitive Ability: Analysis
Client Needs: Physiological Integrity
Integrated Process: Nursing Process/
Planning
Content Area: Delegating/Prioritizing

Answer: 1
Rationale: Bleomycin sulfate (Blenoxane), an antineoplastic medication, can cause interstitial pneumonitis that can progress to pulmonary fibrosis. Pulmonary function studies along with hematological, hepatic, and renal function tests need to be monitored. The nurse needs to monitor for dyspnea and monitor lung sounds for adventitious sounds that indicate pulmonary toxicity. Also the nurse needs to notify the physician immediately if pulmonary toxicity occurs. Alopecia (hair loss) can occur, but monitoring for it is not a priority intervention. Changing the client's position and monitoring for anorexia are important but are not the priority.

Test-Taking Strategy: Note the strategic word *priority* and use the ABCs—airway, breathing, and circulation. Select option 1 because it relates to airway. Review the interventions associated with caring for the client receiving bleomycin sulfate and the test-taking strategies for answering pharmacology questions and prioritizing questions if you had difficulty with this question.

Tip for the Beginning Nursing Student: Chemotherapy is the use of medications in the treatment of cancer that kill cancer cells. A concern with the use of chemotherapy is that it also affects and destroys normal cells. This is what causes the side and adverse effects of the medications. Many chemotherapeutic agents cause nausea, vomiting, and alopecia (hair loss), among other effects. Also some chemotherapeutic medications affect specific cells in certain organs. Bleomycin sulfate (Blenoxane) is one of these medications and can cause interstitial pneumonitis that can progress to pulmonary fibrosis. Pneumonitis refers to inflammation of the lungs; and pulmonary fibrosis refers to the formation of scar tissue in the connective tissue of the lungs. You will learn about this medication and other chemotherapeutic medications in a pharmacology course or in your medical-surgical nursing course when you study oncologic disorders.

Reference
Hodgson, B., & Kizior, R. (2009). *Saunders nursing drug handbook 2009* (p. 145). Philadelphia: Saunders.

---

155. Quinapril hydrochloride (Accupril) is prescribed as an adjunctive therapy in the treatment of heart failure. After administering the first dose, the nurse monitors which of the following most closely?
  1 Respirations
  2 Urine output
  3 Lung sounds
  4 Blood pressure

Level of Cognitive Ability: Application
Client Needs: Physiological Integrity
Integrated Process: Nursing Process/ Assessment/Data Collection
Content Area: Delegating/Prioritizing

Answer: 4
Rationale: Quinapril hydrochloride (Accupril) is an angiotensin-converting enzyme (ACE) inhibitor. It is used in the treatment of hypertension and as adjunctive therapy in the treatment of heart failure. Excessive hypotension ("first-dose syncope") can occur in clients with heart failure or in clients who are severely salt or volume depleted. Although lung sounds, urine output, and respirations would be monitored, the nurse would most closely monitor the client's blood pressure.

Test-Taking Strategy: Focus on the name of the medication, and note the strategic words *most closely.* This tells you that all options may be correct and that you must prioritize. Recall that most ACE inhibitor names end with the letters -*pril* and that these medications are used to treat hypertension. Review the adverse and toxic effects of quinapril hydrochloride (Accupril) and the test-taking strategies for answering pharmacology questions if you had difficulty with this question.

Tip for the Beginning Nursing Student: Quinapril hydrochloride (Accupril) is a medication that is primarily used to treat hypertension and manage heart failure. This medication is classified as an angiotensin-converting enzyme (ACE) inhibitor and antihypertensive. A priority nursing intervention when a medication with antihypertensive effects is administered is to monitor the client's blood pressure. Additional important interventions include client teaching related to safety because of the hypotensive effects of the medication. One important point to teach the client is to rise slowly from a lying to sitting position and to permit the legs to dangle from the bed momentarily before standing. You will learn about this medication in a pharmacology course or in your medical-surgical nursing course when you study cardiovascular disorders.

Reference
Hodgson, B., & Kizior, R. (2009). *Saunders nursing drug handbook 2009* (p. 988). Philadelphia: Saunders.

---

156. A nurse is preparing a plan of care for a postoperative client who is receiving morphine sulfate by continuous intravenous infusion for pain. The nurse includes monitoring of which factor as a priority nursing action in the plan of care?

Answer: 4
Rationale: Morphine sulfate suppresses respirations and decreases the client's blood pressure; therefore monitoring for both decreased respirations and blood pressure are priority nursing actions. Although monitoring of options 1, 2, and 3 may be a component of the plan of care for this client, option 4 identifies the priority nursing action.

1 Constipation
2 Urine output
3 Temperature
4 Blood pressure

Level of Cognitive Ability: Application
Client Needs: Physiological Integrity
Integrated Process: Nursing Process/
Planning
Content Area: Delegating/Prioritizing

Test-Taking Strategy: Note the strategic word *priority*. Use the ABCs—airway, breathing, and circulation—to direct you to the correct option. Monitoring blood pressure determines the circulatory status of the client. Review the effects of morphine sulfate and the test-taking strategies for answering pharmacology questions and prioritizing questions if you had difficulty with this question.

Tip for the Beginning Nursing Student: Morphine sulfate is an opiate analgesic that is used to alleviate pain in a client. It is used to treat pain that occurs in many types of disorders and is frequently used to alleviate pain in the postoperative client or the client with cancer. Because it is an opiate analgesic it will cause a decrease in vital signs, specifically respirations and blood pressure. Monitoring vital signs, specifically respirations and blood pressure, is a critical nursing intervention. You will learn about this medication and other opiate analgesics in a pharmacology course or in your medical-surgical nursing course.

Reference
Hodgson, B., & Kizior, R. (2009). *Saunders nursing drug handbook 2009* (p. 787). Philadelphia: Saunders.

---

157. A postoperative client who underwent pelvic surgery suddenly develops dyspnea and tachypnea. The nurse suspects that the client has a pulmonary embolism and prepares to take which action first?
1 Insert a urinary (Foley) catheter.
2 Administer low-flow oxygen through a nasal cannula.
3 Obtain an intravenous (IV) infusion pump to administer heparin.
4 Increase the rate of the IV fluids infusing to prevent hypotension.

Level of Cognitive Ability: Application
Client Needs: Physiological Integrity
Integrated Process: Nursing Process/
Implementation
Content Area: Delegating/Prioritizing

Answer: 2
Rationale: Pulmonary embolism is a life-threatening emergency. Maintenance of cardiopulmonary stability is the first priority. Low-flow oxygen by nasal cannula is administered first. Hypotension is treated with fluids. IV anticoagulation is initiated, and bicarbonate may be administered to correct acidosis. Some clients may require endotracheal intubation to maintain an adequate PaO$_2$. A perfusion scan among other tests may be performed, and the electrocardiogram (ECG) is monitored for the presence of dysrhythmias. In addition, a urinary catheter may be inserted. However, the first nursing action is to administer oxygen.

Test-Taking Strategy: Note the strategic word *first*. Use of the ABCs—airway, breathing, and circulation—will direct you to option 2. Review the immediate nursing actions when pulmonary embolism occurs and the test-taking strategies for answering prioritizing questions if you had difficulty with this question.

Tip for the Beginning Nursing Student: Pulmonary embolism is characterized by the blockage of a pulmonary artery by fat, air, tumor tissue, or a thrombus that usually arises from a peripheral vein. It is characterized by dyspnea, tachycardia, anxiety, sudden chest pain, shock, and cyanosis. It is a life-threatening condition and requires immediate and aggressive treatment. Airway, however, is the priority. You will learn about pulmonary embolism in your medical-surgical nursing course when you study respiratory and cardiovascular disorders.

Reference

deWit, S. (2009). *Medical-surgical nursing: Concepts & practice* (p. 342). St. Louis: Saunders.

Ignatavicius, D., & Workman, M. (2010). *Medical-surgical nursing: Patient-centered collaborative care* (6th ed., p. 680). Philadelphia: Saunders.

---

158. A client returns to the nursing unit from the postanesthesia care unit (PACU) following a transurethral resection of the prostate. The nurse does which of the following first?

1 Checks the client's respirations

2 Checks the color of the client's urine

3 Checks the urinary (Foley) catheter for patency

4 Reads the nursing notes written by the PACU nurse

Level of Cognitive Ability: Application
Client Needs: Physiological Integrity
Integrated Process: Nursing Process/ Implementation
Content Area: Delegating/Prioritizing

Answer: 1

Rationale: The first action of the nurse is to assess the patency of the airway, and the nurse would observe the client and assess the breathing pattern and respirations. If the airway is not patent and the client is not breathing, immediate measures must be taken for the survival of the client. The nurse then assesses cardiovascular function, the condition of the surgical site, the tubes or drains for patency and drainage, and function of the central nervous system. The PACU nurse normally provides a verbal report. Even so, reading the nursing notes would not be the first action.

Test-Taking Strategy: Note the strategic word *first.* Use the ABCs—airway, breathing, and circulation. This will direct you to option 1. Airway patency and respirations are the priority. Review priority nursing assessments in the postoperative client and the test-taking strategies for answering prioritizing questions if you had difficulty with this question.

Tip for the Beginning Nursing Student: A transurethral resection of the prostate is a surgical procedure in which a cystoscope (an instrument used for examining and treating lesions of the urinary tract) is passed through the urethra to resect (remove tissue from) the prostate. An important point to remember is that airway is always the priority in the care of a client. You will learn about this surgical procedure when you study renal disorders in your medical-surgical nursing course, and you will learn about perioperative care in your fundamentals of nursing course.

References

deWit, S. (2009). *Medical-surgical nursing: Concepts & practice* (p. 982). St. Louis: Saunders.

Ignatavicius, D., & Workman, M. (2010). *Medical-surgical nursing: Critical thinking for collaborative care* (6th ed., p. 289). Philadelphia: Saunders.

---

159. A child with a diagnosis of pertussis (whooping cough) is being admitted to the pediatric unit. As soon as the child arrives on the unit, the nurse would first:

1 Weigh the child.

2 Take the child's temperature.

3 Place the child on a pulse oximeter.

4 Administer the prescribed antibiotic.

Answer: 3

Rationale: To adequately determine if the child is getting enough oxygen, the child is placed on a pulse oximeter. The pulse oximeter will then provide ongoing information on the child's oxygen level. The child is also immediately placed on a cardiorespiratory monitor to provide early identification of periods of apnea and bradycardia. The nurse would then perform an assessment, including taking the child's temperature and weight and asking the parents about the child. An antibiotic may be prescribed, but the child's airway status needs to be assessed first.

Level of Cognitive Ability: Application
Client Needs: Physiological Integrity
Integrated Process: Nursing Process/
   Implementation
Content Area: Delegating/Prioritizing

Test-Taking Strategy: Note the strategic word *first*. Focus on the child's diagnosis, and use the ABCs—airway, breathing, and circulation. This will direct you to option 3. Review care of the child with pertusis and the test-taking strategies for answering prioritizing questions if you had difficulty with this question.

Tip for the Beginning Nursing Student: Pertussis is an acute, highly contagious respiratory disease characterized by coughing and a loud whooping inspiration that occurs primarily in infants and children. Pulse oximetry uses a clip-like device that measures the amount of saturated hemoglobin in the tissue capillaries and thus the percentage of oxygen saturation in the blood. An important point to remember is that airway is always the priority in the care of a client. You will learn about pertussis in your pediatrics nursing course when you study respiratory disorders, and you will learn about measuring oxygenation using pulse oximetry in your fundamentals of nursing course.

References

Price, D., & Gwin, J. (2008). *Pediatric nursing: An introductory text* (10th ed., p. 267). St. Louis: Saunders.
Hockenberry, M., & Wilson, D. (2007). *Nursing care of infants and children* (8th ed., pp. 672-673). St. Louis: Mosby.

---

160. A nurse is preparing to perform oral suctioning on a client who has coughed resulting in secretions in the mouth and is unable to spit out the secretions adequately. The nurse determines that there is a physician's order for the procedure and explains the procedure to the client. List in order of priority the actions that the nurse would take to perform this procedure safely. Number 1 is the first action.
___Washes hands
___Applies a face shield
___Removes the client's oxygen mask
___Places the oxygen mask on the client
___Applies a clean disposable glove to the dominant hand and attaches the suction catheter to the connecting tubing
___Inserts the catheter into the client's mouth and moves the catheter around the mouth, pharynx, and gum line until secretions are cleared

Answer: 1, 2, 4, 6, 3, 5

Rationale: The nurse always washes the hands before performing any procedure, applies a face shield because suctioning may cause splashing of body fluids, and then dons a clean glove. A clean rather than a sterile glove can be used in this procedure because the oral cavity is not sterile. The nurse then completes preparation by attaching the suction catheter to the connecting suction tubing. The nurse removes the oxygen mask just before implementing the procedure so that the client is oxygenated as much as possible (remember that suctioning can deplete oxygen). The catheter is then inserted into the client's mouth until secretions are cleared. If the client is not tolerating the procedure, then the catheter is removed and the oxygen mask is reapplied. The nurse next encourages the client to cough because coughing moves secretions from the lower to upper airways into the mouth. At this point, suctioning is repeated if necessary. The oxygen mask is then reapplied.

Test-Taking Strategy: The best strategy to use to answer this question is to first focus on the data in the question and then to visualize the procedure. Remember that hands are always washed first. Next remember that any preparation activities are done before removing the client's oxygen mask and that the client's oxygen is reapplied after completion of the procedure. Review the procedure for oral suctioning and the test-taking strategies for answering prioritizing questions if you had difficulty with this question.

Level of Cognitive Ability: Application
Client Needs: Safe and Effective Care Environment
Integrated Process: Nursing Process/ Implementation
Content Area: Delegating/Prioritizing

Tip for the Beginning Nursing Student: Suctioning is a procedure that is used to remove accumulated secretions from the oral cavity or respiratory tract when the client is unable to effectively cough them out. It is a sterile procedure when done to remove secretions from the respiratory tract and is a nonsterile procedure when suctioning secretions from the oral cavity. It requires specific actions to prevent trauma to the mucosa of the oral cavity or respiratory tract and to prevent hypoxia. You will learn about the procedure for suctioning in your fundamentals of nursing course and in your medical-surgical nursing course when you study respiratory disorders.

References
deWit, S. (2009). *Medical-surgical nursing: Concepts & practice* (pp. 310-311). St. Louis: Saunders.
Potter, P., & Perry, A. (2009). *Fundamentals of nursing* (7th ed., pp. 931, 936). St. Louis: Mosby.

---

161. A nurse hears the alarm sound on the telemetry monitor, quickly looks at the monitor, and notes that a client is in ventricular tachycardia. The nurse rushes to the client's room, and, on reaching the client's bedside, the nurse performs the following actions. List in order of priority the actions that the nurse would take, with number 1 being the first action.

___Opens the airway
___Delivers two breaths
___Determines breathlessness
___Begins cardiac compressions
___Determines unresponsiveness
___Checks for a pulse at the carotid artery

Level of Cognitive Ability: Application
Client Needs: Physiological Integrity
Integrated Process: Nursing Process/ Implementation
Content Area: Delegating/Prioritizing

Answer: 2, 4, 3, 6, 1, 5

Rationale: Determining unresponsiveness is the first action to take. When a client is in ventricular tachycardia, there is a significant decrease in cardiac output. However, assessing for unresponsiveness ensures that the client is affected by the decreased cardiac output. If the client is unresponsive the nurse proceeds through the ABCs— airway, breathing, and circulation—of cardiopulmonary resuscitation (CPR), remembering that the nurse would assess before taking an action.

Test-Taking Strategy: Note the strategic words *in order of priority.* Use the steps of basic life support to answer the question. Remember that determining unresponsiveness is the first action, followed by the ABCs—airway, breathing, and circulation. Also remember that assessment comes before implementation. Review the priority nursing actions if a client experiences ventricular tachycardia and the test-taking strategies for answering prioritizing questions if you had difficulty with this question.

Tip for the Beginning Nursing Student: Ventricular tachycardia means that the ventricles are beating at a rate greater than 100 beats/min. If the client experiencing ventricular tachycardia is unresponsive, CPR may need to be initiated because ventricular tachycardia can progress to ventricular fibrillation, another life-threatening situation. You will learn about cardiac dysrhythmias and their treatment in your medical-surgical nursing course when you study cardiac disorders.

References
deWit, S. (2009). *Medical-surgical nursing: Concepts & practice* (pp. 472-473, 478). St. Louis: Saunders.
Monahan, F., Sands, J., Marek, J., Neighbors, M., & Green, C. (2007). *Phipps' medical-surgical nursing: Health and illness perspectives* (8th ed., pp. 785-786). St. Louis: Mosby.

162. A nurse is assessing a client with a diagnosis of bulimia nervosa who has problems with nutrition. The nurse would obtain information from the client about which of the following first?

1 Lack of control

2 Previous and current coping skills

3 Feelings about self and body weight

4 Eating patterns, food preferences, concerns about eating

Level of Cognitive Ability: Application
Client Needs: Physiological Integrity
Integrated Process: Nursing Process/ Assessment/Data Collection
Content Area: Delegating/Prioritizing

Answer: 4

Rationale: The nurse would first identify the client's eating patterns, food preferences, and concerns about eating when caring for the client with bulimia nervosa. The nurse would also obtain information about the client's feelings about self and body weight, previous and current coping skills, and lack of control, but this information is secondary to eating patterns and food preferences.

Test-Taking Strategy: Note the strategic word *first.* Use Maslow's Hierarchy of Needs theory to prioritize. Option 4 is the only option that relates to a physiological need. Review care for the client with bulimia nervosa and the test-taking strategies for answering prioritizing questions if you had difficulty with this question.

Tip for the Beginning Nursing Student: Bulimia nervosa is a disorder characterized by a craving for food and continuous eating followed by purging. It is also known as binge eating. The condition can lead to severe nutritional deficiencies, self-deprivation, and depression. You will learn about bulimia when you study eating disorders in a medical-surgical nursing course or in a psychiatric/mental health nursing course.

References

deWit, S. (2009). *Medical-surgical nursing: Concepts & practice* (pp. 1114-1116). St. Louis: Saunders.

Ignatavicius, D., & Workman, M. (2010). *Medical-surgical nursing: Patient-centered collaborative care* (6th ed., p. 1393). Philadelphia: Saunders.

---

163. A community health nurse is assisting residents involved in a hurricane and flood. Many of the older residents are emotionally despondent and refuse to evacuate their homes. With regard to rescue and relocation of the older residents the nurse plans to first:

1 Contact families.

2 Attend to emotional needs.

3 Attend to nutritional and basic needs.

4 Arrange for transportation to shelters.

Level of Cognitive Ability: Application
Client Needs: Physiological Integrity
Integrated Process: Nursing Process/ Planning
Content Area: Delegating/Prioritizing

Answer: 3

Rationale: Attending to people's basic needs of food, shelter, and clothing is the priority. Options 1, 2, and 4 may or may not be needed at a later date.

Test-Taking Strategy: Note the strategic word *first,* and use Maslow's Hierarchy of Needs theory. Option 3 addresses basic physiological needs. Options 1, 2, and 4 address psychosocial needs and may be appropriate at a later date. Review the nurse's role in the event of a disaster and the test-taking strategies for answering prioritizing questions if you had difficulty with this question.

Tip for the Beginning Nursing Student: A disaster is any human-made or natural event that causes destruction and devastation that require assistance from others. In regard to a health care agency, a disaster can be external or internal. External disasters include those that occur outside the agency, and internal disasters include those that occur inside the agency. A disaster preparedness plan is a formal plan of action for coordinating the response of a health care agency's staff in the event of a disaster in the health care agency or surrounding community. You will learn about disasters and a disaster preparedness plan in many of your nursing courses, including fundamentals, medical-surgical, leadership and management, and community.

References

deWit, S. (2009). *Medical-surgical nursing: Concepts & practice* (p. 1056). St. Louis: Saunders.

Ignatavicius, D., & Workman, M. (2009). *Medical-surgical nursing: Patient-centered collaborative care* (5th ed., pp. 163-164). Philadelphia: Saunders.

---

164. An antepartum client at 32 weeks' gestation positioned herself supine on the examination table to await the obstetrician. The nurse enters the examination room, and the client says, "I'm feeling a little lightheaded and sick to my stomach." The nurse recognizes that the client may be experiencing vena caval syndrome (hypotensive syndrome) and takes which immediate action?

1 Gives the client an emesis basin

2 Places a cool cloth on the client's forehead

3 Calls the obstetrician to see the client immediately

4 Places a folded towel or sheet under the client's right hip

Level of Cognitive Ability: Application
Client Needs: Physiological Integrity
Integrated Process: Nursing Process/ Implementation
Content Area: Delegating/Prioritizing

Answer: 4

Rationale: Lying supine (on the back) applies additional gravity pressure on the abdominal blood vessels (iliac vessels, inferior vena cava, and ascending aorta), increasing compression and impeding blood flow and cardiac output. This results in hypotension, dizziness, nausea, pallor, clammy (cool, damp) skin, and sweating. Raising one hip higher than the other reduces the pressure on the vena cava, restoring the circulation and relieving the symptoms. Although an emesis basin and a cool cloth placed on the forehead may be helpful these are not the immediate actions. It is not necessary to call the obstetrician immediately unless the client's complaints are unrelieved following repositioning.

Test-Taking Strategy: Note the strategic word *immediate.* Focus on the information in the question and the goals of care. In other words, think about what complications that you want to prevent. Remember that if a question requires you to prioritize and one of the options relates to positioning a client, that option may be the correct one. Review care of the client experiencing vena caval syndrome and the test-taking strategies for answering prioritizing questions if you had difficulty with this question.

Tip for the Beginning Nursing Student: Vena caval syndrome, also know as supine hypotension, is a condition in which a fall in blood pressure occurs when a pregnant woman is lying on her back. It is caused by impaired venous return that results from pressure of the gravid uterus on the vena cava. Therefore raising one hip higher than the other reduces the pressure on the vena cava, restoring the circulation and relieving the symptoms. You will learn about vena caval syndrome in your maternity nursing course.

References

Leifer, G. (2007). *Introduction to maternity and pediatric nursing* (5th ed., pp. 52-53). Philadelphia: Saunders.

Wong, D., Perry, S., Hockenberry, M., Lowdermilk, D., & Wilson, D. (2006). *Maternal-child nursing care* (3rd ed., p. 286). St. Louis: Mosby.

165. A client is hospitalized with chest pain, and myocardial infarction is suspected. The client tells the nurse that the chest pain has returned, and the nurse administers one 0.4-mg nitroglycerin tablet sublingually as prescribed. What does the nurse do next before administering another sublingual nitroglycerin tablet if the pain is not relieved?
1 Notifies the physician
2 Checks the client's blood pressure
3 Encourages the client to deep breathe
4 Places the client in Trendelenburg's position

Level of Cognitive Ability: Application
Client Needs: Physiological Integrity
Integrated Process: Nursing Process/ Implementation
Content Area: Delegating/Prioritizing

Answer: 2
Rationale: Nitroglycerin tablets are administered one every 5 minutes, not exceeding three tablets, for chest pain as long as the client maintains a systolic blood pressure of 100 mm Hg or above. The nurse would check the client's blood pressure before administering a second nitroglycerin tablet. The physician is notified if the chest pain is not relieved after administering three tablets. If there is a sudden drop in blood pressure, the client is placed in Trendelenburg's (head-lowered) position and the physician is notified. Deep breathing will not relieve the chest pain that occurs as a result of myocardial infarction.

Test-Taking Strategy: Note the strategic word *next.* Use the ABCs—airway, breathing, and circulation. This will direct you to option 2. Checking the blood pressure is a means of assessing the client's circulatory status. Review care of the client experiencing chest pain and the test-taking strategies for answering pharmacology questions if you had difficulty with this question.

Tip for the Beginning Nursing Student: A myocardial infarction is also known as a heart attack and results in necrosis of cardiac muscle caused by an obstruction in a coronary artery. When a client experiences chest pain and a cardiac problem is suspected, nitroglycerin is administered. Nitroglycerin is a coronary vasodilator that acts by dilating the coronary vessels, and thus increased blood flow and oxygenation ensue. You will learn about myocardial infarction and nitroglycerin in your medical-surgical nursing course when you study cardiovascular disorders.

References
deWit, S. (2009). *Medical-surgical nursing: Concepts & practice* (p. 493). St. Louis: Saunders.
Hodgson, B., & Kizior, R. (2009). *Saunders nursing drug handbook 2009* (p. 841). Philadelphia: Saunders.

166. A client receiving a blood transfusion develops signs of a blood transfusion reaction. List in order of priority the actions that the nurse will take. Number 1 is the first nursing action.
___Document the occurrence.
___Stop the blood transfusion.
___Check the client's vital signs.
___Maintain a patent intravenous (IV) line with normal saline solution.
___Send the blood bag and tubing to the blood bank for examination.
___Check the client's urine output, and obtain a urine specimen for analysis.

Answer: 6, 1, 3, 2, 5, 4
Rationale: If a transfusion reaction is suspected, the transfusion is stopped and then normal saline is infused pending further physician orders. This maintains a patent IV access line and aids in maintaining the client's intravascular volume. The physician and blood bank are notified immediately. The nurse would monitor the client's vital signs and urine output and would obtain a urine specimen for analysis to check for hemolysis of red blood cells. The nurse then sends the blood bag and tubing to the blood bank for examination and documents the occurrence on the transfusion report and in the client's chart.

Test-Taking Strategy: The best strategy to use to answer this question is to visualize the occurrence. Stopping the blood is the first action; and because the IV line needs to remain patent, normal saline solution needs to be infused. Next use the ABCs—airway, breathing, and circulation—to

Level of Cognitive Ability: Application
Client Needs: Physiological Integrity
Integrated Process: Nursing Process/
   Implementation
Content Area: Delegating/Prioritizing

determine that the client's vital signs need to be monitored. Then select monitoring urine output and obtaining a urine specimen because this action relates to a physiological need. From the remaining interventions, select documentation last because all interventions, including that the nurse sent the blood bag and tubing to the blood bank for examination, need to be documented. Review interventions if a transfusion reaction occurs and the test-taking strategies for answering prioritizing questions if you had difficulty with this question.

Tip for the Beginning Nursing Student: A blood transfusion involves the administration of whole blood or a component of blood, such as packed red blood cells. It is prescribed to replace blood lost as a result of trauma, surgery, or disease. A major concern associated with the administration of blood is a blood transfusion reaction, and the nurse monitors the client very closely for this life-threatening complication. It is important to know the signs of a transfusion reaction and the nursing interventions if a transfusion reaction occurs. You will learn about the administration of blood transfusions and the associated complications in your medical-surgical nursing course when you study hematological disorders.

References

Christensen, B., & Kockrow, E. (2006). *Adult health nursing* (5th ed., p. 581). St. Louis: Mosby.

Lewis, S., Heitkemper, M., Dirksen, S., & Bucher, L. (2007). *Medical-surgical nursing: Assessment and management of clinical problems* (7th ed., pp. 732-734). St. Louis: Mosby.

Linton, A. (2007). *Introduction to medical-surgical nursing* (4th ed., p. 581). Philadelphia: Saunders.

---

167. A client with a diagnosis of sickle cell crisis is being admitted to the hospital. The nurse anticipates that which priority intervention will be prescribed?
1 Laboratory studies
2 Genetic counseling
3 Oxygen administration
4 Electrolyte replacement therapy

Level of Cognitive Ability: Analysis
Client Needs: Physiological Integrity
Integrated Process: Nursing Process/
   Planning
Content Area: Delegating/Prioritizing

Answer: 3

Rationale: Oxygen, intravenous fluids, pain medication, and red blood cell transfusions are the primary interventions for treating sickle cell crisis. Laboratory studies may also be prescribed but are not the priority in the care of the client. Electrolyte replacement therapy may be necessary, but this treatment would be based on the results of laboratory studies. Genetic counseling is recommended but not during the acute phase of illness.

Test-Taking Strategy: Note the strategic word *priority.* Option 2 can be eliminated first using Maslow's Hierarchy of Needs theory because this option addresses a psychosocial need not a physiological one. From the remaining options use the ABCs—airway, breathing, and circulation—to direct you to option 3. Review care of the client in sickle cell crisis and the test-taking strategies for questions that require prioritizing if you had difficulty with this question.

Tip for the Beginning Nursing Student: Sickle cell anemia is a severe, chronic, and incurable anemic condition characterized by abnormal hemoglobin (Hgb S) that results in distortion and fragility of the erythrocytes (sickled shape).

Sickle cell crisis is an acute episodic condition that can occur when an individual has sickle cell anemia and results in the aggregation and clumping of the distorted erythrocytes, leading to occlusion and ischemia of tissue. You will learn about sickle cell crisis in your pediatric nursing course and in your medical-surgical nursing course when you study hematological disorders.

References
Christensen, B., & Kockrow, E. (2006). *Adult health nursing* (5th ed., p. 303). St. Louis: Mosby.

Ignatavicius, D., & Workman, M. (2010). *Medical-surgical nursing: Patient-centered collaborative care* (6th ed., p. 897). Philadelphia: Saunders.

---

168. A nurse is planning the client assignments for the day. Which of the following clients would the nurse assign to the nursing assistant?
1 A client on strict bedrest
2 A client scheduled for discharge to home
3 A client scheduled for a cardiac catheterization
4 A postoperative client who had an emergency appendectomy

Level of Cognitive Ability: Application
Client Needs: Safe and Effective Care Environment
Integrated Process: Nursing Process/ Implementation
Content Area: Delegating/Prioritizing

Answer: 1

Rationale: The nurse is legally responsible for client assignments and must assign tasks based on the guidelines of nurse practice acts and the job descriptions of the employing agency. A client scheduled for discharge to home, a postoperative client who had an emergency appendectomy, or a client scheduled for a cardiac catheterization has both physiological and psychosocial needs that require care by a licensed nurse. The nursing assistant has been trained to care for a client on bedrest. The nurse provides instructions to the nursing assistant, but the tasks required are within the role description of a nursing assistant.

Test-Taking Strategy: Note that the question asks for the assignment to be delegated to the nursing assistant. When asked questions related to delegation, think about the role description of the employee and the needs of the client. This will direct you to option 1. Review the principles for planning client assignments and the test-taking strategies for answering delegation questions if you had difficulty with this question.

Tip for the Beginning Nursing Student: Delegating and assignment making are responsibilities of the nurse; and it is important that you assign tasks and activities that are appropriate based on the individual's educational experience, nurse practice acts, and the health care agency's policies and procedures. When you need to assign a task or activity to a nursing assistant, think about the word *noninvasive*. Select the task or activity that is a noninvasive one. You will learn about delegating and assignment making in your leadership and management course or in another nursing course that addresses these guidelines and principles.

References
Linton, A. (2007). *Introduction to medical-surgical nursing* (4th ed., p. 44). Philadelphia: Saunders.

Potter, P., & Perry, A. (2009). *Fundamentals of nursing* (7th ed., pp. 309-311). St. Louis: Mosby.

169. A hospitalized client with type 1 diabetes mellitus tells the nurse that she feels like she is having a hypoglycemic reaction. The nurse would first:

1 Obtain a blood glucose reading.
2 Give the client 4 oz of orange juice.
3 Prepare to administer 50% dextrose intravenously.
4 Prepare to administer subcutaneous glucagon hydrochloride.

Level of Cognitive Ability: Application
Client Needs: Physiological Integrity
Integrated Process: Nursing Process/ Implementation
Content Area: Delegating/Prioritizing

Answer: 1

Rationale: Management of hypoglycemia depends on the severity of the reaction. To reverse mild hypoglycemia, a 15-g simple carbohydrate is given and works quickly to increase blood glucose levels. However, a blood glucose test (with a glucose meter) should be performed first as soon as manifestations begin. If a meter is not available, it is safest to treat the hypoglycemia. Fifty-percent dextrose and glucagon hydrochloride are used to treat severe hypoglycemia particularly in the unconscious client.

Test-Taking Strategy: Note the strategic word *first,* and note that the client is hospitalized. Use the steps of the nursing process, and note that option 1 is the only option that addresses assessment/data collection. Review care of the client experiencing a hypoglycemic reaction and the test-taking strategies for answering prioritizing questions if you had difficulty with this question.

Tip for the Beginning Nursing Student: Diabetes mellitus is a disorder of carbohydrate, fat, and protein metabolism that is primarily the result of a deficiency or complete lack of insulin secretion by the beta cells of the pancreas or resistance to insulin. The client is treated with exogenous insulin, and both hypoglycemia (a low blood glucose level) and hyperglycemia (a high blood glucose level) are complications. It is important to know the signs of each complication and how to treat them. It is also important to teach the client these signs and their treatment. If a low blood glucose level occurs the client is treated with a 15-g simple carbohydrate to increase blood glucose levels. You will learn about diabetes mellitus and its complications in your medical-surgical nursing course when you study endocrine disorders.

References

Christensen, B., & Kockrow, E. (2006). *Adult health nursing* (5th ed., p. 559). St. Louis: Mosby.

Monahan, F., Sands, J., Marek, J., Neighbors, M., & Green, C. (2007). *Phipps' medical-surgical nursing: Health and illness perspectives* (8th ed., p. 1160). St. Louis: Mosby.

170. A client is admitted to the emergency department with complaints of severe, radiating chest pain, and a myocardial infarction (heart attack) is suspected. The nurse immediately applies oxygen to the client and plans to take which action next?

1 Obtain a 12-lead electrocardiogram (ECG).
2 Call radiology to order a chest radiograph.
3 Call the laboratory to order stat blood work.

Answer: 1

Rationale: The initial action is to apply oxygen, because the client may be experiencing myocardial ischemia. Based on the options provided, an ECG will be done next because this test can provide evidence of cardiac damage and the location of myocardial ischemia. Vital signs are also measured and may be done just before obtaining the ECG or quickly thereafter. Nitroglycerin, a coronary artery vasodilator, may also be administered. The nurse would then obtain blood work because it can assist in determining the choice of treatment. Although the chest radiograph may show cardiac enlargement, it does not influence the immediate treatment. Notifying the coronary care unit to inform them that the client will need admission would be done

4 Notify the coronary care unit to inform them that the client will need admission.

Level of Cognitive Ability: Application
Client Needs: Physiological Integrity
Integrated Process: Nursing Process/ Implementation
Content Area: Delegating/Prioritizing

once the diagnosis is confirmed and admission is deemed necessary.

Test-Taking Strategy: Note the strategic word *next*. Remember that the immediate goal of therapy is to prevent myocardial ischemia. Use knowledge regarding the procedures for determining treatment to answer this question. Review care of the client with chest pain and the test-taking strategies for answering prioritizing questions if you had difficulty with this question.

Tip for the Beginning Nursing Student: A myocardial infarction is also known as a heart attack and results in necrosis of cardiac muscle caused by an obstruction in a coronary artery. Chest pain is a significant characteristic of a heart attack. In fact, whenever a client complains of chest pain, the nurse should suspect the presence of a heart attack and act quickly until this diagnosis can be ruled out. You will learn about myocardial infarction and its immediate treatment in your medical-surgical nursing course when you study cardiovascular disorders.

References

deWit, S. (2009). *Medical-surgical nursing: Concepts & practice* (p. 420). St. Louis: Saunders.

Lewis, S., Heitkemper, M., Dirksen, S., & Bucher, L. (2007). *Medical-surgical nursing: Assessment and management of clinical problems* (7th ed., p. 806). St. Louis: Mosby.

---

171. A nurse is caring for a client with a brainstem injury. The nurse monitors which of the following as the priority?
  1 Urine output
  2 Electrolyte results
  3 Peripheral vascular status
  4 Respiratory rate and rhythm

Level of Cognitive Ability: Application
Client Needs: Physiological Integrity
Integrated Process: Nursing Process/ Assessment/Data Collection
Content Area: Delegating/Prioritizing

Answer: 4
Rationale: The respiratory center is located in the brainstem. Monitoring the respiratory status is a priority in a client with a brainstem injury, although the nurse may also monitor laboratory results, urine output, and peripheral vascular status.

Test-Taking Strategy: Use the ABCs—airway, breathing, and circulation. Option 4 relates to airway. Also, recalling the anatomical location of the respiratory center will direct you to the correct option. Review care of the client with a brainstem injury and the test-taking strategies for prioritizing questions if you had difficulty with this question.

Tip for the Beginning Nursing Student: The brainstem is made up of several structures, including the midbrain, pons, and medulla oblongata. The vital centers of cardiac, respiratory, and vasomotor control are located in the medulla oblongata. If injury occurs to the brainstem, the nurse would monitor the respiratory status as a priority, followed by the cardiac status and vasomotor status. You will learn about brainstem injuries and their complications in your medical-surgical nursing course when you study neurological disorders.

References

deWit, S. (2009). *Medical-surgical nursing: Concepts & practice* (pp. 523-524). St. Louis: Saunders.

Lewis, S., Heitkemper, M., Dirksen, S., & Bucher, L. (2007). *Medical-surgical nursing: Assessment and management of clinical problems* (7th ed., p. 1486). St. Louis: Mosby.

---

172. A client is scheduled for a diagnostic procedure requiring the injection of a radiopaque dye. The nurse checks which most critical information before the procedure?

  1 Intake and output
  2 Height and weight
  3 Baseline vital signs
  4 History of allergy to iodine or shellfish

Level of Cognitive Ability: Application
Client Needs: Physiological Integrity
Integrated Process: Nursing Process/Assessment/Data Collection
Content Area: Delegating/Prioritizing

Answer: 4

Rationale: Procedures that involve the injection of a radiopaque dye require an informed consent. The risk for allergic reaction exists if the client has an allergy to iodine or shellfish. The risk of allergic reaction and possible anaphylaxis must be determined before the procedure. Although options 1, 2, and 3 identify information obtained before the procedure, these items are not the most critical.

Test-Taking Strategy: Note the strategic words *most critical.* Use the ABCs—airway, breathing, and circulation. The risk for an allergic reaction and anaphylaxis makes option 4 correct. Review the complications associated with injection of a radiopaque dye and the test-taking strategies for answering prioritizing questions if you had difficulty with this question.

Tip for the Beginning Nursing Student: Many diagnostic tests may require injection of a radiopaque dye. This type of dye, which contains properties of iodine, is used for diagnosis to provide better visualization of body structures. Whenever a radiopaque dye is used, the nurse needs to assess the client for an allergy to both iodine and shellfish. You will learn about diagnostic tests and the important associated nursing responsibilities in preparing the client for these tests in your fundamentals of nursing course and in other nursing courses.

References

Christensen, B., & Kockrow, E. (2006). *Foundations of nursing* (5th ed., p. 486). St. Louis: Mosby.

Potter, P., & Perry, A. (2009). *Fundamentals of nursing* (7th ed., pp. 1474-1475). St. Louis: Mosby.

---

173. A nurse is developing a plan of care for a client in Buck's skin traction. The nurse identifies which nursing diagnosis as the priority?

  1 *Social isolation*
  2 *Risk for loneliness*
  3 *Deficient diversional activity*
  4 *Risk for impaired skin integrity*

Level of Cognitive Ability:
  Comprehension
Client Needs: Physiological Integrity

Answer: 4

Rationale: Buck's skin traction is a type of traction in which weights are attached to the skin with the use of a boot or elastic bandage. The priority nursing diagnosis for the client is *Risk for impaired skin integrity.* Risk for altered neurovascular status is also a concern. Options 1, 2, and 3 may also be appropriate for the client in Buck's skin traction, but *Risk for impaired skin integrity* presents the greatest risk.

Test-Taking Strategy: Note the strategic word *priority.* Use Maslow's Hierarchy of Needs theory. The only option that indicates a physiological need is option 4. Options 1, 2, and

Integrated Process: Nursing Process/
  Planning
Content Area: Delegating/Prioritizing

3 indicate psychosocial needs. Review care to the client in Buck's extension traction and the test-taking strategies for answering prioritizing questions if you had difficulty with this question.

Tip for the Beginning Nursing Student: Traction may be used to treat fractures; it provides immobilization to hold the broken bone fragments in contact with each other or in very close approximation until healing takes place. The two types of traction are skin and skeletal. Skin traction is achieved by applying a boot, wrap, or a commercially pre-pared device directly to the skin, which is then attached to weights. Skeletal traction is attached directly to bone. You will learn about the various types of traction and the asso-ciated nursing care in your medical-surgical nursing course when you study musculoskeletal disorders.

References
Ignatavicius, D., & Workman, M. (2010). *Medical-surgical nursing: Patient-centered collaborative care* (6th ed., pp. 1189-1190). Philadelphia: Saunders.
Linton, A. (2007). *Introduction to medical-surgical nursing* (4th ed., p. 923). Philadelphia: Saunders.

---

174. A nurse is reviewing the plan of care for a child with juvenile idio-pathic arthritis (JIA). The nurse determines that which of the following is a priority nursing diagnosis?
  1 *Acute pain*
  2 *Risk for injury*
  3 *Disturbed body image*
  4 *Bathing/hygiene self-care deficit*

Level of Cognitive Ability:
  Comprehension
Client Needs: Physiological Integrity
Integrated Process: Nursing Process/
  Planning
Content Area: Delegating/Prioritizing

Answer: 1
Rationale: All the nursing diagnoses are appropriate for the child with JIA. The priority nursing diagnosis relates to pain. *Acute pain* needs to be managed before other prob-lems can be addressed.

Test-Taking Strategy: Note the strategic word *priority.* Use Maslow's Hierarchy of Needs theory, remembering that physiological needs (option 1) receive highest priority. Option 2 addresses safety and security needs and is also a risk (potential), not an actual, problem. Option 3 addresses self-esteem needs. Option 4 is less of a priority as compared with acute pain. Review care of the child with JIA and the test-taking strategies for answering prioritizing questions if you had difficulty with this question.

Tip for the Beginning Nursing Student: Arthritis is an inflammatory condition of the joints characterized by pain, swelling, heat, redness, and limitation of movement. It can affect the client's ability to perform activities of daily living. It can also result in debilitation. It can occur in childhood or adulthood. You will learn about arthritis and its compli-cations in your pediatric nursing course and in your medical-surgical nursing course.

References
Hockenberry, M., & Wilson, D. (2007). *Nursing care of infants and children* (8th ed., p. 1791). St. Louis: Mosby.
Price, D., & Gwin, J. (2008). *Pediatric nursing: An introductory text* (10th ed., pp. 314, 317). St. Louis: Saunders.

175. A client has been newly diagnosed with diabetes mellitus. The nurse does which of the following as the first step in teaching the client about the disorder?

1 Decide on the teaching approach.
2 Plan for the evaluation of the session.
3 Gather all available resource materials.
4 Identify the client's knowledge and needs.

Level of Cognitive Ability: Application
Client Needs: Health Promotion and Maintenance
Integrated Process: Teaching and Learning
Content Area: Delegating/Prioritizing

Answer: 4

Rationale: Determining what to teach a client begins with an assessment of the client's own knowledge and learning needs. Once these have been determined, the nurse can effectively plan a teaching approach, the actual content, and resource materials that may be needed. The evaluation is done after teaching is completed.

Test-Taking Strategy: Note the strategic word *first.* Use the steps of the nursing process to remember that data collection and assessment are the first step. Review teaching and learning principles and the test-taking strategies for answering prioritizing questions if you had difficulty with this question.

Tip for the Beginning Nursing Student: Diabetes mellitus is a disorder of carbohydrate, fat, and protein metabolism that is primarily the result of a deficiency or complete lack of insulin secretion by the beta cells of the pancreas or resistance to insulin. Treatment includes diet, medication, and exercise. The client needs to be taught about the disorder and needs to understand how to care for self to maintain normal blood glucose levels and to prevent complications of the disease. Teaching is a very important role of the nurse for all clients, and teaching and learning principles are used to guide the nurse. You will learn about teaching and learning principles in your fundamentals of nursing course and you will learn about diabetes mellitus in your medical-surgical nursing course when you study endocrine disorders.

References

Ignatavicius, D., & Workman, M. (2010). *Medical-surgical nursing: Patient-centered collaborative care* (6th ed., p. 1475). Philadelphia: Saunders.
Linton, A. (2007). *Introduction to medical-surgical nursing* (4th ed., pp. 1020-1021). Philadelphia: Saunders.

19 Chapter

Leadership/Management Questions

176. A charge nurse is observing a new nursing graduate perform an ear irrigation to remove impacted cerumen from the client's ear. The charge nurse intervenes during the procedure if the new nursing graduate did which of the following?

1 Washed her hands before performing the procedure

2 Positioned the client with the affected side up following the irrigation

3 Warmed the irrigating solution to a temperature that is close to body temperature

4 Directed a slow steady stream of irrigation solution toward the upper wall of the ear canal

Level of Cognitive Ability: Application
Client Needs: Safe and Effective Care Environment
Integrated Process: Nursing Process/Implementation
Content Area: Leadership/Management

Answer: 2

Rationale: During the irrigation the client is positioned sitting with an ear basin under the ear. Irrigation solutions that are not close to the client's body temperature can be uncomfortable and may cause injury, nausea, and vertigo. A slow steady stream of solution should be directed toward the upper wall of the ear canal and not toward the tympanic membrane. Following the irrigation the client should lie on the affected side for a time to finish the drainage of the irrigating solution and to allow gravity to assist in the removal of the earwax and solution. Too much force could cause the tympanic membrane to rupture.

Test-Taking Strategy: Note the strategic word *intervenes.* This word indicates a negative event query and that you are looking for an incorrect nursing action. Visualizing this procedure will assist in directing you to option 2. Review this procedure and the various test-taking strategies if you had difficulty with this question.

Tip for the Beginning Nursing Student: An ear irrigation is the instillation of water or a saline solution into the ear and is usually done to remove excess cerumen from the ear. Ear irrigations are not done if a perforated tympanic membrane is suspected. It is important for the nurse to know the procedure for performing an ear irrigation to prevent complications of the procedure, such as rupture of the tympanic membrane. You will learn about the procedure for performing ear irrigations and the role of the nurse as a teacher and supervisor in your fundamentals of nursing course or in your leadership/management course.

References
deWit, S. (2009). *Medical-surgical nursing: Concepts & practice* (p. 656). St. Louis: Saunders.
Monahan, F., Sands, J., Marek, J., Neighbors, M., & Green, C. (2007). *Phipps' medical-surgical nursing: Health and illness perspectives* (8th ed., p. 1850). St. Louis: Mosby.

177. The nurse is supervising a nursing assistant performing mouth care on an unconscious client. The nurse would intervene if the nurse noted the nursing assistant doing which of the following?
1 Turning the client's head to one side
2 Using small volumes of fluid to rinse the mouth
3 Using a gloved finger to open the client's mouth
4 Placing an emesis basin under the client's mouth

Level of Cognitive Ability: Application
Client Needs: Safe and Effective Care Environment
Integrated Process: Nursing Process/ Implementation
Content Area: Leadership/ Management

Answer: 3
Rationale: The client who is unconscious is at great risk for aspiration. The nursing assistant turns the client's head to the side and places an emesis basin underneath the mouth. A bite stick or a padded tongue blade is used to open the mouth, not a gloved finger, to prevent injury to the caregiver. Small volumes of fluids are used to rinse the mouth.

Test-Taking Strategy: Note the strategic word *intervene.* This word indicates a negative event query and that you are looking for the option that is incorrect. Visualize this procedure, and remember that the nurse never places a finger into a client's mouth. Review the procedure for administering mouth care to the client who is unconscious and the various test-taking strategies if you had difficulty with this question.

Tip for the Beginning Nursing Student: Unconsciousness is a state of complete or partial unawareness or lack of response to stimuli. It can be caused by a variety of conditions, such as shock, hypoxia, or brain attack (stroke). The client who is unconscious requires complete care including mouth care. Depending on the state of unawareness, the client may exhibit some responses to stimuli, such as bearing down with the teeth if an object is placed in the mouth. It is extremely important to remember that you should never insert a finger into a client's mouth regardless of the state of consciousness. You will learn about the procedure for performing mouth care and the role of the nurse as a teacher and supervisor in your fundamentals of nursing course or in your leadership/ management course.

References
deWit, S. (2009). *Medical-surgical nursing: Concepts & practice* (p. 532). St. Louis: Saunders.
Potter, P., & Perry, A. (2009). *Fundamentals of nursing* (7th ed., pp. 888-890). St. Louis: Mosby.

---

178. A nurse is observing a student donning a pair of sterile gloves and preparing a sterile field. The nurse intervenes if the student:
1 Puts the right glove on and then the left glove
2 Dons the sterile gloves without washing the hands
3 Uses the inner wrapper of the gloves as a sterile field
4 Touches the gloves on the overbed table, removes them, and dons another sterile pair

Level of Cognitive Ability: Application
Client Needs: Safe and Effective Care Environment

Answer: 2
Rationale: Hands must always be washed (even though sterile gloves are used) to keep germs from spreading. The inside wrapper provides an excellent area for usage because it is sterile. Gloves that touch anything unsterile must be considered contaminated, and a new package of gloves must be obtained and used. The order of placing gloves on is up to the individual as long as sterile technique is not broken.

Test-Taking Strategy: Note the strategic word *intervenes.* This word indicates a negative event query and that you are looking for the option that identifies an incorrect action. Visualize each option keeping the principles of sterile technique in mind. Noting the words *without washing the hands* in option 2 will direct you to this option. Review sterile

Integrated Process: Nursing Process/
Implementation
Content Area: Leadership/
Management

technique for donning gloves and the various test-taking strategies if you had difficulty with this question.

Tip for the Beginning Nursing Student: Sterile technique, also know as aseptic technique, is the use of special procedures to prevent contamination of the nurse, object, or area by microorganisms. A sterile field is an area that the nurse prepares that is considered free of microorganisms. Sterile technique and a sterile field are used to perform various procedures, such as changing a wound dressing. Handwashing is always done before any procedure even if the nurse plans to don gloves. You will learn about sterile technique, the procedure for donning sterile gloves and setting up a sterile field, and the role of the nurse as a teacher and supervisor in your fundamentals of nursing course or in your leadership/management course.

References

deWit, S. (2009). *Medical-surgical nursing: Concepts & practice* (p. 120). St. Louis: Saunders.
Potter, P., & Perry, A. (2009). *Fundamentals of nursing* (7th ed., p. 665). St. Louis: Mosby.

---

179. A nurse reviews the laboratory results of a client receiving chemotherapy and notes that the white blood cell count is extremely low. The nurse asks a nursing student assigned to care for the client to place the client on neutropenic precautions. The nurse determines the need to review the procedures for neutropenic precautions with the student nurse if which of the following was noted?
1 The water pitcher is removed from the client's room.
2 Fresh cut flowers were removed from the client's room.
3 A box of face masks was placed at the entrance to the client's room.
4 Bananas and apples brought to the client by a family member were left in the client's room.

Level of Cognitive Ability: Analysis
Client Needs: Safe and Effective Care Environment
Integrated Process: Teaching and Learning
Content Area: Leadership/
Management

Answer: 4
Rationale: In the immunocompromised client a low-bacteria diet is necessary. This includes avoiding fresh fruits and vegetables. Thorough cooking of all food is also required. Anyone who enters the client's room should perform strict and thorough handwashing and wear a mask. Cut flowers or any standing water is removed from the room because it tends to harbor bacteria.

Test-Taking Strategy: Note the strategic words *determines the need to review the procedures.* These words indicate a negative event query and that you are looking for the action that is incorrect. Recall that neutropenic precautions are implemented when a client is at high risk for contracting an infection. Next look for the action that places the client at risk for infection. This will direct you to option 4. Review interventions for the client on neutropenic precautions and the various test-taking strategies if you had difficulty with this question.

Tip for the Beginning Nursing Student: Neutropenia is an abnormal decrease in the number of neutrophils in the blood that places the client at risk for infection. Therefore neutropenic precautions are instituted. This type of precautions focuses on protecting the client from infection, and any potential source of infection is avoided in the client's environment or in the care of the client. You will learn about neutropenic precautions and the role of the nurse as a teacher and supervisor in your fundamentals of nursing course or in your leadership/management course.

References

Lewis, S., Heitkemper, M., Dirksen, S., & Bucher, L. (2007). *Medical-surgical nursing: Assessment and management of clinical problems* (7th ed., p. 715). St. Louis: Mosby.

Linton, A., & Maebius, N. (2007). *Introduction to medical-surgical nursing* (4th ed., p. 602). Philadelphia: Saunders.

---

180. A nurse is observing a nursing student perform nasotracheal suctioning on an adult client. The nurse would intervene if the nursing student:

1 Set the wall suction pressure at 140 mm Hg

2 Inserted the catheter during client inhalation

3 Encouraged the client to cough after suctioning

4 Applied intermittent suction for up to 10 to 15 seconds

Level of Cognitive Ability: Application

Client Needs: Safe and Effective Care Environment

Integrated Process: Nursing Process/ Implementation

Content Area: Leadership/ Management

Answer: 1

Rationale: When suctioning an adult client, the wall suction should be set at 80 to 120 mm Hg (portable suction is set at 7 to 15 mm Hg). Elevated suction pressure settings can increase the risk of trauma to the mucosa and can induce greater hypoxia. Options 2, 3, and 4 are correct steps in performing this procedure.

Test-Taking Strategy: Note the strategic words *would intervene.* These words indicate a negative event query and that you are looking for an incorrect action. Visualizing this procedure will assist in eliminating options 2, 3, and 4. Review suctioning procedures and the various test-taking strategies if you had difficulty with this question.

Tip for the Beginning Nursing Student: Suctioning is a procedure that is used to remove accumulated secretions from the respiratory tract when the client is unable to effectively cough them out. It is a sterile procedure and requires specific actions to prevent trauma to the mucosa of the respiratory tract and to prevent hypoxia. You will learn about the procedure for suctioning and the role of the nurse as a teacher and supervisor in your fundamentals of nursing course or in your leadership/management course.

References

Christensen, B., & Kockrow, E. (2006). *Adult health nursing* (5th ed., p. 218). St. Louis: Mosby.

Potter, P., & Perry, A. (2009). *Fundamentals of nursing* (7th ed., p. 935). St. Louis: Mosby.

---

181. A nurse is preparing to administer a medication to a client and notes that the dose prescribed is higher than the recommended dosage. The nurse calls the physician to clarify the order, and the physician instructs the nurse to administer the dose as prescribed. Which of the following actions would the nurse take?

1 Call the pharmacy.

2 Contact the nursing supervisor.

3 Call the medical director on call.

4 Administer the dose as prescribed.

Answer: 2

Rationale: If the physician writes an order that requires clarification it is the nurse's responsibility to contact the physician for clarification. If there is no resolution regarding the order because the order remains as it was written after talking with the physician, or because the physician cannot be located, the nurse should then contact the nurse manager or supervisor for further clarification as to what the next step should be. Under no circumstances should the nurse proceed to carry out the order until clarification is obtained. Calling the pharmacy is a resource action that will confirm that the dose of medication prescribed is inappropriate, but this action will not resolve the problem facing the nurse. Option 3 is a premature action.

Test-Taking Strategy: Eliminate option 4 first because this is an unsafe action. Option 3 is a premature action

Level of Cognitive Ability: Application
Client Needs: Safe and Effective Care Environment
Integrated Process: Nursing Process/ Implementation
Content Area: Leadership/ Management

and should be eliminated next. Eliminate option 1 next because this action will not resolve the problem. Also recall that the nurse should follow the organizational chain of command and seek assistance from the nursing supervisor. Review nursing responsibilities related to physicians' orders and the various test-taking strategies if you had difficulty with this question.

Tip for the Beginning Nursing Student: The client's physician will document specific orders or prescriptions regarding the client's care in the medical record, and the nurse needs to follow the orders unless the nurse deems that an order may harm the client. If the order can cause harm to the client, the nurse needs to contact the physician to change the order. If the physician does not change the order or if the nurse is unable to locate the physician, the nurse would follow the chain of command in the health care organization. In this situation the nurse would contact the nursing supervisor. Under no circumstances would a nurse implement an order that could cause harm to the client. You will learn about physicians' orders and the associated legal responsibilities in your fundamentals of nursing course or in your leadership/management course.

References

Christensen, B., & Kockrow, E. (2006). *Foundations of nursing* (5th ed., pp.703-705). St. Louis: Mosby.
Linton, A., & Maebius, N. (2007). *Introduction to medical-surgical nursing* (4th ed., p. 33). Philadelphia: Saunders.
Potter, P., & Perry, A. (2009). *Fundamentals of nursing* (7th ed., pp. 336, 704-705). St. Louis: Mosby.

---

182. The charge nurse is observing a new nursing graduate insert an indwelling urinary (Foley) catheter. The charge nurse intervenes if the new nursing graduate begins to do which of the following?
   1 Lubricates the catheter before inserting it
   2 Cleans the area around the urinary meatus before inserting the catheter
   3 Inflates the balloon to test patency before inserting the catheter
   4 Inflates the balloon as soon as urine begins to flow through the catheter tubing

Level of Cognitive Ability: Application
Client Needs: Safe and Effective Care Environment

Answer: 4
Rationale: After urine begins to flow, the catheter is inserted 2.5 cm (1 inch) more. Doing so ensures that the balloon is in the bladder, not the urethra. Options 1, 2, and 3 identify correct procedure.

Test-Taking Strategy: Note the strategic word *intervenes.* This word indicates a negative event query and tells you that you are looking for the option that identifies an incorrect action by the new nursing graduate. Visualizing this procedure and reading each option carefully will direct you to option 4. Review this procedure and the various test-taking strategies if you had difficulty with this question.

Tip for the Beginning Nursing Student: A Foley catheter is a rubber tube with a balloon tip that is filled with a sterile liquid after it is inserted in the bladder. It is connected to a bag that collects urine draining from the bladder. Sterile technique is used to insert this catheter. This type of catheter is used when continuous drainage of the bladder is needed, such as during a surgical procedure. You will learn about this type of catheter and the procedure for its inser-

Integrated Process: Nursing Process/ Implementation
Content Area: Leadership/ Management

tion in your fundamentals of nursing course. You will learn about the role of the nurse as a supervisor and teacher in your leadership/management course.

References
Linton, A., & Maebius, N. (2007). *Introduction to medical-surgical nursing* (4th ed., p. 848). Philadelphia: Saunders.
Monahan, F., Sands, J., Marek, J., Neighbors, M., & Green, C. (2007). *Phipps' medical-surgical nursing: Health and illness perspectives* (8th ed., pp. 993-994). St. Louis: Mosby.
Potter, P., & Perry, A. (2009). *Fundamentals of nursing* (7th ed., pp. 1159-1161). St. Louis: Mosby.

183. A hospitalized client tells his evening nurse that he has received pain medication at 10:00 AM and again at 2:00 PM and that the medication provided no relief from the pain. The client says to the nurse, "Whenever that daytime nurse takes care of me and gives me pain medication it never works! I am so glad that you are here so that I can get some relief from this pain." The nurse has observed this same occurrence with other clients who were cared for by this same daytime nurse and suspects that the daytime nurse is self-abusing drugs. The nurse implements which action?

1 Reports the information to the nursing supervisor
2 Calls the impaired nurse organization and reports the daytime nurse
3 Talks with the daytime nurse who gave the medication to the client
4 Reports the information about the daytime nurse to the police department

Level of Cognitive Ability: Application
Client Needs: Safe and Effective Care Environment
Integrated Process: Nursing Process/ Implementation
Content Area: Leadership/ Management

Answer: 1
Rationale: If the nurse suspects that another nurse is self-abusing drugs, the nurse needs to report the suspicion to the nursing supervisor. Factual information such as that described by the client and specific information related to the nurse's observations need to be reported. The nurse would not confront the nurse who is suspected of self-abusing drugs because this may lead to a conflict. The nurse would follow the organizational chain of communication of the institution to report the incident. The suspicion needs to be reported to the nursing supervisor, who will then report to the board of nursing. The board of nursing has jurisdiction over the practice of nursing and may develop plans for treatment and supervision.

Test-Taking Strategy: Eliminate options 2 and 4 first because they are comparable or alike and both relate to reporting the incident to agencies outside the hospital. From the remaining options recall that agency channels of communication are used when reporting an incident. Also the action in option 3 can lead to a conflict. Review nursing responsibilities related to reporting incidents and the various test-taking strategies if you had difficulty with this question.

Tip for the Beginning Nursing Student: Drug abuse is the use of drugs illegally. If a nurse is suspected of drug abuse and is taking drugs intended for use by the client, the other nurse needs to report such suspicion. Failure to provide a client with required and needed treatment is harmful to the client and is illegal. You will learn about drug abuse and the impaired nurse and associated nursing responsibilities in your fundamentals of nursing course or in your leadership/management course.

References
deWit, S. (2009). *Medical-surgical nursing: Concepts & practice* (p. 1134). St. Louis: Saunders.
Ignatavicius, D., & Workman, M. (2010). *Medical-surgical nursing: Patient-centered collaborative care* (6th ed., p. 82). Philadelphia: Saunders.

184. A nurse determines that a client with a brain attack (stroke) is experiencing difficulty with fine motor coordination when performing activities of daily living. The nurse suggests that the client be referred to a:
 1 Physical therapist
 2 Speech pathologist
 3 Recreational therapist
 4 Occupational therapist

Level of Cognitive Ability: Application
Client Needs: Safe and Effective Care Environment
Integrated Process: Nursing Process/ Implementation
Content Area: Leadership/ Management

Answer: 4
Rationale: The occupational therapist provides assistance with developing methods that assist in managing difficulty with fine motor coordination when performing activities of daily living. Although a physical therapist may also address fine motor activities, the focus is primarily on gross motor skills and the development of muscle strength. Speech pathologists and recreational therapists do not address this aspect of care.

Test-Taking Strategy: Focus on the subject—fine motor coordination when performing activities of daily living. This will assist in eliminating options 2 and 3. From the remaining options, noting the words *activities of daily living* will direct you to option 4. Review the roles of the health care members identified in the options and the various test-taking strategies if you had difficulty with this question.

Tip for the Beginning Nursing Student: A brain attack (stroke) is an abnormal condition of the brain that is characterized by occlusion by a clot, hemorrhage, or vasospasm that results in ischemia of the brain tissues. Paralysis, weakness, sensory changes, speech defects, or even death can occur. The client who experiences a stroke will require rehabilitative services that will assist the client to relearn activities to promote independence. You will learn about strokes in your medical-surgical nursing course when you study neurological disorders, and you will learn about the roles of various health care team members in your fundamentals of nursing course or in your leadership/management course.

References
Ignatavicius, D., & Workman, M. (2010). *Medical-surgical nursing: Patient-centered collaborative care* (6th ed., p. 96). Philadelphia: Saunders.
Linton, A., & Maebius, N. (2007). *Introduction to medical-surgical nursing* (4th ed., p. 886). Philadelphia: Saunders.

185. A nurse notes that a nursing assistant dons clean gloves but did not wash her hands before taking an oral temperature on a client. The nurse implements a teaching session for nursing assistants incorporating which of the following principles?
 1 Learning is a cognitive, passive process.
 2 Learning involves a change of behavior.
 3 Nursing assistants need constant supervision when caring for clients.
 4 Negative rewards reduce undesirable behavior and should be used when an error is seen.

Answer: 2
Rationale: The nurse assumes leadership for improving client care by implementing a teaching session that has the potential for changing behavior. Persons who change their behavior have internalized information and apply it to their actions. Options 3 and 4 use negative strategies to change behavior, and this is not usually successful. Option 1 views the learner as not being actively involved in the teaching and learning process.

Test-Taking Strategy: Eliminate options 3 and 4 first because they do not provide a positive view of learners. Eliminate option 1 because learning should be an active not a passive process. Review teaching and learning principles and the various test-taking strategies if you had difficulty with this question.

Level of Cognitive Ability: Application
Client Needs: Safe and Effective Care Environment
Integrated Process: Teaching and Learning
Content Area: Leadership/ Management

Tip for the Beginning Nursing Student: Handwashing is always done before and after every client contact even if the nurse intends to don gloves for client care. If the nurse observes an incorrect action by another health care provider it is the nurse's responsibility to teach correct procedure to ensure client safety and a safe environment. Learning involves acquiring knowledge about a skill and changing behavior as a result of the training. Teaching is a responsibility of the nurse, and you will learn about this role and the teaching and learning process in your fundamentals of nursing course or in your leadership/ management course.

Reference

Potter, P., & Perry, A. (2009). *Fundamentals of nursing* (7th ed., pp. 363-364, 380). St. Louis: Mosby.

---

186. A physician has prescribed a cleansing enema for an adult client. The nurse provides directions to a nursing assistant who is trained and certified to administer enemas and tells the nursing assistant that the maximum volume of fluid that can be administered is:
    1 100 mL
    2 300 mL
    3 500 mL
    4 1000 mL

Level of Cognitive Ability: Application
Client Needs: Safe and Effective Care Environment
Integrated Process: Nursing Process/ Implementation
Content Area: Leadership/ Management

Answer: 4

Rationale: Cleansing enemas promote complete evacuation of feces from the colon. They act by stimulating peristalsis through the infusion of a large volume of solution or through local irritation of the colon's mucosa. For an adult client, 750 to 1000 mL is used. Therefore the maximum volume of solution for an adult is 1000 mL.

Test-Taking Strategy: Note the strategic words *maximum volume,* and note that the question addresses an adult client. Recalling the anatomy of the colon in an adult client and the procedure for administering a cleansing enema will direct you to option 4. Review this procedure and the various test-taking strategies if you had difficulty with this question.

Tip for the Beginning Nursing Student: An enema is the introduction of solution into the rectum for cleansing the bowel. Cleansing of the bowel may be prescribed to treat constipation or may be prescribed as a preprocedure treatment, such as before a diagnostic test or surgical procedure involving the colon. You will learn about the procedure for administering an enema in your fundamentals of nursing course. You will also learn about the role of the nurse as a teacher and supervisor in your leadership/management course.

References

Christensen, B., & Kockrow, E. (2006). *Foundations of nursing* (5th ed., pp. 598-599). St. Louis: Mosby.

Potter, P., & Perry, A. (2009). *Fundamentals of nursing* (7th ed., p. 1200). St. Louis: Mosby.

187. A client requires a partial bed bath. The nurse gives instructions to a nursing assistant about the partial bed bath and tells the nursing assistant to:

1 Just wash the client's hands and face.

2 Provide mouth care and perineal care only.

3 Let the client decide what she wants washed.

4 Be sure to bathe the client's body parts that would cause discomfort or odor if left unbathed.

Level of Cognitive Ability: Application
Client Needs: Safe and Effective Care Environment
Integrated Process: Nursing Process/ Implementation
Content Area: Leadership/ Management

Answer: 4

Rationale: A partial bed bath involves bathing the body parts that would cause discomfort or odor if left unbathed. This may include the axillary areas, perineal areas, and any skin fold areas. Options 1, 2, and 3 do not completely address a partial bed bath.

Test-Taking Strategy: Note the strategic words *partial bed bath.* Eliminate option 1 because of the word *just* and option 2 because of the word *only.* From the remaining options, recalling the definition of a partial bed bath will direct you to option 4. Review the components of a partial bed bath and the various test-taking strategies if you had difficulty with this question.

Tip for the Beginning Nursing Student: Bathing a client is an important role of the nurse and is necessary for hygienic purposes and to prevent infection, maintain skin integrity, stimulate circulation, and provide comfort. Several types of baths may be given, including a bed bath, tub bath, shower, complete bath, or partial bath. You will learn about bathing a client in your fundamentals of nursing course. You will also learn about the role of the nurse as a teacher and supervisor in your leadership/management course.

Reference
Potter, P., & Perry, A. (2009). *Fundamentals of nursing* (7th ed., pp. 865, 867). St. Louis: Mosby.

---

188. A charge nurse is observing a new nursing graduate insert a nasal trumpet airway into a client. The nurse would intervene if the new nursing graduate did which of the following?

1 Checks the nose for septal deviation

2 Uses a nasal trumpet that is slightly larger than the nares

3 Inserts the nasal trumpet gently following the contour of the nasopharyngeal passageway

4 Lubricates the nasal trumpet with a water-soluble lubricant jelly containing a local anesthetic

Level of Cognitive Ability: Application
Client Needs: Safe and Effective Care Environment
Integrated Process: Nursing Process/ Implementation
Content Area: Leadership/ Management

Answer: 2

Rationale: The nurse would select a nasal trumpet airway that is slightly smaller than the nares and slightly larger than the suction catheter to be used to suction the client. Options 1, 3, and 4 are correct actions for inserting a nasal trumpet airway.

Test-Taking Strategy: Note the strategic words *nurse would intervene.* These words indicate a negative event query and indicate that you are looking for the option that indicates an incorrect action by the new nursing graduate. Noting the words *slightly larger than the nares* and visualizing this procedure will direct you to option 2. Review the procedure for inserting a nasal trumpet and the various test-taking strategies if you had difficulty with this question.

Tip for the Beginning Nursing Student: A nasal trumpet is a tube that is inserted into one of the client's nostrils to provide assistance in maintaining the client's airway and to provide a route for suctioning secretions from the client. You will learn about a nasal trumpet and the procedure for its insertion in your fundamentals of nursing course. You will learn about the role of the nurse as a teacher and supervisor in your leadership/management course.

References

Christensen, B., & Kockrow, E. (2006). *Foundations of nursing* (5th ed., p. 560). St. Louis: Mosby.

Perry, A. & Potter, P. (2010). *Clinical nursing skills & techniques* (7th ed., pp. 632, 635). St. Louis: Mosby.

Potter, P., & Perry, A. (2009). *Fundamentals of nursing* (7th ed., p. 1203). St. Louis: Mosby.

---

189. A nurse is observing a nursing assistant measuring the blood pressure (BP) of a client. The nurse intervenes if which action was observed that would interfere with accurate measurement of the BP?

1 Positions the client's arm at heart level

2 Exposes the extremity fully by removing constricting clothing

3 Explains the procedure to the client and asks the client to rest for 5 minutes

4 Palpates the radial artery and places the cuff of the sphygmomanometer 1 inch above the brachial artery

Level of Cognitive Ability: Application
Client Needs: Safe and Effective Care Environment
Integrated Process: Nursing Process/ Implementation
Content Area: Leadership/ Management

Answer: 4

Rationale: When taking a BP, the brachial artery is palpated and the cuff of the sphygmomanometer is positioned 1 inch above this site of pulsation. Options 1, 2, and 3 are correct actions when taking a BP.

Test-Taking Strategy: Note the strategic words *nurse intervenes.* These words indicate a negative event query and that you need to select the option that indicates an incorrect action by the nursing assistant. Visualizing this procedure will assist in eliminating options 1, 2, and 3. Review the principles related to BP measurement and the test-taking strategies for answering negative event queries if you had difficulty with this question.

Tip for the Beginning Nursing Student: Blood pressure is the amount of pressure exerted on the walls of the arteries and veins and the heart chambers by the circulating volume of blood. This pressure is measured by taking the client's BP. To ensure accuracy of the measurement a specific procedure is followed. You will learn about the procedure for taking the client's BP in your fundamentals of nursing course and about the role of the nurse as a teacher and supervisor in your leadership/management course.

References

deWit, S. (2009). *Medical-surgical nursing: Concepts & practice* (p. 421). St. Louis: Saunders.

Potter, P., & Perry, A. (2009). *Fundamentals of nursing* (7th ed., pp. 538-539). St. Louis: Mosby.

---

190. A nurse is reviewing the preprocedure care for a client scheduled to have an echocardiogram following a myocardial infarction. The nurse determines that the student nurse understands the preprocedure instructions if the student nurse stated that the client needs to be told that:

1 He needs to sign an informed consent.

2 He cannot eat or drink anything for 4 hours before the procedure.

Answer: 3

Rationale: Echocardiography uses ultrasound to evaluate the heart's structure and motion. It is a noninvasive, risk-free, pain-free test that involves no special preparation. It is commonly done at the bedside or on an outpatient basis. The client must lie quietly for 30 to 60 minutes while the procedure is being performed. Options 1, 2, and 4 are incorrect.

Test-Taking Strategy: Focus on the diagnostic test being performed. Recalling that echocardiography uses ultrasound and that ultrasound is noninvasive will assist in eliminating options 1, 2, and 4. Review this procedure and the various test-taking strategies if you had difficulty with this question.

3 The procedure is painless and takes 30 to 60 minutes to complete.

4 An allergy to iodine or shellfish is a contraindication to having the procedure.

Level of Cognitive Ability: Analysis
Client Needs: Safe and Effective Care Environment
Integrated Process: Teaching and Learning
Content Area: Leadership/ Management

Tip for the Beginning Nursing Student: Diagnostic uses of an echocardiogram include the detection of atrial or other tumors, measurement of the heart chambers, and evaluation of valve and chamber function. You will learn about various diagnostic tests in your fundamentals of nursing course; an important point to remember is that an informed consent is needed if the test is invasive. Another important point is that the nurse must ensure that the client understands the test to be done and its purpose and teaches the client about the test. You will also learn about the role of the nurse as a client teacher in your fundamentals of nursing course or in your leadership/management course.

References

Chernecky, C., & Berger, B. (2008). *Laboratory tests and diagnostic procedures* (5th ed., pp. 459-460). Philadelphia: Saunders.

Ignatavicius, D., & Workman, M. (2010). *Medical-surgical nursing: Patient-centered collaborative care* (6th ed., p. 725). Philadelphia: Saunders.

Linton, A. (2007). *Introduction to medical-surgical nursing* (4th ed., p. 637). Philadelphia: Saunders.

---

191. A nurse is reviewing the preprocedure care for a client who is scheduled for a cardiac catheterization with a nursing student. The nurse determines that the student needs supervision while preparing the client if the nursing student stated that the client needs to be told that:

1 The procedure takes about 5 hours.

2 He may experience flushing feelings during the procedure.

3 The blood vessels and flow of blood will be assessed with this procedure.

4 There is little to no pain with catheter insertion because a local anesthetic is used.

Level of Cognitive Ability: Analysis
Client Needs: Safe and Effective Care Environment
Integrated Process: Teaching and Learning
Content Area: Leadership/ Management

Answer: 1

Rationale: A cardiac catheterization is a diagnostic test that assesses the coronary arteries and the flow of blood through them. The procedure is done in a darkened cardiac catheterization room in the radiology department. A local anesthetic is used so there is little to no pain with catheter insertion. The procedure may take approximately 1 to 3 hours, during which the client may feel various sensations, such as a feeling of warmth or flushing, with catheter passage and dye injection.

Test-Taking Strategy: Note the strategic words *that the student needs supervision.* These words indicate a negative event query and that you need to select the incorrect statement by the nursing student. Recalling the purpose of the procedure will assist in eliminating option 3. Next recalling that a dye is injected will assist in eliminating options 2 and 4. Also noting the words *5 hours* in option 1 will direct you to this option. Review the procedure for a cardiac catheterization and the test-taking strategies for answering negative event queries if you had difficulty with this question.

Tip for the Beginning Nursing Student: Cardiac catheterization is a common test performed to assess the status of the coronary arteries or the presence of congenital heart disease, stenosis, or valvular disease. Risks associated with the procedure include dysrhythmias, infection, and thrombosis and the nurse needs to monitor the client closely following the procedure. You will learn about cardiac catheterization in your medical-surgical nursing course when you study cardiovascular disorders. You will also learn about the role of the nurse as a client teacher in your fundamentals of nursing course or in your leadership/management course.

References

Chernecky, C., & Berger, B. (2008). *Laboratory tests and diagnostic procedures* (5th ed., p. 297). Philadelphia: Saunders.

deWit, S. (2009). *Medical-surgical nursing: Concepts & practice* (p. 413). St. Louis: Saunders.

---

192. A nurse has instructed a nursing assistant in the procedure for collecting a 24-hour urine specimen from a client. The nurse determines that the nursing assistant understands the directions if the nursing assistant states to:

1 Keep the specimen at room temperature.

2 Save the first urine specimen collected at the start time.

3 Discard the last voided specimen at the end of the collection time.

4 Ask the client to void, discard the specimen, and note the start time.

Level of Cognitive Ability: Analysis

Client Needs: Safe and Effective Care Environment

Integrated Process: Teaching and Learning

Content Area: Leadership/Management

Answer: 4

Rationale: Because a 24-hour urine specimen is a timed quantitative determination, the test must be started with an empty bladder. Therefore the first urine is discarded. Fifteen minutes before the end of the collection time, the client should be asked to void and this specimen is added to the collection. The urine collection should be refrigerated or placed on ice to prevent changes in urine composition.

Test-Taking Strategy: Note that options 2 and 4 are opposite, which is an indication that one of them is likely to be the correct option. Recalling that the 24-hour urine specimen is a timed quantitative determination will assist in directing you to option 4. Review the procedure for collecting a 24-hour urine specimen and the various test-taking strategies if you had difficulty with this question.

Tip for the Beginning Nursing Student: Urine specimens may be collected to diagnose various conditions. These specimens may be prescribed to be collected as a random specimen, a sterile specimen, or a 24-hour urine collection. An important point to remember is that the procedure for its collection needs to be followed to ensure accurate results. You will learn about collecting urine specimens in your fundamentals of nursing course. You will also learn about the role of the nurse as a teacher and supervisor in your fundamentals of nursing course or in your leadership/management course.

References

deWit, S. (2009). *Medical-surgical nursing: Concepts & practice* (p. 821). St. Louis: Saunders.

Ignatavicius, D., & Workman, M. (2010). *Medical-surgical nursing: Patient-centered collaborative care* (6th ed., p. 1540). Philadelphia: Saunders.

---

193. A nurse is teaching a nursing assistant how to measure a carotid pulse. The nurse tells the nursing assistant to measure the pulse on only one side of the client's neck primarily:

1 Because the pulse rate will be easier to count

2 To prevent dizziness and a drop in the heart rate

Answer: 2

Rationale: Applying pressure to both carotid arteries at the same time is contraindicated. Excess pressure to the baroreceptors in the carotid vessels could cause the heart rate and blood pressure to reflexively drop and cause syncope. In addition, the manual pressure could interfere with the flow of blood to the brain.

Test-Taking Strategy: Note the strategic word *primarily*. Note that option 2 describes the greatest danger to the

3 So that the client will not feel a sense of choking

4 Because it will provide a more accurate determination of the quality of the pulse

Level of Cognitive Ability: Application
Client Needs: Safe and Effective Care Environment
Integrated Process: Teaching and Learning
Content Area: Leadership/ Management

client. Review the function and location of baroreceptors in the carotid vessels and the various test-taking strategies if you had difficulty with this question.

Tip for the Beginning Nursing Student: The carotid artery is located in the neck region and is one of the major arteries supplying blood to the head. It is one of the pulse points in the body that can be palpated to check a client's pulse. You will learn about palpation of this artery in your fundamentals of nursing course or in a physical assessment course. You will also learn about the role of the nurse as a teacher and supervisor in your fundamentals of nursing course or in your leadership/management course.

Reference
Potter, P., & Perry, A. (2009). *Fundamentals of nursing* (7th ed., p. 521). St. Louis: Mosby.

---

194. A nurse is supervising a nursing student who is performing a pulse oximetry measurement on a client with peripheral vascular disease. The nurse determines that the nursing student is performing the procedure accurately if the student places the oximetry probe on which anatomical area?
  1 Left thumb
  2 One of the toes
  3 Right index finger
  4 Bridge of the nose

Level of Cognitive Ability: Analysis
Client Needs: Safe and Effective Care Environment
Integrated Process: Nursing Process/ Evaluation
Content Area: Leadership/ Management

Answer: 4
Rationale: If the client has peripheral vascular disease, the pulse oximetry probe would be placed on the earlobe or bridge of the nose because peripheral vasoconstriction or inadequate blood flow to the peripheral areas of the body will interfere with the oxygen saturation measurement. Placing the probe on the anatomical areas noted in options 1, 2, and 3 will not provide an accurate measurement of the oxygen saturation.

Test-Taking Strategy: Focus on the client's diagnosis—peripheral vascular disease—and recall the pathophysiology associated with the disease. Note that options 1, 2, and 3 are comparable or alike in that they indicate using a peripheral body area. Review the procedure for pulse oximetry measurement and the various test-taking strategies if you had difficulty with this question.

Tip for the Beginning Nursing Student: Peripheral vascular disease is an abnormal condition that affects the blood vessels leading to decreased blood to the body part. Pulse oximetry uses a clip-like device that measures the amount of saturated hemoglobin in the tissue capillaries and thus the percentage of oxygen saturation in the blood. You will learn about peripheral vascular disease in your medical-surgical nursing course when you study cardiovascular disorders and about measuring oxygenation using pulse oximetry in your fundamentals of nursing course. You will also learn about the role of the nurse as a teacher and supervisor in your fundamentals of nursing course or in your leadership/management course.

Reference
Jarvis, C. (2008). *Physical examination and health assessment* (5th ed., p. 169). Philadelphia: Saunders.

195. A nursing student is preparing a client who will have spinal anesthesia for surgery. The nurse in charge asks the nursing student to identify which of the following as the highest priority data to report to the nurse on the next shift who will care for the client postoperatively?

1 Voided 300 mL preoperatively
2 Pulse rate of 78 beats/min
3 Blood pressure of 126/78 mm Hg
4 Presence of weakness in the left lower extremity

Level of Cognitive Ability: Analysis
Client Needs: Safe and Effective Care Environment
Integrated Process: Communication and Documentation
Content Area: Leadership/Management

Answer: 4
Rationale: It is important to document and report any preoperative weakness or impaired movement of a lower extremity in the client who is to have spinal anesthesia because it causes temporary paralysis of the lower extremities. When the client's function returns, the preoperative weakness or impairment will not be misinterpreted as a complication of anesthesia. Options 1, 2, and 3 may be documented and reported, but they are not the highest priority.

Test-Taking Strategy: Note the strategic words *spinal anesthesia* and *highest priority.* Note the relationship between the words *spinal anesthesia* and option 4. Also note that the data in options 1, 2, and 3 are normal findings. Review care of the preoperative client and the test-taking strategies for answering prioritizing questions if you had difficulty with this question.

Tip for the Beginning Nursing Student: Spinal anesthesia is done by an injection into the subarachnoid cerebrospinal fluid space. It produces a state of lack of sensation in the lower part of the body. An important nursing responsibility in the postoperative period is to monitor for the return of sensation in the lower body. If sensation does not return or is altered in any way, the surgeon is notified. You will learn about spinal anesthesia in your fundamentals of nursing course and about the role of the nurse as a teacher and supervisor in this course or in your leadership/management course.

References
Ignatavicius, D., & Workman, M. (2010). *Medical-surgical nursing: Patient-centered collaborative care* (6th ed., pp. 289-290). Philadelphia: Saunders.
Linton, A. (2007). *Introduction to medical-surgical nursing* (4th ed., p. 259). Philadelphia: Saunders.

196. A client comes to the hospital emergency department with complaints of severe right lower abdominal pain characteristic of appendicitis. The client does not have any health insurance. The nurse understands that legally the hospital must:

1 Refer the client to the nearest public hospital.
2 Have a physician see the client before admission.
3 Provide uncompensated care in emergency situations.
4 Respect the family's requests to admit their family member to the hospital.

Answer: 3
Rationale: Federal law and many state laws require that hospitals must provide emergency care. The client can be transferred only after the client has been medically screened and stabilized. The client must give consent for the transfer, and there must be a facility that will accept the client. Options 1, 2, and 4 do not fully address the legal requirements for emergency care.

Test-Taking Strategy: Note the strategic words *does not have any health insurance* and the word *legally.* Noting that the situation presented is an emergency one will direct you to option 3. Option 3 addresses the legal scope of providing emergency care. Review the legal issues related to providing emergency care and the various test-taking strategies if you had difficulty with this question.

Level of Cognitive Ability:
Comprehension
Client Needs: Safe and Effective Care
Environment
Integrated Process: Nursing
Process/Planning
Content Area: Leadership/
Management

Tip for the Beginning Nursing Student: You will learn about various types of health insurance plans and the issues associated with health insurance in your fundamentals of nursing course or in your leadership/management course. An important point to remember is that the client is the priority. If an emergency condition exists the health care agency must provide care regardless of the client's insurance status. Appendicitis is an acute inflammation of the appendix that if left untreated can lead to perforation and peritonitis, which is life threatening. You will learn about appendicitis in your pediatrics course and your medical-surgical nursing course when you study gastrointestinal disorders.

Reference
Potter, P., & Perry, A. (2009). *Fundamentals of nursing* (7th ed., pp. 327-328). St. Louis: Mosby.

---

197. The nurse tells a nursing assistant that a client recovering from a myocardial infarction requires a complete bed bath. During the bath the nurse would intervene if the nurse observed the nursing assistant:
1 Washing the client's chest
2 Giving the client a back rub
3 Asking the client to wash his legs
4 Washing the client's perineal area

Level of Cognitive Ability: Application
Client Needs: Safe and Effective Care
Environment
Integrated Process: Nursing Process/
Implementation
Content Area: Leadership/
Management

Answer: 3
Rationale: A complete bed bath is for clients who are totally dependent and require total hygiene care. Total care may be necessary for a client recovering from a myocardial infarction to conserve the client's energy and reduce oxygen requirements. The nurse would intervene if the nurse observed the nursing assistant asking the client to wash his legs. Options 1, 2, and 4 are components of providing a complete bed bath.

Test-Taking Strategy: Note the words *the nurse would intervene.* These words indicate a negative event query and that you need to select the option that identifies an incorrect action by the nursing assistant. Focusing on the words *complete bed bath* will direct you to option 3 because in this option the nurse asks the client to participate in the bathing process. Review the procedure for giving a complete bed bath and the various test-taking strategies if you had difficulty with this question.

Tip for the Beginning Nursing Student: Bathing a client is an important role of the nurse and is necessary for hygienic purposes and to prevent infection, maintain skin integrity, stimulate circulation, and provide comfort. Several types of baths may be given, including a bed bath, tub bath, shower, complete bath, or partial bath. You will learn about bathing a client in your fundamentals of nursing course. You will also learn about the role of the nurse as a teacher and supervisor in your leadership/management course.

References
Christensen, B., & Kockrow, E. (2006). *Foundations of nursing* (5th ed., pp. 444, 452-453). St. Louis: Mosby.
Potter, P., & Perry, A. (2009). *Fundamentals of nursing* (7th ed., pp. 865, 867). St. Louis: Mosby.

198. A nurse is observing a nursing student auscultating the breath sounds of a client. The nurse would intervene if the nursing student did which of the following?
1 Used the diaphragm of the stethoscope
2 Placed the stethoscope directly on the client's skin
3 Asked the client to breathe slowly and deeply through the mouth
4 Asked the client to lie flat on the right side and then on the left side

Level of Cognitive Ability: Application
Client Needs: Safe and Effective Care Environment
Integrated Process: Nursing Process/ Implementation
Content Area: Leadership/ Management

Answer: 4
Rationale: The client ideally should sit up and breathe slowly and deeply through the mouth. The diaphragm of the stethoscope, which is warmed before use, is placed directly on the client's skin, not over a gown or clothing.

Test-Taking Strategy: Note the strategic words *nurse would intervene.* These words indicate a negative event query and that you are looking for the option that gives an incorrect action by the nursing student. Noting the words *lie flat* will direct you to option 4. Review the procedure for auscultating breath sounds and the various test-taking strategies if you had difficulty with this question.

Tip for the Beginning Nursing Student: A breath sound is the sound of air passing in and out of the lungs as heard with a stethoscope. Normal breath sounds include vesicular, bronchovesicular, and bronchial sounds. Auscultating breath sounds is a part of a nursing assessment, and you will learn about this procedure and evaluating breath sounds in your fundamental of nursing course or in a physical assessment course. You will also learn about the role of the nurse as a teacher and supervisor in your fundamentals of nursing course or in your leadership/ management course.

References
deWit, S. (2009). *Medical-surgical nursing: Concepts & practice* (p. 293). St. Louis: Saunders.
Potter, P., & Perry, A. (2009). *Fundamentals of nursing* (7th ed., pp. 595-596). St. Louis: Mosby.

---

199. A nurse is observing a nursing assistant talking to a client who is hearing impaired. The nurse would intervene if the nursing assistant did which of the following during communication with the client?
1 Spoke in a normal tone
2 Spoke clearly to the client
3 Faced the client when speaking
4 Spoke directly into the impaired ear

Level of Cognitive Ability: Application
Client Needs: Safe and Effective Care Environment
Integrated Process: Communication and Documentation
Content Area: Leadership/ Management

Answer: 4
Rationale: When communicating with a hearing impaired client, the nurse should speak in a normal tone to the client and should not shout. The nurse should talk directly to the client while facing the client and speak clearly. If the client does not seem to understand what is said, the nurse should express the statement differently. Moving closer to the client and toward the better ear may facilitate communication, but the nurse should avoid talking directly into the impaired ear.

Test-Taking Strategy: Note the strategic words *the nurse would intervene.* These words indicate a negative event query and that you are looking for the option that gives an incorrect action by the nursing assistant. Noting the words *directly into the impaired ear* will direct you to option 4. Review care of the hearing impaired client and the various test-taking strategies if you had difficulty with this question.

Tip for the Beginning Nursing Student: Special communication techniques are needed when caring for a hearing impaired client. Some of these include facing the client when speaking; enunciating words slowly, clearly, and in a normal voice; avoiding placing the hands over the mouth when speaking so that the client can lip-read; and avoiding speaking into the impaired ear. It is important for the nurse to know these techniques because the nurse needs to use them to communicate with the hearing impaired client to prevent social isolation. In addition, teaching and supervising others are roles of the nurse, and the nurse needs to intervene if he or she observes incorrect communication techniques performed by another health care team member. You will learn about communication techniques for clients with hearing impairment and the role of the nurse as a teacher and supervisor in your fundamentals of nursing course or in your leadership/management course.

References

Ignatavicius, D., & Workman, M. (2010). *Medical-surgical nursing: Patient-centered collaborative care* (6th ed., p. 1135). Philadelphia: Saunders.

Linton, A. (2007). *Introduction to medical-surgical nursing* (4th ed., p. 1198). Philadelphia: Saunders.

---

200. A nurse administers a fatal dose of morphine sulfate to a client. During the subsequent investigation of error, it is determined that the nurse did not check the client's respiratory rate before administering the medication. Failure to adequately assess the client is addressed under which function of the nurse practice act?

1 Defining the specific educational requirements for licensure in the state
2 Describing the scope of practice of licensed and unlicensed care providers
3 Recommending specific terms of incarceration for nurses who violate the law
4 Identifying the process for disciplinary action if standards of care are not met

Level of Cognitive Ability: Analysis
Client Needs: Safe and Effective Care Environment
Integrated Process: Nursing Process/ Assessment/Data Collection
Content Area: Leadership/ Management

Answer: 4

Rationale: In this situation, acceptable standards of care were not met (the nurse failed to adequately check the client before administering a medication). Option 4 refers specifically to the situation described in the question, whereas options 1, 2, and 3 do not.

Test-Taking Strategy: Note the relationship between the words *failure to adequately assess the client* in the question and *standards of care are not met* in option 4. Review the legal implications related to medication errors and the various test-taking strategies if you had difficulty with this question.

Tip for the Beginning Nursing Student: A nurse practice act is a statute enacted by the legislation of a state. Nurse practice acts may vary from state to state but generally include educational requirements of the nurse, distinguish between nursing practice and medical practice, and define the scope of practice for the nurse. Additional issues that may be covered in the act include grounds for disciplinary action and the rights of the nurse if disciplinary action is taken. All nurses are responsible for knowing the provisions of the act in the state in which they work. You will learn about the nurse practice act in your fundamentals of nursing course or in your leadership/management course.

References

Linton, A. (2007). *Introduction to medical-surgical nursing* (4th ed., pp. 31-32). Philadelphia: Saunders.

Potter, P., & Perry, A. (2009). *Fundamentals of nursing* (7th ed., p. 629). St. Louis: Mosby.

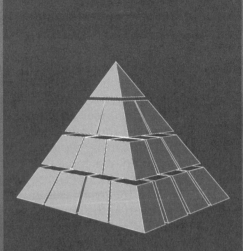

Part IV

Appendices

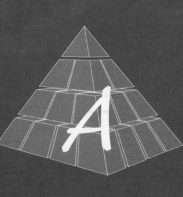

Pyramid Points for Using Test-Taking Strategies

APPENDIX A-1: QUESTIONS THAT REQUIRE PRIORITIZING

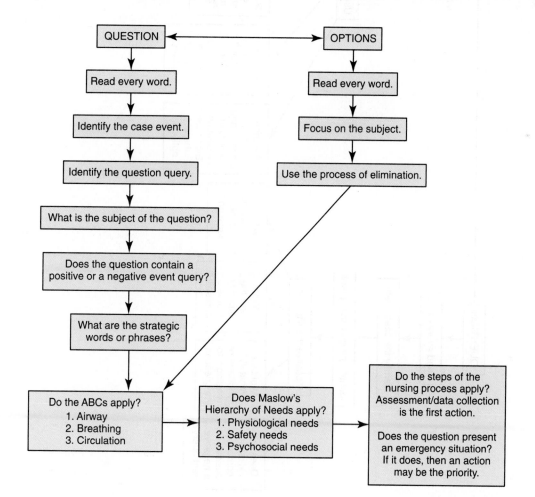

APPENDIX A-2: THE QUESTION AND THE OPTION

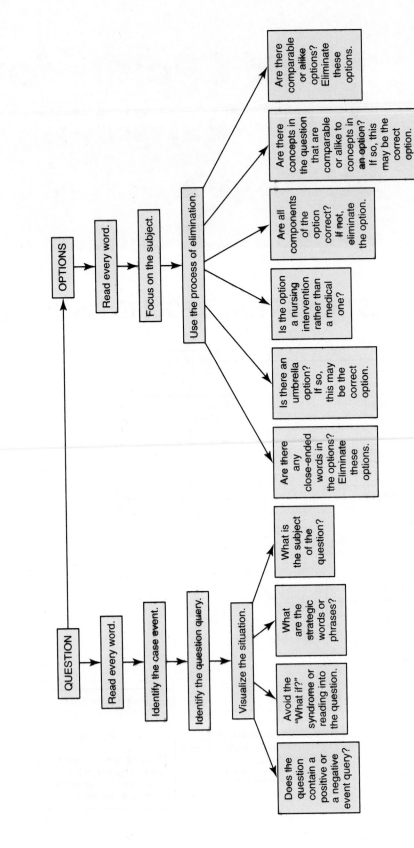

QUESTION

Read every word.

Identify the case event.

Identify the question query.

Visualize the situation.

- Does the question contain a positive or a negative event query?
- Avoid the "What if?" syndrome or reading into the question.
- What are the strategic words or phrases?
- What is the subject of the question?

OPTIONS

Read every word.

Focus on the subject.

Use the process of elimination.

- Are there any close-ended words in the options? Eliminate these options.
- Is there an umbrella option? If so, this may be the correct option.
- Is the option a nursing intervention rather than a medical one?
- Are all components of the option correct? If not, eliminate the option.
- Are there concepts in the question that are comparable or alike to concepts in an option? If so, this may be the correct option.
- Are there comparable or alike options? Eliminate these options.

APPENDIX A-3: THE SUBJECT OF THE QUESTION

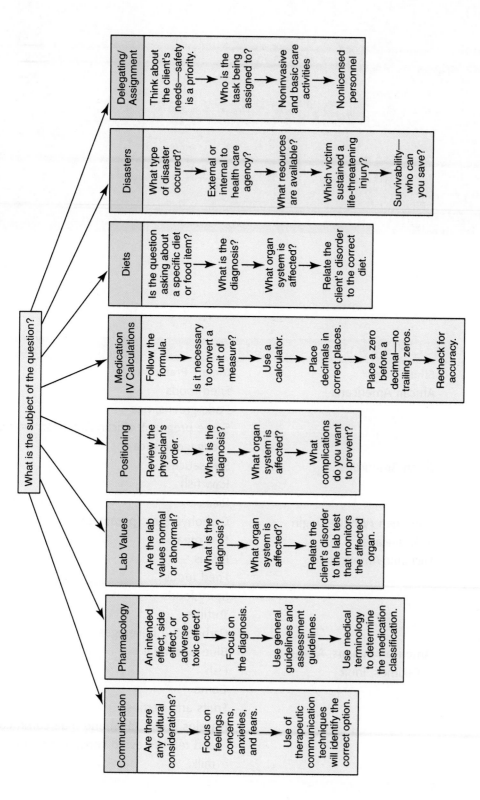

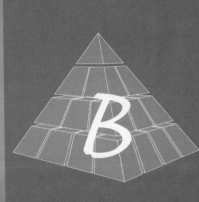

Cultural Characteristics and Practices

ETHNICITY AND DIETARY PREFERENCES

Ethnic Group	Dietary Preference
African Americans	Fried foods
	Pork, greens, rice
	Some pregnant African-American women engage in pica
Asian Americans	Soy sauce
	Raw fish
	Rice
European (White)-Origin Americans	Carbohydrates (potatoes)
	Red meat
Hispanic Americans	Beans
	Fried foods
	Spicy foods
	Tortillas
	Carbonated beverages
American Indians, Aleuts, Eskimos, Inuit	Blue cornmeal
	Fish
	Game
	Fruits and berries
	Navajos prefer meat and blue cornmeal and tend to avoid consumption of milk

RELIGION AND DIETARY PREFERENCES

Religious Group	Dietary Preference
Seventh-Day Adventist (Church Of God)	Alcohol and caffeinated beverages prohibited
	Many are lacto-ovo vegetarians; those who eat meat avoid pork
	Overeating prohibited; 5-6 hr between meals without snacking
Buddhism	Alcohol prohibited
	Many are lacto-ovo vegetarians
	Some eat fish, and some avoid only beef
Roman Catholicism	Avoid meat on Ash Wednesday and Fridays of Lent
	Optional fasting practiced during Lent season
	Children, pregnant women, and the ill exempt from fasting
Church of Jesus Christ of Latter-Day Saints (Mormon)	Alcohol and caffeinated beverages prohibited
	Consumption of meat limited
	First Sunday of the month optional for fasting
Hinduism	Many individuals vegetarians
	Limit consumption of meat with abstinence from some types of meat
	Fasting rituals vary
	Children not allowed to participate in fasting
Islam	Pork, birds of prey, alcohol, and any meat product not ritually slaughtered prohibited
	During month of Ramadan, fasting during daytime hours
Jehovah's Witness	Any foods to which blood has been added prohibited
	Can consume animal flesh that has been drained
Judaism	Dietary kosher laws must be followed by Orthodox believers
	Meats allowed include animals that are vegetable eaters, cloven-hoofed animals, and animals that are ritually slaughtered
	Fish that have scales and fins allowed
	Any combination of meat and milk prohibited
	During Yom Kippur, 24-hr fasting observed
	Pregnant women and those who are seriously ill exempt from fasting
	During Passover, only unleavened bread eaten
Pentecostal (Assembly of God)	Alcohol prohibited
	Avoid consumption of anything to which blood has been added
	Some individuals avoid pork
Eastern Orthodox	During Lent all animal products including dairy products are forbidden
	Fasting during Advent
	Exceptions from fasting include illness and pregnancy

RELIGION AND END-OF-LIFE CARE PRACTICES

Religious Group	End-of-Life Care Practice
Catholic and Eastern Orthodox	Anointing of the sick done by a priest
	Other sacraments before death include reconciliation and holy communion
Protestant	No last rites (anointing of the sick accepted by some groups)
	Prayers given to offer comfort and support
Church of Jesus Christ of Latter-Day Saints (Mormon)	May administer a sacrament if the client requests
Jehovah's Witness	Do not believe in sacraments
	Will be excommunicated if they receive a blood transfusion
Islam	Second-degree male relatives, such as cousins or uncles, should be contact persons and determine whether client and/or family should be given information about the client
	Client may choose to face Mecca (west or southwest in the United States)
	The head should be elevated above the body
	Discussions about death not usually welcomed
	Stopping medical treatment is against the will of Allah (Arabic word for God)
	Grief may be expressed through slapping or hitting the body
	If possible, only a same-gender Muslim should handle the body after death; if not possible, non-Muslims should wear gloves so as not to touch the body
Judaism	Prolongation of life important (life support must be maintained for a client until death)
	A dying person should not be left alone (a rabbi's presence is desired)
	Autopsy and cremation forbidden
Hinduism	Rituals: tying a thread around the neck or wrist of the dying person, sprinkling the person with special water, or placing a leaf of basil on the tongue
	After death, sacred threads are not removed and body is not washed
Buddhism	A shrine to Buddha may be placed in client's room
	Time for meditation at the shrine is important and should be respected
	Clients may refuse medications that could alter their awareness (e.g., opioids)
	After death, a monk may recite prayers for 1 hr (need not be done in the presence of the body)

THE AMISH SOCIETY: BELIEFS AND PRACTICES

Maintain a culture distinct and separate from the non-Amish.

Usually speak a German dialect called Pennsylvania Dutch.

German language used during worship; English learned in school.

Men follow the laws of the Hebrew Scriptures with regard to beards (mustaches not grown because of the long association of mustaches with the military).

Men usually dress in a plain, dark suit; women usually wear a plain dress with long sleeves, bonnet, and apron.

Women are not allowed to hold positions of power in the congregational organization.

Marriage outside the faith is not allowed.

Family life has patriarchal structure.

Although roles of the women are considered equally important to those of men, they are very unequal in terms of authority.

Unmarried women remain under the authority of their father.

Wives submissive to their husbands.

Generally remain separate from rest of the world, physically and socially.

Reject materialism and worldliness.

Some Amish prefer not to be photographed.

Value living simply; may choose to avoid technology, such as electricity and cars.

Highly value responsibility, generosity, and helping others.

Often work as farmers, builders, quilters, and homemakers.

May use traditional health care and alternative health care, such as healers, herbs, and massage.

Believe that health is a gift from God but that clean living and a balanced diet help maintain it.

Amish have lower risk factors for disease than the general population because of their work in manual labor, consumption of fresh foods, and rare consumption of tobacco and alcohol.

Many choose not to have health insurance and maintain mutual aid funds for Amish members to help with medical costs.

Funerals conducted in the home without a eulogy, flower decorations, or any other display; plain and simple caskets without adornment.

At death, women usually buried in their bridal dress.

ONE IS BELIEVED TO LIVE ON AFTER DEATH, WITH EITHER ETERNAL REWARD IN HEAVEN OR PUNISHMENT IN HELL.

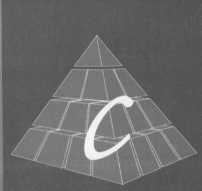

Pharmacology Strategies for Answering Test Questions

GENERAL PHARMACOLOGY GUIDELINES TO FOLLOW

1. Medication absorption, distribution, metabolism, and excretion are affected by age and physiological processes; the older client and the neonate and infant are at greater risk for toxicity than the adult.
2. Many medications are contraindicated in pregnancy and during breast-feeding.
3. Antacids are not usually administered with medication because the antacid will affect the absorption of the medication.
4. Grapefruit juice is not usually administered with medication because it contains a substance that affects the absorption of the medication.
5. Enteric-coated and sustained-release tablets should not be crushed; also, capsules should not be opened.
6. Nursing interventions always include monitoring for intended effects, side effects, adverse effects, or toxic effects of the medication.
7. Nursing interventions always include client education.
8. The nurse or client should never adjust or change a medication dose, abruptly stop taking a medication, or discontinue a medication.
9. The nurse may withhold a medication if he or she suspects that the client is experiencing an adverse or toxic effect of a medication; the nurse must immediately contact the physician if either effect occurs.
10. The client needs to avoid taking any over-the-counter medications or any other medications, such as herbal preparations, unless they are approved for use by the health care provider.
11. The client must know how to correctly administer the medication.
12. The client needs to be aware of the side effects of medications and how to check his or her own temperature, pulse, and blood pressure.
13. The client needs to take the prescribed dose for the prescribed length of therapy and understand the necessity of compliance.
14. The client needs to avoid consuming alcohol and to avoid smoking.
15. The client should wear a Medic-Alert bracelet if he or she is taking medications, such as but not limited to anticoagulants, oral hypoglycemics or insulin, certain cardiac medications, corticosteroids and glucocorticoids, antimyasthenic medications, anticonvulsants, and monoamine oxidase inhibitors.
16. The client must follow up with a health care provider as prescribed.

DETERMINING THE MEDICATION CLASSIFICATION: COMMONALITIES IN MEDICATION NAMES

1. Androgens: Most medication names end with the letters -*terone*, such as testosterone (Androderm, Testoderm).
2. Angiotensin-converting enzyme (ACE) inhibitors: Most medication names end with the letters -*pril*, such as enalapril (Vasotec).
3. Antidiuretic hormones: Most medication names end with the letters -*pressin*, such as desmopressin (DDAVP).
4. Antilipemic medications: Most medication names end with the letters -*statin*, such as atorvastatin (Lipitor).
5. Antiviral medications: Most antiviral medications contain *vir* in their names, such as ritonavir (Norvir).
6. Benzodiazepines: Benzodiazepines include alprazolam (Xanax), chlordiazepoxide (Librium), clorazepate (Tranxene), estazolam (ProSom), and triazolam (Halcion); most other benzodiazepines names end with the letters -*pam*, such as diazepam (Valium).
7. β-Adrenergic blockers: Most medication names end with the letters -*lol*, such as atenolol (Tenormin).
8. Calcium channel blockers: Most medication names end with the letters -*pine*, such as amlodipine (Norvasc); some exceptions include diltiazem (Cardizem, Cardizem SR) and verapamil (Calan, Isoptin).
9. Carbonic anhydrase inhibitors: Most medication names end with the letters -*mide*, such as acetazolamide (Diamox).
10. Estrogens: Most estrogen medications contain *est* in their names, such as conjugated estrogen (Premarin).
11. Glucocorticoids and corticosteroids: Most medication names end with the letters -*sone*, such as prednisone (Deltasone).
12. Histamine H_2–receptor antagonists: Most medication names end with the letters -*dine*, such as cimetidine (Tagamet).
13. Nitrates: Most medications contain *nitr* in their names, such as nitroglycerin (Nitrostat).
14. Pancreatic enzyme replacements: Most medications contain *pancre* in their names, such as pancrelipase (Pancrease).
15. Phenothiazines: Most phenothiazine medication names end with the letters -*zine*, such as chlorpromazine (Thorazine).
16. Proton pump inhibitors: Most medication names end with the letters -*zole*, such as lansoprazole (Prevacid).
17. Sulfonamides: Most medications include *sulf* in their names, such as sulfasalazine (Azulfidine).
18. Sulfonylureas: Most medication names end with the letters -*mide*, such as chlorpropamide (Diabinese).
19. Thiazide diuretics: Most medication names end with the letters -*zide*, such as hydrochlorothiazide (HydroDIURIL).
20. Thrombolytic medications: Most medication names end with the letters -*ase*, such as alteplase (Activase).
21. Thyroid hormones: Most medications contain *thy* in their names, such as levothyroxine (Synthroid).
22. Xanthine bronchodilators: Most medication names end with the letters -*line*, such as theophylline.

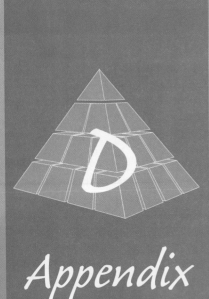

Commonly Used Units of Measure and Medication and Intravenous Calculation Formulas

METRIC SYSTEM
Abbreviations

gram: g, gm, Gm
kilogram: kg, Kg
liter: L
meter: m
microgram: mcg
milligram: mg
milliliter: mL

Equivalents

1 g = 1000 mg
1 kg = 1000 g or 2.2 lb
1 mg = 1000 mcg or 0.001 g
1000 mL = 1 L

HOUSEHOLD SYSTEMS
Household (Volume)

1 gallon = 4 quarts
1 quart = 2 pints or 1 liter
1 pint = 500 milliliters
1 cup = 240 milliliters or 8 fluid ounces
2 tablespoons = 30 milliliters
30 milliliters = 1 fluid ounce
1 tablespoon = 15 milliliters or 3 teaspoons
1 teaspoon = 4-5 milliliters or 60 drops
60 microdrops = 1 milliliter

Household (Weight)

1 pound = 16 ounces
2.2 pounds = 1 kilogram

Household (Length)

1 inch = 2.5 centimeters

CONVERSION BETWEEN METRIC UNITS
Problem 1

Convert 3 grams (g) to milligrams (mg).

Solution

Change a larger unit to a smaller unit.
3.000 g = 3000 mg (moving decimal three places to right)

Problem 2

Convert 500 milliliters (mL) to liters (L).

Solution

Change a smaller unit to a larger unit.
500 mL = 0.5 L (moving decimal three places to left)

CELSIUS AND FAHRENHEIT TEMPERATURE
Converting Fahrenheit (F) to Celsius (C)

To convert Fahrenheit to Celsius, subtract 32 and divide result by 1.8.

Formula

$$C = (F - 32) \text{ divided by } 1.8$$

Converting Celsius (C) to Fahrenheit (F)

To convert Celsius to Fahrenheit, multiply by 1.8 and add 32.

Formula

$$F = (1.8 \times C) + 32$$

FORMULA FOR CALCULATING A MEDICATION DOSAGE

$$\frac{D \text{(Desired)}}{A \text{(Available)}} \times Q \text{(Quantity)} = X$$

D (Desired) = Dosage that the physician ordered
A (Available) = Dosage strength as stated on the medication label
Q (Quantity) = Volume or form in which the dosage strength is available, such as tablets, capsules, or milliliters

FORMULAS FOR INTRAVENOUS CALCULATIONS

Flow Rates

$$\frac{\text{Total volume} \times \text{drop (gt) factor}}{\text{Time in minutes}} = \text{drops (gtt)/min}$$

Infusion Time

$$\frac{\text{Total volume to infuse}}{\text{mL/hr being infused}} = \text{Infusion time}$$

Number of mL/hr

$$\frac{\text{Total volume in mL}}{\text{No. of hr}} = \text{No. of mL/hr}$$

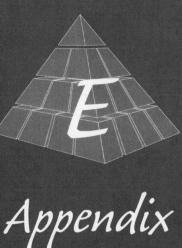

Laboratory Values

Laboratory Test	Normal Value
Arterial blood gases	pH: 7.35-7.45
	P_{CO_2}: 35-45 mm Hg
	HCO_3^-: 22-27 mm Hg
	P_{O_2}: 80%-100%
	Sa_{O_2}: 96%-100%
Blood urea nitrogen (BUN)	8-25 mg/dL
Creatinine	0.6-1.3 mg/dL
Cholesterol	Total: 140-199 mg/dL
	High-density lipoprotein (HDL): 30-70 mg/dL
	Low-density lipoprotein (LDL): <130 mg/dL
Triglycerides	<200 mg/dL
Glucose	70-110 mg/dL
Hemoglobin A_{1c}	<7.5%
Hemoglobin	Female: 12-15 g/dL
	Male: 14-16.5 g/dL
Hematocrit	Female: 35%-47%
	Male: 42%-52%
Platelets	150,000-400,000 cells/mm^3
Red blood cells	Female: 4-5.5 million cells/μL
	Male: 4.5-6.2 million cells/μL
Electrolytes	Potassium: 3.5-5.1 mEq/L
	Sodium: 135-145 mEq/L
	Chloride: 98-107 mEq/L
	Bicarbonate: 22-27 mEq/L
Erythrocyte sedimentation rate (ESR)	0-30 mm/hr
White blood cells	4500-11,000 cells/mm^3

Laboratory Test	Normal Value
Protein	6-8 g/dL
Uric acid	Female: 2.5-6.2 mg/dL
	Male: 4.5-8 mg/dL
Albumin	25-151 units/L
Lipase	10-140 units/L
Ammonia	35-65 mcg/dL
Alkaline phosphatase	4.5-13 King-Armstrong units/dL
Bilirubin (total)	<1.5 mg/dL
Bleeding time	1-9 min
Clotting time	8-15 min
Activated partial thromboplastin time (aPTT)	20-36 sec
Prothrombin time (PT)	9.5-11.8 sec
International normalized ratio (INR)	2-3 (standard warfarin therapy)
Creatine kinase (CK)	CK-MB: 0%-5% of total CK value
	CK-MM: 95%-100% of total CK value
	CK-BB: 0% of CK value
Lactate dehydrogenase	140-280 units/L
Lactate dehydrogenase isoenzymes	LDH_1: 14%-26%
	LDH_2: 29%-39%
	LDH_3: 20%-26%
	LDH_4: 8%-16%
	LDH_5: 6%-16%
Troponin	<0.6 ng/mL
Troponin I	>1.5 ng/mL indicates myocardial infarction
Troponin T	>0.1-0.2 ng/mL indicates myocardial infarction
Myoglobin	<90 mcg/L; elevation could indicate myocardial infarction
Magnesium	1.6-2.6 mg/dL
Phosphorus	2.7-4.5 mg/dL
Calcium	8.6-10 mg/dL

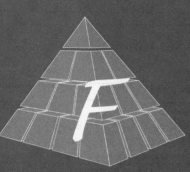

Guidelines Related to Positioning

Appendix

Always review physician's orders!
Focus on the client's diagnosis!
Identify the anatomical location of the client's diagnosis!
Consider the pathophysiology of the disorder and the goals of care!
Think about the complications that you want to prevent!

1. Elevation of an affected body part reduces edema.
2. Clients who have had neck or head surgery are placed in semi-Fowler's or Fowler's position.
3. Following a liver biopsy, the client is placed in a right lateral (side-lying) position to provide pressure to the site and prevent bleeding.
4. Clients receiving irrigations or feeding through a nasogastric, gastrostomy, or jejunostomy tube are placed in semi-Fowler's or Fowler's position to prevent aspiration.
5. Left Sims' position is used to administer a rectal enema or irrigation to allow the solution to flow by gravity in the natural direction of the colon.
6. Clients with a respiratory disorder or cardiovascular disorder are placed in semi-Fowler's or Fowler's position.
7. Clients with peripheral arterial disease may be advised to elevate their feet and legs at rest because swelling can prevent arterial blood flow, but they should not raise their legs above the level of the heart because extreme elevation slows arterial blood flow; some clients may be advised to maintain a slightly dependent position to promote perfusion.
8. Clients with peripheral venous disease are usually advised to elevate their feet and legs.
9. Clients with a head injury are placed in semi-Fowler's or Fowler's position.

10. If a client develops autonomic dysreflexia the head of the bed is elevated.

11. In clients with hemorrhagic strokes, the head of the bed is usually elevated to 30 degrees to reduce intracranial pressure and to facilitate venous drainage.

12. For clients with ischemic strokes, the head of the bed is usually kept flat.

13. Following craniotomy the client should NOT be positioned on the site that was operated on, especially if the bone flap has been removed, because the brain has no bony covering on the affected site; semi-Fowler's or Fowler's position is maintained with the head in a midline, neutral position to facilitate venous drainage from the head, and extreme hip and neck flexion is avoided.

14. With increased intracranial pressure the client is placed in semi-Fowler's or Fowler's position; the head is maintained in a midline, neutral position to facilitate venous drainage from the head, and extreme hip and neck flexion is avoided.

15. In a spinal cord injury the client is immobilized on a spinal backboard, with the head in a neutral position, to prevent incomplete injury from becoming complete; head flexion, rotation, or extension is avoided and the client is logrolled.

16. In the client who underwent a total hip replacement, positioning will depend on the surgical techniques used, the method of implantation, the prosthesis, and physician's preference; extreme internal and external rotation and adduction are avoided and side-lying on the operative side is not allowed (unless specifically prescribed by the physician).

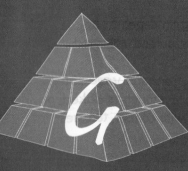

Therapeutic Diets

G

Appendix

Diet	Indications	Nursing Considerations
Clear liquid diet	Serves a primary function of providing fluids and electrolytes to prevent dehydration Initial feeding after complete bowel rest Used initially to feed malnourished person or person who has not had any oral intake for some time Bowel preparation for surgery or tests Postsurgical diet To treat diarrhea	Clear liquid is deficient in energy and most nutrients The body digests and absorbs clear liquids easily Contributes to little or no residue in gastrointestinal (GI) tract Can be unappetizing and boring Client should not stay on clear liquid diet for more than 1-2 days Consists of foods that are relatively transparent to light, are clear, and liquefy at body or room temperature Includes items such as water, bouillon, clear broth, carbonated beverages, gelatin, hard candy, lemonade, Popsicles, and regular or decaffeinated coffee or tea Limit amount of caffeine consumed by client because caffeine can cause an upset stomach and sleeplessness Client may have salt or sugar Dairy products not allowed
Full liquid diet	May be used as second diet after clear liquids following surgery or for client who is unable to chew or swallow	Nutritionally deficient in energy and most nutrients Includes both clear and opaque liquid foods and those that liquefy at body temperature Includes all clear liquids and items such as plain ice cream, sherbet, breakfast drinks, milk, pudding and custard, strained soups, and strained vegetable juices

Diet	Indications	Nursing Considerations
Sodium-restricted diet	Hypertension, heart failure, renal disease, cardiac disease, and cirrhosis of liver	Individualized and can include 4 g of sodium daily (no–added salt diet), 2-3 g of sodium daily (moderate restriction), 1 g of sodium daily (strict restriction), or 500 mg of sodium daily (severe and seldom prescribed) Encourage intake of fresh, rather than processed, foods, which have higher amounts of sodium Canned, frozen, instant, smoked, pickled, and boxed items usually contain higher amounts of sodium Lunch meats, soy sauce, salad dressings, fast foods, soups, and snacks such as potato chips and pretzels contain large amounts of sodium Certain medications contain significant amounts of sodium May use salt substitutes to improve palatability; most salt substitutes contain large amounts of potassium and should not be used by clients with renal disease
Protein-restricted diet	Acute renal failure, chronic renal disease, cirrhosis of liver, and hepatic coma	Provides enough protein to maintain nutritional status but not an amount that will allow buildup of waste products from protein metabolism (40-60 g of protein daily) The smaller the amount of protein allowed, the more important it becomes that all protein included in the diet be of high quality Adequate total energy intake from foods is critical for clients on protein-restricted diets (protein will be used for energy, rather than for protein synthesis) Special low-protein products, such as pastas, bread, cookies, wafers, and gelatin made with wheat starch, can improve energy intake and add variety to the diet Carbohydrates in powdered or liquid form can also provide additional energy Vegetables and fruits contain some protein; for very low-protein diets, these foods must be calculated into the diet Foods are limited from milk, meat, bread, and starch exchange
Renal diet	Used for client with acute and chronic renal failure and those requiring hemodialysis or peritoneal dialysis	Controlled amounts of protein, sodium, phosphorus, calcium, potassium, and fluids may be prescribed; may also need modification in fiber, cholesterol, and fat, based on individual requirements Most clients receiving dialysis need to restrict fluids

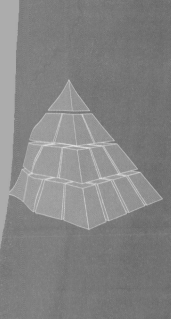

Index

Diet	Indications	Nursing Considerations
Vegetarian diets—cont'd	*Lacto vegetarian:* consumes dairy products but excludes eggs, meat, poultry, and seafood	Potential deficiencies in vegetarian diets: energy, protein, vitamin B$_{12}$, zinc, iron, calcium, omega-3 fatty acids, and vitamin D (if limited exposure to sunlight)
	Vegan: refrains from eating animal products	To enhance absorption of iron, vegetarians should include good source of iron and vitamin C with each meal
	Pesco vegetarian: consumes seafood, but excludes meat, poultry, eggs, and dairy products	Foods commonly eaten: tofu, tempeh, soy milk and soy products, meat analogues, legumes, nuts and seeds, sprouts, and variety of fruits and vegetables
		Soy protein considered equivalent in quality to animal proteins
Enteral nutrition	When GI tract is functional but oral intake is not feasible	Clients with lactose intolerance (diarrhea, bloating, cramping) need to be placed on lactose-free formulas
	Used for clients with swallowing problems, burns, major trauma, liver failure, or severe malnutrition	
Parenteral nutrition (PN)	Clients with severely dysfunctional or nonfunctional GI tracts who are unable to process nutrients may benefit from PN	Always check solution with physician's order to ensure that prescribed components are contained in the solution
	Clients who can take some oral nutrition but not enough to meet their nutrient requirements may benefit from PN	To prevent infection and solution incompatibility, IV medications and blood not given through the PN line
	Clients with multiple GI surgeries, GI trauma, severe intolerance to enteral feedings, or intestinal obstructions or who need to rest the bowel for healing may benefit from PN	Monitor partial thromboplastin time and prothrombin time for clients receiving anticoagulants
		Monitor electrolytes, albumin, and liver and renal function studies
		In severely dehydrated clients, albumin level may drop initially as treatment restores hydration
	Clients with acquired immunodeficiency syndrome, cancer, burn injuries, malnutrition, or clients receiving chemotherapy may benefit from PN	With severely malnourished clients, monitor for "refeeding syndrome" (rapid drop in potassium, magnesium, and phosphate serum levels)
		Abnormal liver function values may indicate excess of or intolerance to fat emulsion or problems with metabolism with glucose and protein
	PN is least desirable form of nutrition and is used when there is no other nutritional alternative	Abnormal renal function tests may indicate excess of amino acids
		PN solutions should be stored under refrigeration and administered within 24 hr from the time that they were prepared (remove from refrigerator 0.5-1 hr before use)
		PN solutions that are cloudy or darkened should not be used and should be returned to the pharmacy
		Additions to PN solutions should be made in the pharmacy and not on the nursing unit

Diet	Indications	Nursing Considerations
Potassium-modified diet	Low-potassium diet indicated for hyperkalemia, which may be due to impaired renal function, hypoaldosteronism, Addison's disease, angiotensin-converting enzyme inhibitor medications, immunosuppressive medications, potassium-sparing diuretics, and chronic hyperkalemia High-potassium diet indicated for hypokalemia, which may be due to renal tubular acidosis, GI losses (diarrhea, vomiting), intracellular shifts, potassium-wasting diuretics, antibiotics, mineralocorticoid or glucocorticoid excess from primary or secondary aldosteronism, Cushing's syndrome, or exogenous steroid use	Foods low in potassium: applesauce, green beans, cabbage, lettuce, peppers, grapes, blueberries, cooked summer squash, cooked turnip greens, fresh pineapple, and raspberries Foods high in potassium: avocado, bananas, cantaloupe, carrots, fish, mushrooms, oranges, pork, beef, veal, potatoes, raisins, spinach, strawberries, tomatoes
High-calcium diet	Calcium needed during bone growth and in adulthood to prevent osteoporosis and to facilitate vascular contraction and vasodilation, muscle contraction, and nerve transmission	Primary dietary sources of calcium are dairy products Clients with lactose intolerance need to incorporate sources of calcium other than dairy products into their dietary patterns regularly Foods high in calcium: broccoli, carrots, cheese, collard greens, green beans, milk, rhubarb, spinach, tofu, low-fat yogurt
Low-purine diet	Used to treat gout, kidney stones, and elevated uric acid levels	Purine is precursor for uric acid, which forms stones and crystals Foods to restrict: anchovies, herring, mackerel, sardines, scallops, glandular meats, gravies, meat extracts, wild game, goose, and sweetbreads
High-iron diet	Used in anemia	Replaces iron deficit from inadequate intake or loss Includes organ meats, meat, egg yolks, whole-wheat products, dark green leafy vegetables, dried fruit, legumes
Vegetarian diets	Types of vegetarian diets *Lacto-ovo vegetarian:* consumes eggs and dairy products but excludes meat, poultry, and seafood	Ensure that client eats sufficient amount of varied foods to meet normal nutrient and energy needs Educate client about consuming complementary proteins over course of each day, to ensure all essential amino acids are provided